SCIENTIFIC AMERICAN
MOLECULAR
ONCOLOGY

SCIENTIFIC AMERICAN Introduction to Molecular Medicine
Edward D. Rubenstein, M.D., Series Editor

SCIENTIFIC AMERICAN Molecular Oncology
Edited by J. Michael Bishop, M.D., and Robert A. Weinberg, Ph.D.

Previously Published
SCIENTIFIC AMERICAN Molecular Cardiovascular Medicine
Edited by Edgar Haber, M.D.

SCIENTIFIC AMERICAN Introduction to Molecular Medicine
*Edited by Philip Leder, M.D., David A. Clayton, Ph.D., and
Edward Rubenstein, M.D.*

Forthcoming
SCIENTIFIC AMERICAN Molecular Neurology
Edited by Joseph B. Martin, M.D., Ph.D.

SCIENTIFIC AMERICAN

MOLECULAR ONCOLOGY

Edited by

J. Michael Bishop, M.D.
University Professor
University of California, San Francisco

and

Robert A. Weinberg, Ph.D.
Member, Whitehead Institute for Biomedical Research
Professor of Biology, Massachusetts Institute of Technology

Scientific American, Inc., New York

Cover Illustration by Seward Hung
A Mitogenic Pathway Involving $G_{s\alpha}$, *from Chapter 5.*

Library of Congress Cataloging-in-Publication Data

Scientific American molecular oncology/edited by J. Michael Bishop
and Robert A. Weinberg.
p. cm.—(Scientific American introduction to molecular medicine)
Includes index.
ISBN 0-89454-023-8
1. Cancer—Molecular aspects. I. Bishop, J. Michael, 1936– . II. Weinberg, Robert A. (Robert
Allan), 1942– . III. Scientific American, Inc. IV. Series.
[DNLM: 1. Neoplasm—etiology. 2. Neoplasms—genetics. 3. Oncogenes—physiology.
QZ 202 S414 1996]
RC268.4.S37—1996
616.99'407—dc20
DNLM/DLC   96-29150
for Library of Congress   CIP

Editorial Director	Aileen M. McHugh
Publishing Director	Linnéa C. Elliott
Project Editor	Ozzievelt Owens
Director of Art and Design	Elizabeth Klarfeld
Vice President, Associate Publisher/Production	Richard Sasso
Production Manager	Christina Hippeli
Electronic Composition	Diane Joiner
	Carol Hansen

ISBN: 0-89454-023-8

Scientific American, Inc., 415 Madison Avenue, New York, NY 10017

Contributors

J. Michael Bishop, M.D.   University Professor, University of California, San Francisco

Eric R. Fearon, M.D., Ph.D.   Associate Professor of Internal Medicine, Human Genetics, and Pathology, Division of Molecular Medicine and Genetics, University of Michigan Medical School

Hidesaburo Hanafusa, Ph.D.   Leon Hess Professor; Head, Laboratory of Molecular Oncology, The Rockefeller University, New York

Douglas Hanahan, Ph.D.   Professor of Biochemistry; Associate Director, Hormone Research Institute, University of California, San Francisco

Mark A. Israel, M.D.   Professor, Department of Neurological Surgery and Department of Pediatrics, University of California, San Francisco

José F. Leis, M.D., Ph.D.   Instructor in Medicine, Dana-Faber Cancer Institute, Brigham and Women's Hospital, and Harvard Medical School

David M. Livingston, M.D.   Emil Frei Professor of Medicine, Dana-Farber Cancer Institute and Harvard Medical School

Douglas R. Lowy, M.D.   Chief, Laboratory of Cellular Oncology, National Cancer Institute, National Institutes of Health

G. Steven Martin, Ph.D.   Professor of Biochemistry and Molecular Biology, Department of Molecular and Cell Biology, University of California at Berkeley

Tony Pawson, Ph.D.   Senior Scientist, Programme in Molecular Biology and Cancer, Samuel Lunenfeld Research Institute, Mount Sinai Hospital, Toronto

Robert A. Weinberg, Ph.D.   Member, Whitehead Institute for Biomedical Research; Professor of Biology, Massachusetts Institute of Technology

Preface

T his book is the third in a series from SCIENTIFIC AMERICAN *Medicine* that is meant to describe the molecular underpinnings of human disease. No disease is more amenable to such description than cancer, as our distinguished group of authors make clear in the chapters that follow.

We have endeavored to make the text accessible to the practicing physician and the resident, who might have no more than a passing knowledge of cells, genes, and macromolecules, yet sufficiently informative to be useful as an initial source for the specialist as well. We have also labored to eliminate redundancy among the chapters. Where we have not done so, it is because the authors convinced us that certain redundancies preserved the internal coherence of chapters and would serve the purposes of readers who might be using the book as an occasional reference.

The recent progress in our understanding of cancer offers many lessons. Preeminent among these are the continuing value of fundamental research that may have no immediate reference to disease and the broad-ranging impact of findings about rare diseases such as inherited cancers. If we have succeeded in making these lessions clear, we will have achieved our purpose for creating this book. We are grateful to the renowned scientists who wrote the text and endured our persistent queries. And we thank Hilary Evans, who recruited us to this endeavor and provided gentle encouragement during fallow periods.

J. M. Bishop, M.D.
R. A. Weinberg, Ph.D.

Contents

CHAPTER 1

Introduction

J. Michael Bishop, M.D., Robert A. Weinberg, Ph.D.

It has been axiomatic among the medical profession that cancer is not one disease but many. This is a reasonable view for the pathologist, who sees the diversity of cellular abnormalities that cancers present; for the epidemiologist, who knows the great number (albeit not necessarily the identities) of agents that cause cancer; and for the oncologist, who must cope with the heterogeneous response of cancers to therapy. For molecular and cellular biologists, however, a different image holds sway. All types of cancer cells share certain fundamental disturbances. Surely a unifying explanation for this commonality must exist.

There is now good reason to believe that a unifying explanation for cancer has been found. No matter what form cancer takes, it remains a malady of genes, and most, if not all, causes of cancer act by damaging genes directly or indirectly. This genetic paradigm has greatly enhanced our understanding of cancer and now guides most research on the disease. The major purposes of this book are to demonstrate how the genetic paradigm for cancer was formed, to explain how it illuminates our understanding of cancer, and to anticipate what it offers for the future management of the disease.

The authors of this book work with the faith that an understanding of the pathogenesis of cancer at the molecular level is a prerequisite to the development of new types of diagnostics and more effective therapeutics. This faith largely remains to be fulfilled. Although the past decade has seen penetrating discoveries about the molecular basis of cancer, these discoveries have yet to be substantially translated into diagnosis and treatment. Nevertheless, there can be no doubt that this translation will come and that when it does come, it will be based on the progress in fundamental research described in this book.

Two Approaches to Cancer

The appearance of a book like this is testimony to the broad-ranging revolution that has swept through biomedical research during the past two decades. This revolution has been based principally on the newfound ability to isolate genes through the use of recombinant DNA, to determine the chemical sequence of such genes, and to remodel their function. These tactics have produced, among many other marvels, an unprecedented grasp on the fundamental mechanisms by which cancer arises.

The research responsible for these breakthroughs was based on two concepts. First, cancer is fundamentally a disease of individual cells. Hence, we should be able to understand most, if not all, of the properties of malignant tumors if we understand the properties of their individual cellular components. That conviction has fueled decades of work that has attempted to recapitulate the events of tumorigenesis in cell culture [*see Chapter 3*]. Second, the behavior of cells and, by extension, complex tissues can be understood in terms of the genes operating within these cells. Indeed, the complexity of cancer can be understood only through attention to genes; cancer is a perversion of cellular phenotype, and genes are the determinants of that phenotype.

The cellular and genetic views of cancer have become interwoven into a single fabric that offers a unified view of cancer. Our purpose in this introductory chapter is to provide a brief account of how the fabric was woven. We do so in the hope that our account will allow readers to better appreciate the ensuing chapters.

The Cellular Lineage of Cancer

Rudolph Virchow dimly perceived the heritable nature of the neoplastic phenotype well before the end of the 19th century. He noted a resemblance between the cellular components of metastases and those of the primary tumor. This resemblance, he suggested, sustained the newly emerged theory of the cell, which proposed that all cells come from other cells.

Then Virchow made another, more daring, proposal. If all the cells of a tumor are relatives, perhaps they all originate from a single progenitor. This may have been the earliest proposal of what we now take to be a fundamental property of most, if not all, tumors: they are clonal—the entire mass of tumor cells originates from a single wayward progenitor [*see Chapter 3*].

The proposal of clonality had a powerful implication, which Virchow was not in a good position to understand. The neoplastic phenotype must be remarkably stable because it persists through the countless cell divisions required for the generation of a tumor from a single progenitor cell. In other words, the phenotype of tumor cells must be heritable. This notion leads to the suspicion that the abnormalities of cancer cells are based on genetic change. The cancer scientists of our century were remarkably slow to recognize the validity of this simple deduction.

The External Causes of Cancer

If cancer begins as a single cell that eventually progresses to a full-blown malignancy, what initiates the deadly sequence? For more than two centuries, the focus has been on external causes [*see Chapter 2*]. What are those causes? That question sired two competing views, which emerged more or less in concert at the turn of this century. One view held that chemical and physical agents were mainly responsible for cancer; the other looked to viruses as the principal agents of the disease. Both contributed vital pieces to the solution of the cancer puzzle.

The realization that cancers can be triggered by chemical and physical agents reaches back to 1761, when John Hill, of London, suggested that the inhalation of snuff might cause nasal cancer. Fourteen years later, Percival Pott achieved lasting fame when he reported that the chimney sweeps of Britain were prone to cancer of the scrotum. Pott attributed the cancers to exposure to soot from incompletely burned coal.

The general significance of these early inferences went unappreciated until the late 19th century. Then, industrial exposures to large quantities of noxious agents brought paraffin oils, mining dust, arsenic, and aniline dyes under suspicion. At the same time, it became apparent that the newly discovered x-rays and their seemingly benevolent cousin, sunlight, could be carcinogenic.

Epidemiological observations in human populations were soon supplemented with experimental observations. The pioneers were Clunet, who in 1908 demonstrated that x-rays could induce skin cancer in rats, and Yamagiwa and his colleagues, who in 1915 and the years following induced skin cancer by applying coal tar to the ears of rabbits and the backs of mice. These crude beginnings launched a vast array of experimental studies designed to identify chemical carcinogens and to explain their actions—a genre of work that dominated cancer research for many decades.

The list of potential carcinogens has now expanded to include many hundreds of organic compounds, each capable of inducing tumors in one or another laboratory animal. At least one major form of human cancer, carcinoma of the lung, has been attributed persuasively to the complex mixture of chemical carcinogens found in the smoke of cigarettes. This principal cause of lung cancer would have come as no surprise to King James I of England, who in 1604 issued a royal edict entitled "Counterblast to Tobacco" and encouraged the public display of human lungs blackened by tobacco smoke in the hope of discouraging the use of tobacco.

The competing view held that most cancers were caused by viruses. This idea emerged under the influence of the "germ theory" of disease, which by the end of the 19th century had acquired sweeping scope—owing mainly to the work of Robert Koch, in Germany, and Louis Pasteur, in France. It seemed as if all diseases might have microbial causes. Thus, it was only natural that the discovery of viruses in the period from 1898 to 1900 would immediately lead to inquiries about whether these agents might cause cancer.

The first durable connection between viruses and cancer came from the pioneering work of Peyton Rous, who, in the years after 1909, described a virus that could induce sarcomas in chickens and could transmit the disease in the manner of an infectious agent. Ironically, Rous abandoned the study of the virus he had discovered after failing to find similar viruses in the tumors of rodents. He reasoned that if the phenomenon was not universal, it was not worthy of pursuit.

Rous was perhaps correct in principle, but he was wrong in reality. In the decades that followed, a series of hard-fought intellectual battles established the point that a diversity of viruses are capable of causing cancer in either experimental or natural circumstances. Of particular note were the discoveries of the Shope papilloma of rabbits, the mammary carcinoma virus of mice, the leukemia viruses of mice, and the papovaviruses known as SV40 and polyoma. Even human adenoviruses were found to be potent tumorigens in rodents; this discovery dramatized the principle that removal of a virus from its natural host could reveal otherwise unrealized tumorigenic potential—in large part because the virus fails to replicate and kill its new host cells [*see Chapter 2*].

Eventually, viruses surfaced as etiologic agents of human cancer also [*see Chapter 2*]. Epstein-Barr virus was for many years the best studied of this group. Its close association with Burkitt's lymphoma in central Africa and nasopharyngeal carcinoma in Asia provided a clear indication that viruses were relevant to the human condition and, thus, represented much more than useful laboratory models. Eventually, human papillomaviruses and hepatitis B virus joined the ranks of culprits; compelling epidemiological evidence now strongly connects the former to cervical and other genitourinary cancers and the latter to liver cancer.

The story came full circle when, in the late 1970s, the discovery of human T cell lymphotropic virus type I provided the first indication that a retrovirus, which was distantly related to Rous's sarcoma virus, could cause a human cancer: the relatively rare adult T cell leukemias seen in southwest Japan, the Caribbean, and smaller, isolated pockets throughout the world. It later became apparent that another retrovirus, human immunodeficiency virus, was at least indirectly involved in the genesis of certain human tumors.

It remains true, however, that most types of human cancer lack the attributes of a transmissible, highly contagious disease. Several explanations can be offered for this inconsistency. First, many human cancers may, in fact, not be caused by viral infection [*see Chapter 2*]. Second, viral infection may initiate the process of tumorigenesis, but progression to overt disease requires the action of additional cofactors [*see Chapters 2 and 8*]. Such a mechanism would leave few epidemiological stigmata of transmissible agents. Third, many tumor viruses have the ability to establish <u>latent, fully inapparent infections,</u> thereby allowing such agents to remain cryptic within a tissue for years or decades, all the while fueling the progression to malignant growth. Again, the resulting pattern of disease may bear little or no resemblance to that of a classic microbial infestation. Given the subtle nature of viral tumorigenesis, it seems reasonable to expect that other viral agents of human cancer may still be hidden from view.

A Genetic Reconciliation

We are now certain that both physicochemical agents and viruses are responsible for various forms of human cancer. Nevertheless, does this fact imply that two unconnected mechanisms of tumorigenesis are operative? Not at all. Instead, as argued repeatedly throughout this volume, both forms of tumorigenesis are based on a common set of genetic mechanisms. The physicochemical agents act by modifying normal genes to become cancer genes; viruses can also be spurs to mutation, and many actually carry pre-formed cancer genes [*see Chapters 2, 3, and 4*].

The first hint of a genetic mechanism for carcinogenesis came in 1928, when, less than 20 years since the recognition that x-rays could be carcino-genic, H. J. Muller discovered that x-rays are mutagenic in fruit flies. At the time, Muller had no apparent scientific interest in cancer, and the connec-tion between his work and malignant disease was overlooked. Nonetheless, his discovery underlies virtually all contemporary thinking about the mech-anisms of tumorigenesis. Within the next decade, the chemical carcinogen 3-methylcholanthrene was shown to be mutagenic in mice. This observa-tion fostered the formal hypothesis that all external carcinogens might be mutagens, and that this property might account for carcinogenicity.

The pursuit of this possibility became mired by two complications. First, some of the identified carcinogens were curiously unreactive in chemical terms. How then could they have biologic effects? The answer lay in the detoxification performed on the chemicals by the liver; in this process, reac-tive intermediates are formed, and these become the actual carcinogens. A second difficulty was the identification of the molecules within cells that served as targets for carcinogens. In this regard, important insight was ob-tained through the use of tumor viruses as models for study of the conver-sion of normal cells to cancerous growth.

A crucial step was taken in the late 1940s, with the demonstration that in tissue culture, some tumor viruses were able to transform normal cells into cells with growth patterns that were reminiscent of those of real tumor cells [*see Chapter 3*]. This transformation was rapid and efficient and thus con-trasted sharply with the effects of chemical or physical carcinogens, which worked only inefficiently, with a long latency, and often only within the confines of living tissues. Transformation of cells in culture demystified the process of tumorigenesis by showing that normal cells can become tumor cells outside the complex environment of a living tissue.

The malignant transformation of cells by tumor viruses led to another seminal insight: the discovery that only one, or at the most several, of the genes carried by tumor viruses were responsible for the transformation [*see Chapters 2, 3, and 4*]. The viral genes responsible for transformation and tu-morigenesis eventually became known as *oncogenes*. The remainder of the genes were devoted exclusively to viral replication. This insight represented a major watershed in our understanding of tumorigenesis because it showed that a small amount of genetic information could dictate the behavior of a genetically complex cell.

Finding the Genetic Targets of Carcinogenesis

The lessons gained from tumor viruses shifted the focus of research on the origins of cancer. Genes came into view as the central mediators of carcino-genesis. Although chemical carcinogens were known to affect a diversity of macromolecules, including proteins, RNA, and DNA, most observers now agreed that DNA was the principal target for carcinogens.

Two schools of thought existed about how carcinogens actually affected DNA. One school proposed that carcinogens affected the expression of genes, causing their selective induction and repression. The process was thought to represent a perversion of the events that occur during embryonic development, when a highly selective readout of specific genes gives rise to differentiated phenotypes. The opposing view was that carcinogens were mutagenic: they damaged genes directly, causing either anomalous activity or loss of function. These genetic abnormalities, in turn, might elicit the profound changes in phenotype that are associated with cancer cells.

The second theory, carcinogen as mutagen, received a strong boost from the work of Bruce Ames and others, who developed convenient tests that allowed the mutagenic potency of chemicals to be measured. The virtue of these tests was that they could be performed with bacterial or vertebrate cells in culture rather than with whole organisms. The results from these tests showed that as long suspected, different chemical species have vastly different potencies as mutagens—varying more than a millionfold.

More important, however, was the fact that strong mutagens were often also potent carcinogens when tested in rodents. Conversely, weak mutagens were often weak carcinogens. Although exceptions to these correlations now abound, an immensely influential theme had been established and still persists: the ability of carcinogens to induce cancer may depend critically on their ability to induce mutations.

Even carcinogens that are not directly mutagenic can be brought into the scheme. By one means or another, these seeming exceptions elicit prolonged cellular proliferation, and this phenomenon in turn favors mutagenesis. Ambiguities about these views still linger, however, causing no end of strife in the statutory world of toxicology, where the identification of potential carcinogens has become a highly controversial and emotionally charged issue.

An entirely different line of inquiry provided further evidence that the genetic apparatus is at fault in tumorigenesis. This evidence came from cytogenetics, which showed that cancer cells frequently harbor abnormal chromosomes. We owe the origin of this idea to Theodor Boveri, who in 1914 used his studies of normal mitosis in sea urchins and worms as a platform for suggesting that cancer might be caused by the abnormal gain or loss of chromosomes. Boveri's prescience would not reach fruition until 1960, when the Philadelphia chromosome was discovered in cells of chronic myelogenous leukemia; this was the first chromosomal anomaly that was specifically implicated in any neoplasm.

The identification of the Philadelphia chromosome opened a floodgate of discovery. Currently, well over 100 different chromosomal translocations are specifically associated with cancer [see Chapters 3 and 8]. The presence of these translocations gives clear evidence of genetic damage in cancer cells, although the techniques of cytogenetics proved too blunt an instrument for deciphering that damage with any precision.

The carcinogen-as-mutagen model clearly implies the presence of mutant genes within the cells of any tumor. These genes must be altered versions of preexisting cellular genes that have been damaged, either by action of carcinogens or by errors intrinsic to the genetic processes of the cell. This idea provided a bridge to the findings of tumor virologists. Perhaps the mutant genes of cancer cells, mysterious as they were at first, would prove to be oncogenes that are functionally akin to those found in many tumor viruses. Indeed, it was the study of tumor viruses that opened the door to the study of cancer genes of vertebrate cells.

Proto-oncogenes

When Peyton Rous first reported the discovery of a sarcoma virus in chickens, he extrapolated the finding to suggest that viruses might account for the development of all cancer, including that of humans. The extrapolation was greeted with disbelief and ridicule. Rous would have to wait more than 50 years for vindication, and when it finally came, it took both expected and unexpected forms. As anticipated by Rous, some human tumors are caused by viruses. Nevertheless, Rous could not have anticipated an additional outcome of his work: his virus would provide the means for prying open a window on the genetic underpinnings of all cancers, irrespective of their cause.

The first step came with the recognition that tumorigenesis by the Rous sarcoma virus could be attributed to a single gene of the virus, eventually called *src* after the tumors (sarcomas) that this virus induces [*see Chapter 4*]. The presence of this gene seemed to have no rhyme or reason because it contributed nothing to the replication of the virus. The puzzle was solved with the discovery that *src* was not a legitimate viral gene at all, but an adventitious passenger in the viral genome. The *src* gene had originated as a gene of normal cells and found its way into Rous sarcoma virus by means of a genetic accident, which is now called *transduction* [*see Chapter 4*].

In due course, it became apparent that the transduction of *src* was only the tip of a genetic iceberg. Several dozen oncogenes of retroviruses have been derived from the genes of normal cells. These normal progenitor genes are known by the generic term *proto-oncogenes*. The conversion of proto-oncogene to viral oncogene can be explained in several ways. For example, the virus may cause the gene to be expressed in excessive amounts or in inappropriate tissues. In addition, the coding domain of the gene may be mutated during the process of transduction or subsequent viral replication, causing the protein product of the gene to malfunction.

Thus, transduction of proto-oncogenes embodies the genetic paradigm of cancer: genes of normal cells can be mutated to tumorigenic forms. But why should aberrations of proto-oncogenes be tumorigenic? The answer came with the discovery that proto-oncogenes encode various components of the signaling pathways by which cells receive and execute commands to proliferate [*see Chapter 5*]. As a result, the mutant versions of proto-oncogenes found in retroviruses can provide cells with illicit, unrelenting stimuli to proliferate. They also provided investigators with an unprecedented access to the details of signaling pathways that operate within cells.

If proto-oncogenes can become outlaws after they are captured by viral genomes, perhaps the same conversion might occur within cells, even without the intervention of a virus. This, too, proved to be the case. The first hint came from the discovery that the DNA of chemically transformed mouse cells carries a potent oncogene that can transform cells in culture [*see Chapter 4*]. This discovery motivated a series of studies that detected biologically active oncogenes in the DNA of many human tumors [*see Chapters 4 and 7*].

By 1983, these oncogenes of human tumors had been identified as mutant alleles of the *ras family* of proto-oncogenes, which was first discovered through their affiliation with a rodent retrovirus. The mutations that caused their activation were reminiscent of those induced by chemical carcinogens. A circle had been closed: the physicochemical agents of carcinogenesis first glimpsed two centuries ago had finally been given at least one precise molecular target. At last, the way in which carcinogens might manipulate the regulatory machinery of human cells became clear.

The role of proto-oncogenes as genetic substrates for tumorigenic damage soon took on an even larger dimension, with the discovery that many of the numerous chromosomal abnormalities found in human tumors affect the function of a proto-oncogene [*see Chapters 4 and 7*]. Many of the afflicted proto-oncogenes were uncovered by the direct excavation of the genome of human tumor cells rather than by the study of retroviruses. As the excavation proceeded, the definition of proto-oncogene changed ever so slightly to include genes that were activated exclusively by chromosomal mutations. Soon, the total repertoire of proto-oncogenes grew to its current number of more than 100 [*see Chapter 4*].

The assortment of proto-oncogenes represented a genetic keyboard on which tumorigenic events of diverse sorts might play. We know of few human tumors in which genetic damage does not affect at least one proto-oncogene [*see Chapter 7*]. Ironically, a mutant form of the archetype *src* has yet to be encountered in human tumors. The laurels of *src* result entirely from its having been a harbinger.

Tumor Suppressor Genes

The discovery of proto-oncogenes revealed a formidable array of genetic substrates for carcinogenic events. At first glance, these genes seemed to suffice to explain all forms of tumorigenesis. However, one observation gave pause. When human tumor cells were fused with normal cells, the resulting hybrids typically lost many of their malignant properties [*see Chapter 6*]. In other words, the malignant phenotype appeared to be genetically recessive and reversible by elements found in normal cells. In contrast, the oncogenes derived from proto-oncogenes were known to be genetically dominant—they exerted their malign effects even in the presence of their normal counterparts.

The results of cell fusions raised the possibility that another sort of gene, whose mechanism of action was quite distinct from that of oncogenes, might be involved in cancer. The representatives of this new class of gene eventually came to be known as *tumor suppressor genes* because they were imagined to be responsible for the suppression of the neoplastic phenotype seen in experiments with cell fusion.

The dominance of oncogenes facilitated their detection by assays in cell culture. Tumor suppressor genes, however, represented another level of difficulty. As recessive elements in tumorigenesis, they were not readily amenable to cell culture assays. Instead, the identity of tumor suppressor genes was teased out through an arduous combination of human genetics, cytogenetics, and molecular cloning [*see Chapter 6*].

The existence and chromosomal location of a recessive cancer gene were first clearly established for the rare tumor of childhood known as *retinoblastoma*. In due course, this tumor yielded the first tumor suppressor gene to be isolated by molecular cloning. Other examples followed, and, at present, more than a dozen tumor suppressor genes have been identified [*see Chapters 6 and 7*]. It seems likely that the number of these genes may eventually equal that of proto-oncogenes.

The elucidation of tumor suppressor genes has illuminated many aspects of tumorigenesis, two of which deserve mention here. First, inheritance of damaged tumor suppressor genes accounts for many forms of familial cancer [*see Chapter 7*]. The inheritance includes a misleading curiosity. Although the inherited mutations are recessive at the cellular level, their pattern of inheritance within families is clearly dominant. This subtle paradox stems from a combination of circumstances: a somatic cell already bearing an inherited defect in one copy of a gene needs to suffer only one additional insult to the second copy in order to uncover the full impact of the recessive damage; the number of cells in most tissues is so large that the necessary second event is virtually certain to occur in at least one cell; and the congruence of two events needs to occur in only one of the cells in order to launch the progression to cancer. Thus, the clonal origin of cancer permits a form of inheritance that is virtually unique among congenital diseases.

Second, if proto-oncogenes can be viewed as accelerators of cellular proliferation, tumor suppressor genes are the countervailing brakes—elements that can inhibit the cell division cycle rather than propel it. Herein lies the explanation for the genetic difference between the two classes of genes. A single jammed accelerator can cause trouble (hence the dominance of oncogenes), whereas both copies of a genetic brake must be inactivated or lost before the full impact is felt (hence the cellular recessiveness of tumor suppressor genes).

The Paradigm Grows More Sophisticated

The discovery that single oncogenes could transform cells in culture and elicit tumors in experimental animals was immensely liberating for investigators of cancer. What had once seemed a hopelessly tangled complexity could now be reduced to the effects of a single gene. However, the liberation was illusory, a departure from the realities of human cancer. The annals of cancer research have long recorded diverse reasons for regarding the genesis of human tumors as a multistep process [*see Chapter 8*]. Thus, it was a misapprehension to think that malfunction of a single proto-oncogene or tumor suppressor gene could suffice to create cancer.

The resolution of this conundrum proved less difficult than might have been expected [*see Chapters 7 and 8*]. As our grasp on cancer genes improved, it became apparent that human tumors contain damage to both proto-oncogenes and tumor suppressor genes (typically, more frequently to the latter than to the former, but almost always a combination of the two). Thus, the multiple individual steps in tumorigenesis may be nothing more than the accretion of genetic lesions involving several genes [*see Chapter 8*], with the sum being a malignant cell.

Nevertheless, important questions remain unanswered. Does each type of tumor require a different, special combination of damaged genes? Must the genes be damaged in a particular order, or is the mere summation of events sufficient to cause malignancy? Decisive answers to these questions are not yet in hand [*see Chapter 7*].

The requirement for multiple genetic lesions in tumorigenesis raises another dilemma. Human cells are remarkably adept at the repair of genetic damage. Moreover, the body is proficient at eliminating individual cells in which this repair has failed. These phenomena result in a net accumulation of mutant cells that is extraordinarily low. No matter how the rate of mutation in human genomes is estimated, cells should not normally accumulate sufficient genetic damage to generate cancer in one lifetime.

This dilemma has now apparently been resolved: during the course of tumorigenesis, the emerging cancer cell becomes more vulnerable to mutagenesis. At least two explanations for this increased mutability exist. First, genes responsible for the repair of DNA become damaged early in the course of tumorigenesis, thereby increasing the risk of stable mutations [*see Chapter 7*]. Second, cells are equipped to kill themselves if genetic damage remains unrepaired, but the equipment necessary to trigger this suicide is impaired during tumorigenesis. The fail-safe device itself fails, thereby facilitating the survival of mutant cells that carry potentially oncogenic lesions in their genomes [*see Chapter 8*].

Molecular Biology and the Management of Cancer

We opened this chapter with the declaration that a molecular understanding of cancer would offer new strategies with which the challenge of cancer can be confronted. We conclude with some indications of how this promise may be realized.

An ugly truth exists about the treatment of cancer: progress in this area has been stalled for several decades. The use of nonspecific cytotoxic drugs and radiation has been pushed to great extremes, yet most solid tumors can be cured only by full surgical excision—a physical impossibility once metastasis has occurred. The genetic paradigm for cancer offers hope for improvement. A molecular enemy is now in view.

Once we understand the growth strategies used by the cancer cell, we may be clever enough to invent specific remedies that thwart them [*see Chapter 9*]. These remedies will be unlike any available before. In addition, the revelations from recent research on the molecular biology of cancer promise to reveal more sensitive means of detection and more exact means of diagnosis [*see Chapter 9*]. When realized, these advances are likely to make current therapies even more effective.

In the final analysis, we would rather prevent cancer than have to treat it. To prevent cancer, we most know its causes. Until now, knowing the causes of cancer has been largely the province of the epidemiologist. Having ferreted out the molecular targets of carcinogenic agents, however, cancer researchers are now able to determine what effect those agents have on their targets. This information may, in turn, lead to algorithms that allow us to reason backward, moving from a description of the chemical and physical damage in cancer genes to the cause itself.

These are all large ambitions. Are they justified? Reasonable? Feasible? We challenge our readers to judge the matter for themselves, once they have perused the remarkable contents of this book.

CHAPTER 2

Normal Cells and Cancer Cells

G. Steven Martin, Ph.D.

In this chapter, the differences between cancer cells and their normal progenitors, and how these differences may account for tumor progression, are discussed. Our understanding of the cellular and molecular differences between normal cells and cancer cells has resulted primarily from studies on the transformation of normal cells into malignant cells in cell culture. This chapter therefore focuses first on the application of cell culture techniques to tumor biology. Then, some of the properties of malignant cells are examined, including their autonomous growth properties and genetic instability, and the alterations in cell differentiation and the cell division cycle that result from malignant transformation are described. Finally, the process of variation and selection that leads to the phenomenon of tumor progression (the evolution of tumor cells into progressively more malignant forms) is described. Although the primary focus of this chapter is on the biologic properties and behavior of cancer cells, the genetic changes in proto-oncogenes or tumor suppressor genes that underlie the altered properties of tumor cells are briefly discussed; these changes are described in detail in the chapters that follow.

Experimental Approaches to Cancer

Cell Culture

The development of cancer in humans is a complex, multistep process. Cancers develop slowly because at the cellular level, each step occurs at a very low frequency. Even in animals exposed to high doses of carcinogens, latency periods lasting months are common. The slow progress of most cancers is fortunate, but it makes experimental approaches to human cancer very difficult. Experimental analysis requires the process of malignant conversion to be a frequent, reproducible event that can be studied by using the tools of cellular and molecular biology. An additional difficulty in studying spontaneous cancers is that identification of the normal cell from which the tumor cells have originated may not be possible. The malignant cells may be derived from a minority population in the normal tissue, for example, a population of dividing precursor cells (stem cells). In extreme cases, the cancer cells may have lost so many markers of differentiation that even the tissue of origin may be difficult to determine. Thus, for human cancers, even a simple comparison between a cancer cell and its normal progenitor is often fraught with difficulty. Moreover, it is extremely difficult to use the tools of cellular and molecular biology to examine or manipulate individual cells of a tumor that is growing in its original host. For all of these reasons, cell cultures are an essential tool of experimental oncology. Under appropriate conditions, normal cells growing in cell culture can be altered into tumorigenic cells that induce tumors when the cells are reinjected into susceptible animal hosts. This process is referred to as *malignant transformation*, or simply *transformation*.

The earliest uses of cell culture date back to Ross Harrison's pioneering studies performed early in this century. By culturing explants of embryonic neural tissue under conditions in which the neurons would extend processes, he was able to confirm the theory of Ramon y Cajal that nerve processes arise as outgrowths from the cell body rather than as products of cell fusion. Subsequently, Alexis Carrel and colleagues were able to show that cells could proliferate in culture if they were stimulated by the appropriate growth factors, which at that time were provided by plasma clots and extracts of embryonic tissues.[1] Tissue culture came into wide and routine use after World War II, with the development of defined media and the discovery of antibiotics that could prevent microbial contamination. The power of cell culture results from the fact that when intact tissues are dissociated, a cell population is generated that can be treated as a population of microorganisms: the cells can be treated with experimental chemicals; exposed to infectious agents, such as tumor viruses; examined by light microscopy while alive; or labeled with radioactive precursors. Most importantly, the progeny of a single cell can be grown into a new population of cells, a process referred to as *cell cloning*[1] (so called to distinguish it from *molecular cloning*, a synonym for recombinant DNA technology). Thus, if a single cell is genetically altered by some cancer-causing agent, its descendants can be grown into mass culture and studied at the biochemical level. Tumors also arise from single cells, so that the generation of cultures of transformed cells by clonal growth from a single altered cell mimics the origination of tumors in vivo.

Cell cultures are initially established by dissociation of a tissue into a single-cell population, usually by treatment with proteolytic enzymes. Cultures established directly from intact tissues in this way are referred to as *primary cultures*. The cells that are most easily cultured are fibroblasts, which proliferate readily after dissociation. In intact tissues, fibroblasts synthesize and organize an extracellular matrix, which is a complex mixture of glycoproteins and carbohydrates that is deposited around the cell and functions as a mechanical support for the tissue. When fibroblasts are dissociated from this matrix, they initially adhere to the plastic or glass surface on which they are plated. However, they rapidly synthesize an extracellular matrix that also adheres to the surface of the tissue culture dish. Proliferation of fibroblasts leads to formation of a layer of cells that covers the surface of the dish. This layer of cells is frequently referred to as a *monolayer* (a somewhat misleading term because the layer of cells may be more than one cell thick). Such a monolayer of cells can in turn be dissociated by treatment with proteolytic enzymes and then be subcultured (or "passaged") to establish fresh cultures. Fibroblast cultures have been used extensively in cancer research because they can be readily transformed into malignant cells by exposure to tumor viruses or chemical carcinogens.

Carcinomas (tumors of ectoderm- or endoderm-derived epithelial cells) are much more common in humans than are sarcomas (tumors of mesodermal or mesenchymal cells). Thus, a tissue culture system that would allow the growth and transformation of epithelial cells would be of considerable utility. However, in contrast to fibroblasts, primary epithelial cells proliferate poorly as single cells. The viability and growth of certain types of epithelial cells may be promoted by allowing the cells to grow on layers of collagen floating on a liquid medium, which permits the cells to reestablish an architecture similar to the one that they adopt in vivo.[2] In a few cases, it has been possible to transform epithelial cells, for example, mouse mammary epithelial cells, but such studies are still in their infancy.

Hematopoietic cells from, for example, bone marrow or yolk sac, can also be cultured and used as substrates for studies on leukemia.[3] Hematopoietic cells are derived from pluripotential stem cells, which proliferate in bone marrow. These cells are the precursors of cells in the lymphoid, myeloid, megakaryocytic, and erythroid lineages. The pluripotential stem cells differentiate into committed progenitor cells, which undergo further proliferation, either in bone marrow, or in the case of lymphoid cells, in peripheral lymphoid organs. Each type of committed progenitor cell gives rise to terminally differentiated cells of a particular class. Pluripotential cells have recently been successfully cultured, but most studies have focused on the more differentiated committed progenitor cells, which can be cultured in semisolid (gelled) media. In such suspension cultures, these progenitor cells undergo several divisions and subsequently differentiate, giving rise to small colonies of differentiated cells. Thus, these committed progenitor cells are sometimes referred to as *colony-forming units*. Cultures containing proliferating progenitor cells have been very useful in studies on leukemic transformation.

The growth of cells in culture, like that of the cells in the original tissues, depends on the presence of appropriate growth factors.[4,5] For routine tissue culture, serum is usually used as a source of growth factors. However, for more controlled analysis, defined growth factors, such as platelet-derived growth factor, epidermal growth factor, and insulin-like growth factor, can be supplied. In some instances, such as when the cultured cells themselves secrete growth factors, cells may be grown in a completely serum-free medium. The growth of fibroblasts or epithelial cells also depends on adhesion to a solid surface. In the case of fibroblasts, this surface is the extracellular matrix that is secreted by the cells themselves; in the case of cultures of epithelial cells that are free of contaminating fibroblasts, the extracellular matrix is provided by the investigator. The adhesion-dependent growth of fibroblasts and epithelial cells in cell culture presumably reflects their behavior in the intact tissue, in which cell growth is dependent on contact with an extracellular matrix or a basement membrane. The biochemical basis for adhesion-dependent growth is not fully understood, but it appears to involve the engagement of cell surface receptors with the extracellular matrix and the generation of an intracellular signal that stimulates cell proliferation.[6] In contrast to fibroblasts and epithelial cells, many types of hematopoietic cells are not adhesion dependent and can be cultured in gelled suspension cultures.

Cells derived by dissociation of normal tissues are referred to as *primary cultures*. As these cultures are passaged, their growth rate progressively declines, and growth eventually ceases, a phenomenon known as *cellular senescence*. This property of limited life span appears to be characteristic of all normal somatic cells.[7] The only clear-cut exception to this rule are the stem cells of the early embryo; these cells are pluripotential and can give rise to cells of both somatic and germ lineages. These cells can give rise to established lines of embryonic stem cells without undergoing any irreversible genetic change. The causes of the limited life span of somatic cells in culture, and the relationship of limited life span in culture to senescence in vivo, are not clearly understood. Recent findings suggest the following, still somewhat speculative, model.[8] The phenomenon may result from alterations in chromosomal DNA that occur during cell proliferation. These alterations may include incomplete replication of chromosome ends[9] or random oxidative damage to bases in DNA.[8] These DNA alterations are believed to result in the activation of a genetic program that arrests growth [*see Chapter 6*]. Whatever its mechanism, escape from this limited life span is a common characteristic of tumor cells.

As cells are passaged, spontaneous variants may appear that do not exhibit this limited life span.[10] These variants are referred to as *established* or *immortalized cell lines*. The frequency of immortalization varies among species: mouse cells invariably give rise to established lines, whereas human cells do not [*see Figure 1*]. Established lines can usually withstand the rigors of growth at a low cell density, which facilitates the process of single-cell cloning, whereas only a small fraction of primary cells can grow as clonal populations. For this reason, established cell lines are frequently preferred for experimental work. However, they invariably have abnormal karyotypes, and thus can be regarded as normal cells only in a limited sense: indeed they are in many respects preneoplastic.[11] Immortalization may involve alterations in tumor suppressor genes [*see Chapter 6*]; in addition, immortalization has been associated with the increased synthesis of telomerase, an enzyme that maintains the ends of intact chromosomes.[9]

Malignant Transformation

When primary fibroblasts or established cell lines are treated with certain types of tumor virus or with physical or chemical carcinogens, altered cells can be isolated that may induce tumors when the cells are injected into ap-

a Human Cells

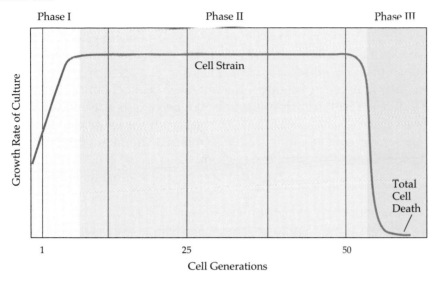

b Mouse Cells

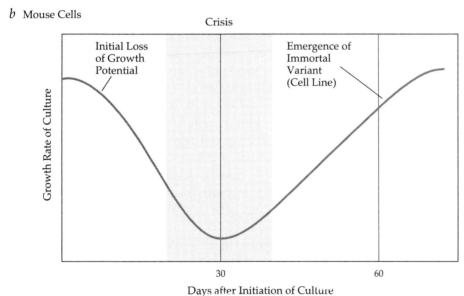

Figure 1 *Stages in the establishment of a cell culture. (a)When an initial explant of human cells is made, some cells die but others grow. During phase I, the growth rate increases. If the remaining cells are continually diluted, the cell strain grows at a constant rate for about 50 cell generations during phase II, after which, growth begins to slow. Ultimately, during phase III, all the cells in the culture die. (b) In a culture prepared from mouse embryo cells, there is initial cell death coupled with the emergence of healthy, growing cells. As these cells are diluted and continue to grow, they begin to lose growth potential. The culture goes into crisis, and most cells die. A small number of cells do not die, but continue growing until their progeny overgrow the culture. These cells constitute a cell line, which will grow as long as it is appropriately diluted and fed with nutrient.*

propriate experimental animals. This type of alteration is referred to as *neoplastic transformation, malignant transformation,* or simply *transformation.* The phenotypic changes that are usually observed in transformed fibroblasts include the acquisition of autonomous or unregulated growth properties. In particular, normal cells cease growing when they are at high population densities or when they are deprived of growth factors; they are said to be quiescent, or in the G_0 stage of the cell cycle [*see* Regulation of the Cell Division Cycle, *below*]. In contrast, transformed cells continue to proliferate under these conditions [*see Figure 2*]. In addition, transformed cells are able to grow in the absence of adhesion to an extracellular matrix ("anchorage-independent growth").[12] Transformed fibroblasts are usually more rounded or "spindly" than their normal precursors [*see Figure 3*]; these morphological changes result from a disruption of the actin cytoskeleton and its trans-

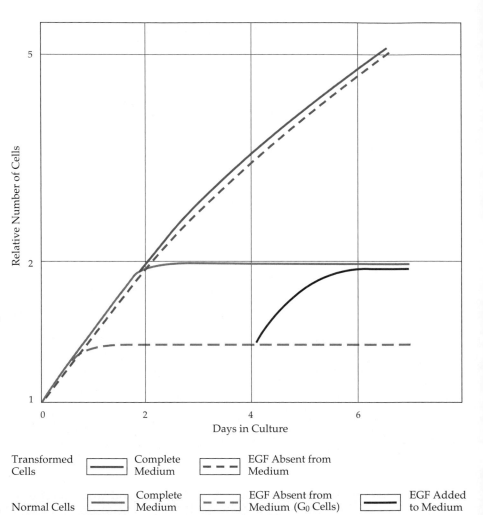

Figure 2 *Differences in the growth of normal and transformed cell cultures. On day 0, equal numbers of normal and transformed cells were plated into a defined medium with or without epidermal growth factor (EGF). Transformed cells grew in the complete medium after normal cells had ceased growth. Transformed cells also grew in the medium without EGF. On day 4, EGF was added to some dishes of normal cells that were initially lacking it. The normal cell cultures responded to the addition of EGF by growing, an indication that without EGF, normal cells can remain viable in a G_0 state.*

membrane linkages to the extracellular matrix and from changes in the structure of the extracellular matrix and matrix receptors.[13,14] In addition, most transformed cells acquire an indefinite life span. The relationship between transformation in cell culture and malignancy in vivo is not a simple one. Thus, cells that are transformed by one or more of the phenotypic criteria described above may nevertheless be unable to induce tumors in vivo, for example, if they are immunogenic and rejected by specific immune mechanisms; for this reason, immunologically compromised ("nude") mice are commonly used in tests of tumorigenicity. Conversely, a cell population that appears to be phenotypically normal may induce tumors in vivo. Despite these complications, and despite the fact that no single phenotypic marker is an infallible indicator of malignancy, each of the alterations associated with transformation apparently can contribute to malignant growth.

When cells are passaged in culture, both transformation and establishment may occur spontaneously. The nature of the processes leading to the appearance of transformed or established cells was studied systematically by Todaro and Green.[10] If mouse cells are serially passaged under conditions, such as high density, that select for the growth of transformed cells, the established cell lines that appear are transformed and induce tumors in animals. If, conversely, the cells are passaged at a low cell density, a condition that does not select for the growth of transformed cells, then the cells that emerge are not phenotypically transformed and are not capable of inducing tumors in vivo. An example of such an established but nontransformed cell line is the mouse 3T3 line (so called because of the particular transfer regimen used to isolate it).[10] Such nontransformed but established lines are much more readily transformed by a variety of agents than are primary cells and have therefore been used extensively in cancer research. However, they may undergo spontaneous transformation, and a subpopulation of transformed malignant cells can arise very readily; indeed, malignant hemangioendotheliomas can be produced by subcutaneous inoculation of 3T3

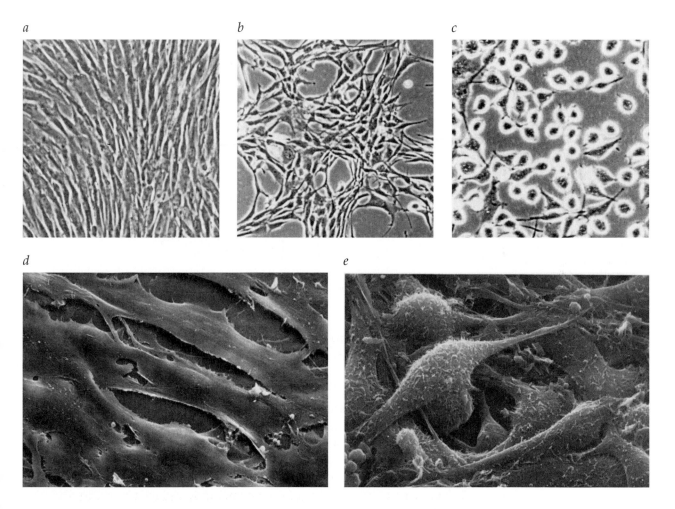

Figure 3   *Morphology of normal and transformed embryo fibroblasts. (a) In cultured normal rat embryo fibroblasts viewed by phase-contrast light microscopy, the cells are aligned and closely packed. (b) In rat embryo fibroblasts that have been transformed by integration of the polyoma virus gene encoding the middle-T antigen, the cells are crisscrossed and chaotic. (c) In rat embryo fibroblasts transformed by the Abelson murine leukemia virus, the cells have lost adherence to the dish and appear almost round. The rounded cells have white halo because they refract light. (d) Scanning electron micrographs of normal 3T3 cells. Each straplike image is a cell. Like the normal rat embryo fibroblasts in (a), the cells are lined up in one direction and are spread out into thin lamellae, with bulges representing the nuclei. (e) Scanning electron micrograph of 3T3 cells transformed by Rous sarcoma virus. The cells are much more rounded, and they are covered with small hairlike processes and bulbous projections. The cells grow one atop the other, and they have lost the side-by-side organization of the normal cells.*

cells attached to glass beads.[11] Thus, established cells are essentially preneoplastic and have undergone some of the steps involved in the generation of a fully malignant cell.

In summary, primary cultures of fibroblasts and established cell lines can be transformed into malignant cells by a variety of agents. Hematopoietic cells can also be transformed in culture. Transformed fibroblasts differ morphologically from their normal progenitors and have acquired growth autonomy (growth factor–independent and anchorage-independent growth); transformed primary cells commonly exhibit an indefinite life span.

Experimental Tumor Virology

Tumor viruses have been isolated from many avian and mammalian species, and some tumor viruses, particularly the papillomaviruses and certain hepatitis viruses, are a significant cause of human cancer [*see Chapter 3*]. Tumor viruses have played a central role in the development of molecular oncology for two reasons. First, cultured cells can be rapidly and reproducibly transformed by certain tumor viruses; therefore, normal and transformed cells can be compared directly, either by cloning transformed cells from an infected cell population or by using a virus that transforms a large fraction of the infected cells. Second, these viruses have relatively simple genomes; thus, the genes responsible for transformation can be identified and characterized. In this respect, two groups of tumor viruses have proved to be particularly informative. The rapidly or acutely transforming retroviruses carry transforming genes that are not required for viral replication; these transforming genes are derived from cellular progenitors, the proto-oncogenes [*see Chapter 4*]. The other group, the papovaviruses, includes the intensively studied monkey virus SV40 and the mouse virus polyoma. These viruses encode replicative proteins that are directly involved in viral DNA replication (the synthesis of progeny viral DNA molecules) and that are also involved in transformation. Many tumor viruses induce tumors in animals but do not transform in cell culture. For example, the nontransforming RNA tumor viruses are retroviruses that induce leukemias or solid tumors after latency periods of months or years; they do not carry transforming genes, and they do not transform cells in culture. Induction of tumors by these viruses results from provirus insertion into, or adjacent to, proto-oncogenes [*see Chapter 4*]. Another group of tumor viruses that do not transform in cell culture are the papillomaviruses; these are papovaviruses that induce tumors in animals and humans, but for which no readily accessible cell culture transformation system exists [*see Chapter 3*]

Transformation by RNA tumor viruses and transformation by DNA tumor viruses have one major feature in common: transformation depends on the integration of viral DNA into the host cell genome. This is a critical step in transformation because the integrated DNA is replicated along with cellular DNA during the cell division cycle; thus, the genome of the virus is perpetuated as the cell multiplies. The persistence of viral DNA allows the continuous expression of viral gene products, which is necessary for the maintenance of the transformed state. The biochemical mechanisms involved in transformation by tumor viruses are described in more detail in later chapters.

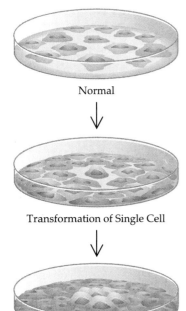

Normal

Transformation of Single Cell

Focus

Figure 4 *Side view of cells growing in a Petri dish. Lacking the contact inhibition of normal cells, transformed cells proliferate to form a thick focus that is visible to the naked eye.*

The retrovirus life cycle is outlined in Chapter 3. In the cytoplasm of the infected cell, the viral reverse transcriptase converts the viral RNA into a linear DNA molecule. The linear DNA then moves to the nucleus, where it becomes integrated into the cellular DNA; the integrated viral DNA is known as the *provirus*. The later steps in the replication cycle, viral assembly and budding, are not cytopathic, that is, the production of virus particles does not kill the infected cell. For this reason, infected cells can continue to proliferate, thereby replicating the proviral DNA along with the cellular DNA. If the virus carries a transforming gene, the cell becomes transformed and produces progeny virus at the same time.

Most studies on transformation by retroviruses have made use of fibroblasts infected by viruses that can transform fibroblasts in cell culture and induce sarcomas in vivo. When the multiplicity of infection—the ratio of infectious virus to susceptible cells—is high, the entire cell population may be transformed, and transformed cells can then be compared with parallel cultures of normal cells.[15] When the multiplicity of infection is low, areas of morphologically distinct transformed cells can be distinguished from a monolayer of morphologically normal cells[16] [*see Figures 4 and 5*]. Each morphologically distinct focus results from the infection of a susceptible cell by a single infectious virus, the division of that infected cell, and the recruitment of neighboring cells to the focus by successive cycles of virus release and reinfection. In addition, transformed cells become anchorage independent and grow into colonies when the cells are suspended in an agarose or methylcellulose medium, whereas normal cells grow for only one or two divisions after suspension [*see Figure 6*]. The development of these assays for transformation by retroviruses, and the development of similar assays for transformation by DNA tumor viruses,[17] represent the foundation of experimental tumor virology.

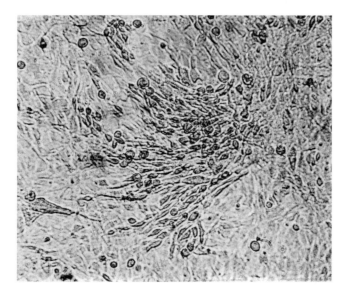

Figure 5 *Chick embryo cells in culture transformed by the Rous sarcoma virus pile up thickly, growing without contact inhibition.*

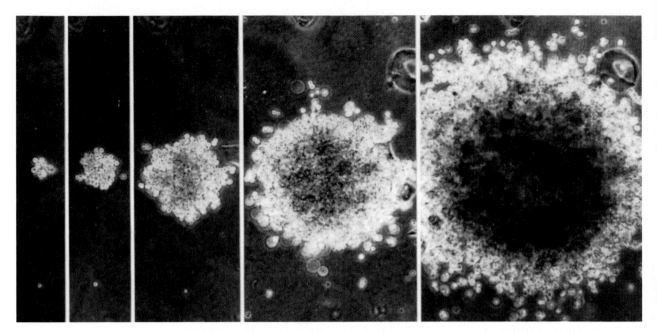

Figure 6 *Unlike normal cells, which cannot grow unless they adhere to a solid substrate, transformed cells are anchorage-independent and thus are able to proliferate into globular colonies within a semiliquid agar suspension. These micrographs, taken at intervals, show the expansion of one such colony of tumor cells.*

Cell types other than fibroblasts can also be transformed by retroviruses. In particular, hematopoietic cells can be transformed by acute leukemia viruses, which induce a rapid leukemia in vivo. When the infected cell suspension is incubated in a gelled medium, the normal target cells proliferate to a limited extent and then undergo terminal differentiation, whereas the transformed cells grow into larger, less differentiated colonies. For example, lymphoid cells can be transformed by Abelson murine leukemia virus,[18] erythroid cells can be transformed by avian erythroblastosis virus,[19,20] and myeloid cells can be transformed by avian myelocytomatosis or myeloblastosis viruses.[19,21] These systems have been very useful for examining the relationship between malignant transformation and cell differentiation [*see* Disturbances of Differentiation, *below*].

In contrast to retroviruses, papovaviruses, such as the monkey virus SV40 and the mouse virus polyoma, are usually cytopathic in their natural hosts. The cells of the natural host are referred to as *permissive cells*, in that they allow viral replication; viral replication in turn leads to cell lysis and release of virus particles. Because these viruses are usually cytopathic in their natural hosts, transformation is generally studied in hosts that do not permit a complete viral replication cycle (although polyoma does induce tumors in its natural host, the mouse, and transformation of mouse cells can be observed under certain circumstances in which virus replication is blocked). The cells of the foreign host are referred to as *nonpermissive cells*. Thus, the monkey virus SV40 replicates in and lyses monkey cells but transforms mouse 3T3 cells. Similarly, the mouse polyoma virus replicates in and lyses mouse 3T3 cells but transforms hamster or rat cells. When nonpermissive cells are infected with a transforming papovavirus, most of the infected cells transiently acquire the properties of transformed cells and grow in an anchorage-independent fashion when they are suspended in gelled medium. The response, referred to as *abortive transformation*, is transient because the DNA of the virus is not replicated and does not persist when the cell proliferates. In a fraction of the infected cell population, however, the DNA becomes integrated into the cellular DNA and is replicated along with the cellular DNA as the cell goes through its division cycle. Integration of the viral DNA therefore results in the stable transformation of some fraction of the infected cells, and these stable transformants can be isolated as morphologically altered clones. Transformation results from the expression, in the nonpermissive cells, of virally encoded proteins, the T (or tumor) antigens. One of the functions of these proteins in the normal host is to promote cellular DNA replication and thus permit viral DNA replication [*see Chapter 3*]. When expressed in the nonpermissive host, the same activities of the T antigens result in transformation.

Experimental Carcinogenesis: Physical and Chemical Agents

Many chemical and physical agents can cause tumors in animals and are carcinogenic in humans [*see Chapter 3*]. Chemical carcinogens include industrial products or byproducts, such as polycyclic aromatic hydrocarbons, aromatic amines, nitrosamines, and halohydrocarbons, and various natural products derived from plant and microbial sources. Many of these chemicals must be activated by metabolic conversion to reactive species; these species are the so-called ultimate carcinogens. The physical carcinogens include both ionizing radiation and ultraviolet radiation. The discovery of these chemical and physical carcinogens and the demonstration that these carcinogens induce transformation by damaging DNA are discussed in Chapter 3; in this chapter, the focus is on the use of these agents in cell culture to examine the mechanisms of carcinogenesis.

Chemical carcinogens can be administered to experimental animals, by administration in the diet, by injection, or by application to the skin; internal organs can be irradiated with ionizing radiation; and ultraviolet-radiation can be used to induce skin cancers. In every case, the appearance of cancers follows the initial insult by months, sometimes years. As the dose of carcinogen is increased, the incidence of cancer increases, and the interval before tumors appear decreases. For these and other reasons, it may be concluded that chemical and physical carcinogenesis involves a series of rare events, the likelihood of which is increased as the dose of carcinogen is increased. More detailed studies have led to a distinction between two phases of carcinogenesis [*see Chapter 3*]. The first phase, or initiation, is typically induced by agents that are mutagenic; therefore, it is believed that these agents are carcinogenic because they induce mutations. The second phase, promotion, is induced by chemical agents known as *tumor promoters*, which promote the growth of the tumor from the initiated (i.e., mutant) cell.

Transformation by chemical and physical carcinogens can also be observed in cell culture.[22] Application of these carcinogens to cultured cell lines usually leads to extensive cell killing, but among the survivors are cells that multiply to form colonies or foci of transformed cells. These transformed cells, like those transformed by tumor viruses, show characteristic differences from their nontransformed progenitors: they are morphologically altered, and their growth becomes autonomous, that is, they lose their dependence on external growth factors and their attachment to a substratum. Moreover, the transformed cells may be capable of forming tumors when these cells are introduced into susceptible host animals. However, the frequency with which these transformed cells arise among the survivors of the carcinogen treatment is usually very low, less than one in 1,000. Furthermore, only established cell lines that are already preneoplastic can be transformed in this way. In many cases, the transformants that arise after the initial carcinogen treatment are only partially autonomous in their growth, and they do not induce tumors in animals; in these cases, further carcinogen treatments or extended periods of growth in culture are required to generate complete transformants.

Thus, striking differences exist between transformation by tumor viruses and transformation by chemical or physical carcinogens. Transformation by tumor viruses that carry a transforming gene is a common event at the cellular level, and most cells that stably incorporate and express the viral genome are transformed: in other words, transformation by tumor viruses is a single-step process. However, some transforming viruses carry more than one transforming gene; in these cases, transformation, although it apparently occurs in one step, depends on more than one biochemical alteration.[23] In contrast, transformation by physical and chemical carcinogens is a multistep process involving a series of rare events. However, at the molecular level, the ultimate biochemical effects of the different carcinogens are similar.

Chromosomal Alterations and the Genetic Stability of Cancer Cells

Another characteristic of cancer cells is their genetic instability and heterogeneity. The cells within a tumor are not genetically identical, even though they are descendants of a single cell [*see* Clonality of Tumors and Tumor Progression, *below*]. This heterogeneity is usually evident when metaphase chromosome spreads are examined or when nuclear DNA content of individual cells is determined by microfluorometry. The development of staining methods that reveal unique banding patterns on individual chromosomes has allowed the detailed analysis of these changes.[24] Tumor cells generally exhibit a variety of departures from the normal diploid karyotype, or chromosome set [*see Figure 7*]: the term *aneuploidy* is used to describe these abnormal and heterogeneous karyotypes, to contrast with the euploid state of normal cells. These abnormalities may take the form of alterations in chromosome number. For example, loss of one of the two members of a pair of homologous chromosomes (i.e., reduction to monosomy) can be important in uncovering the effects of recessive mutations [*see Chapter 6*]. The chromosomal alterations observed in tumor cells may also take the form of structural alterations in individual chromosomes. Reciprocal translocations (reciprocal exchanges between nonhomologous chromosomes without the loss of genetic material) are commonly observed. Deletions within chromosomes (which may result from nonreciprocal exchanges) are also common.

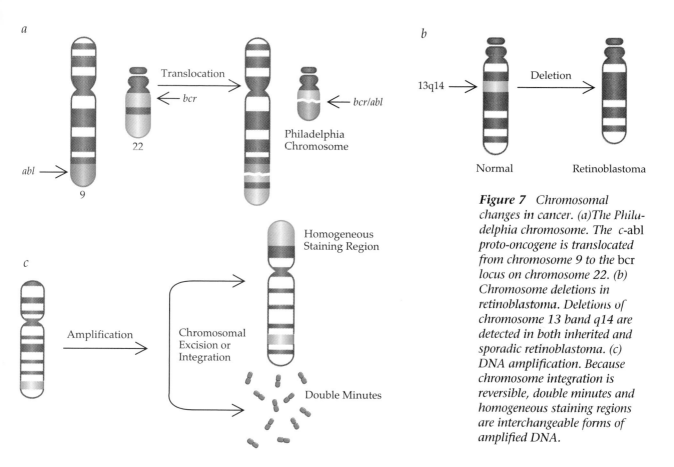

a

Translocation

← *bcr*

22

9

abl →

Philadelphia
Chromosome

← *bcr/abl*

b

13q14 →

Deletion

Normal

Retinoblastoma

c

Amplification

Chromosomal
Excision or
Integration

Homogeneous
Staining Region

Double Minutes

Figure 7 *Chromosomal changes in cancer. (a)The Philadelphia chromosome. The c-abl proto-oncogene is translocated from chromosome 9 to the bcr locus on chromosome 22. (b) Chromosome deletions in retinoblastoma. Deletions of chromosome 13 band q14 are detected in both inherited and sporadic retinoblastoma. (c) DNA amplification. Because chromosome integration is reversible, double minutes and homogeneous staining regions are interchangeable forms of amplified DNA.*

In addition, segments within chromosomes can be selectively amplified, probably as the result of DNA damage (e.g., a double-strand break), followed by some aberrant type of DNA replication, recombination, or repair.[25] Amplified chromosome segments can be cytologically detected as homogeneously stained regions within chromosomes. Alternatively, gene amplification can result in the generation of chromosome fragments that lack spindle attachment points (centromeres); these acentric fragments, referred to as *double minutes*, can replicate independently, but during mitosis, they are distributed to daughter cells at random.

Thus, chromosomal heterogeneity is the norm in cancer, but the origins of this chromosomal heterogeneity are unclear. The maintenance of the normal karyotype depends on the correct function of enzymes involved in the replication of normal DNA complement and in the repair of DNA damage. It also depends on proteins of the mitotic apparatus; these proteins ensure that at cell division, the chromosomes are distributed in an orderly fashion to the daughter cells. In addition, the biochemical machinery that regulates the cell division cycle is itself subject to "checkpoint controls," which ensure that cell division does not occur until DNA replication is completed and DNA damage is repaired [*see* Regulation of the Cell Division Cycle, *below*].[26,27] Defects in any of these processes could give rise to the chromosomal and genetic instability of cancer cells. Evidence indicating that defects in DNA repair play a role in the genesis of cancer has come from studies on certain hereditary cancer syndromes. For example, in xeroderma pigmentosum, which results from defects in excision repair, ultraviolet radiation–induced skin cancers are common.[28] Similarly, hereditary nonpolyposis colon cancer has recently been shown to result from defective DNA mismatch repair.[29] Defects in DNA repair could promote the accumulation of point mutations in the genome, as well as the more cytologically evident chromosomal changes that result in an aneuploid karyotype.

Although little is known about the origins of chromosomal instability, its contributions to tumorigenesis are profound. Amplification of chromosome segments can increase the copy number of proto-oncogenes located within those segments. Translocations can link proto-oncogenes to segments of DNA that affect their function, and chromosome loss or deletion can remove tumor suppressor genes that normally restrain cell proliferation. In addition, chromosomal instability also has important implications for cancer chemotherapy. Chemotherapeutic treatment with cytotoxic drugs often leads to the appearance of drug-resistant cells. These cells may result from the amplification of genes that encode proteins that metabolize the drug or transport it out of the cell. For example, resistance to colchicine or doxorubicin (Adriamycin) usually results from amplification of the *mdr*1 gene, which encodes a transport protein (P-glycoprotein) that pumps cytotoxic drugs out of the cell.[30] These effects of chromosome instability are described in detail in subsequent chapters.

Hormonal Control of Cellular Proliferation

The growth of normal cells is regulated by soluble proteins termed *growth factors* or *cytokines*.[4,5] The first proteins to be identified that convey regulatory information from one cell to another were hormones, which are signaling molecules that are stored in endocrine glands and are secreted when needed into the circulatory system. Hormones can be divided into two general classes. Some are *hydrophilic* (water-soluble) molecules that cannot traverse the cell membrane and must therefore interact with cell surface receptors to induce changes in their target cells. This class includes the protein or peptide hormones and also small molecules, such as catecholamines. Others, such as the steroid hormones, are *hydrophobic* molecules that can cross cell membranes and exert their effects by binding directly to intracellular targets. Hormones of both types can affect cell growth. In addition to the hormones that are stored in endocrine glands, many other regulatory proteins or polypeptides are secreted by various cell types; these proteins can affect the growth of adjacent cells. This type of signaling by polypeptide growth factors or cytokines released from neighboring cells is referred to as *paracrine signaling* (to distinguish it from endocrine regulation by stored hormones). Cells can also secrete growth factors that bind to receptors on the same cells, a type of signaling referred to as *autocrine* signaling.

The first polypeptide growth factor to be recognized was identified in 1954 by Rita Levi-Montalcini. This factor, nerve growth factor, is a neurotrophic factor that affects the differentiation and survival of sensory and sympathetic neurons. A few years later, while trying to purify nerve growth factor, Stanley Cohen identified epidermal growth factor, a factor that promotes the growth of epithelial cells. Since these early studies were performed, many growth factors have been identified that play important roles in the regulation of cell growth and differentiation.[4,5] One growth factor that has been studied extensively is platelet-derived growth factor, which is secreted by platelets after they are activated by their adhesion to a capillary endothelium. Platelet-derived growth factor stimulates the growth of fibroblasts and smooth muscle cells and appears to be involved in wound healing. Vascular endothelial growth factor stimulates the growth of endothelial cells and plays a major role in angiogenesis, the process by which a new capillary supply is formed in developing tissues. Another family of peptide growth factors, the fibroblast growth factor family, regulates the proliferation of many different cell types. Although many growth factors stimulate cell growth, some are inhibitory: tumor growth factor-β, for example, inhibits the growth of epithelial cells and induces terminal differentiation of certain cells, such as myoblasts.

Soluble growth factors play particularly important roles in regulating the proliferation, differentiation, and function of hematopoietic cells, including cells of the immune system. Such growth factors are variously termed *hemopoietins*, *lymphokines*, or *interleukins*. Hemopoietins were originally identified as factors that could induce the formation of colonies of differentiating cells in suspension cultures of hematopoietic tissues, such as the spleen, fetal liver, or yolk sac. For example, colony-stimulating factor 1 stimulates the growth of colonies that contain myeloid cells and macrophages, whereas erythropoietin stimulates the growth of committed erythroid progenitors.[3] Interleukins and lymphokines affect the function of cells of the immune system. Thus, interleukin-2, an autocrine and paracrine factor that is secreted by activated helper T cells, stimulates the growth both of the cells that secrete it as well as the growth of neighboring T and B cells.

Growth factors not only control the proliferation and function of cells in the adult, they also play critical roles in embryogenesis. Growth factors provide inductive signals that regulate the determination and differentiation of embryonic cell lineages. For example, in vertebrate embryos, fibroblast growth factors and members of the tumor growth factor–β family are involved in mesoderm induction and primary embryonic induction—the formation of the embryonic axis.[5] Related growth factors regulate embryonic development in invertebrate embryos.

Thus, in multicellular animals, all aspects of cell function, including cell proliferation, are regulated by intercellular signaling molecules, most of which are protein or peptide growth factors. These growth factors interact with specific protein receptors at the cell surface. Growth factor receptors are generally proteins that traverse the lipid bilayer of the plasma membrane; they contain an external domain, which binds the growth factor, and a cytoplasmic domain, which then triggers further biochemical events within the cell. This process, by which binding of a growth factor (the *ligand*) leads to activation of some intracellular pathway, is known as *signal transduction* [*see Chapter 5*]. The activated receptor induces changes at the cytoplasmic face of the plasma membrane, either by becoming enzymatically active itself or by interacting with other regulatory proteins at the plasma membrane. These changes lead to a series of events in the cytoplasm, such as changes in ion concentration; production of second-messenger molecules, such as cyclic adenosine monophosphate; or activation of protein kinases, which are enzymes that phosphorylate protein substrates. The cytoplasmic signals can then lead to changes in gene expression within the nucleus that may ultimately lead to cell division.

Alterations in growth factor signaling systems underlie the acquisition of growth autonomy by cancer cells. These alterations may affect either the production of growth factors themselves or intracellular signaling pathways within the cancer cells. Tumor cells may secrete increased levels of growth factors to which they themselves respond; such autocrine stimulation can lead to growth factor autonomy. Stimulation of neighboring stromal cells by growth factors that are secreted by carcinoma cells (paracrine signaling) leads to increased proliferation of the stroma; this stromal response may be necessary to support the growth of the tumor epithelial cells. In addition, secretion of fibroblast growth factors and vascular endothelial growth factor by tumors leads to proliferation of endothelial cells and tumor angiogenesis, the invasion of the tumor by a new capillary supply.[31] The growth of solid tumors beyond a certain limiting size is completely dependent on angiogenesis [*see Figure 8*]; increased secretion of angiogenic factors represents a critical step in tumor progression [*see* Clonality of Tumors and Tumor Progression, *below*], and intervention to block tumor angiogenesis may prove to be a useful mode of therapy. Of most relevance to the central theme of this volume, mutations in the intracellular signaling pathways that are activated by growth factors are of central importance in carcinogenesis. These mutations may affect the receptors themselves, the components of the cytoplasmic signaling pathways, or the factors within the nucleus that regulate gene expression [*see Chapter 5*].

Regulation of the Cell Division Cycle

Cell proliferation involves successive cycles of DNA replication and cell division.[32] The term *DNA replication* refers to the enzymatic processes involved in the copying of the two strands of one DNA double helix into two daughter molecules. The terms *cell division* and *mitosis* refer to the processes by which these daughter DNA molecules are separated or segregated into two daughter cells. The coordinated series of events involving successive periods of DNA replication and cell division is referred to as the *cell division cycle*, or simply the *cell cycle*.[32] The exposure of quiescent normal cells to stimulatory growth factors allows the cells to enter the cell division cycle; conversely, when growth factors are withdrawn, normal cells withdraw from the cell cycle. The past 10 years have seen major advances in our understanding of the cell cycle and have led to the realization that disturbances in cell cycle regulation, like disturbances in cell surface signaling, are of major importance in carcinogenesis.

In the early embryo, in which the cytoplasm of the egg is simply divided into smaller and smaller cells, the cell cycle consists simply of successive rounds of DNA replication and mitosis. As the embryo develops and starts to grow in mass as the result of protein synthesis, "G," or "gap," phases are introduced into the cycle [*see Figure 9*]. The gap phases allow time for the cell mass to double in the period between cell divisions. More importantly,

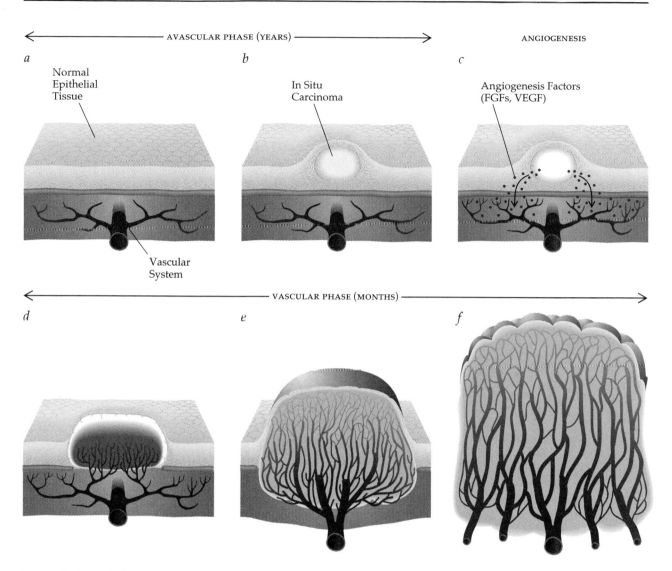

AVASCULAR PHASE (YEARS)   ANGIOGENESIS

a

Normal
Epithelial
Tissue

b

In Situ
Carcinoma

c

Angiogenesis Factors
(FGFs, VEGF)

Vascular
System

VASCULAR PHASE (MONTHS)

d   *e*   *f*

Figure 8 *Vascularization is required to convert an in situ, or dormant, carcinoma into a rapidly growing malignancy that is capable of killing its host. (a) Normal epithelial tissue is isolated from the vascular system by a basement membrane. (b) In the avascular phase, the initial clump of malignant cells may exist as a harmless in situ carcinoma for many years. (c) The tumor must release an angiogenesis factor, such as fibroblast growth factors (FGFs) and vascular endothelial growth factor (VFGF), before nearby blood vessels will send out capillaries that are capable of penetrating the tumor. (d–f) Once the tumor is vascularized, rapid growth follows.*

the introduction of gap phases allows for the regulation of the cell cycle. The first gap phase, G_1, intervenes between mitosis (the M phase) and DNA replication (the "synthesis," or S, phase). The second gap phase, the G_2 phase, occurs between the end of the S phase and the beginning of the M phase. When cells cease to divide, for example, so that they can differentiate into some specialized cell type, they generally do so in the G_1 phase (although occasionally cells can withdraw from the cell cycle when in the G_2 phase). Cells that have withdrawn from the cell cycle in the G_1 phase are said to be in a "G-zero" (G_0) state. In cultures of normal (nontransformed) cells, this state is induced by withdrawal of growth factors; transformed cells in contrast generally do not enter the G_0 state when they are deprived of

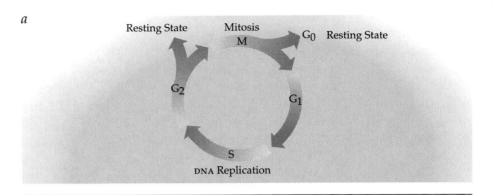

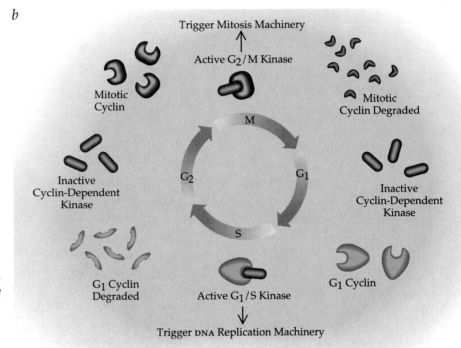

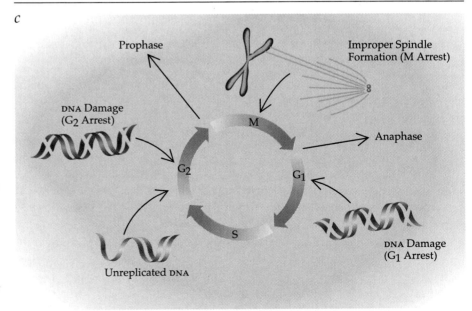

Figure 9 (a) Cell cycle exit in G_1 and G_2. Cells can withdraw from the cell cycle and enter a G_0 or a stable G_2 arrest, in which growth is also halted. (b) The core of the cell cycle control system. A cyclin-dependent kinase associates successively with different cyclins to trigger the downstream processes of the cycle. Kinase activity is terminated by cyclin degradation. (c) Stages at which checkpoint controls can arrest passage through the cell cycle. DNA damage caused by irradiation or chemical modification prevents G_1 cells from entering the S phase and G_2 cells from entering mitosis. Unreplicated DNA prevents entry into mitosis. Defects in assembly of the mitotic spindle or the attachment of kineto-chores to spindle microtubules prevents activation of the system that leads to degrada-tion of mitotic cyclins. Consequently, G_2/M kinase activity remains high, and cells do not enter anaphase.

growth factors [*see Figure 2*].

The major advances in our understanding of the cell cycle have resulted from the identification of the molecular components of the "cell cycle clock" or "cell cycle engine" that drives the progression through the cell cycle. These components are present in all eukaryotic cells, from those in simple unicellular yeasts to those in humans. Two types of proteins are of central importance in the regulation of the cell cycle.[32] One class of proteins is the *cyclins*, so called because they vary in abundance through the cell cycle. The other class of proteins is a family of protein kinases; these kinases are regulated by the binding of cyclins and are therefore known as *cyclin-dependent kinases*. In the simple yeasts, a single cyclin-dependent kinase called Cdc2 regulates both G_1/S and G_2/M transitions. The activity of Cdc2 at the first (G_1/S) transition is activated by one class of cyclins, the so-called G_1 cyclins, and the activity of Cdc2 at the second (G_2/M) transition is regulated by a second class, the mitotic cyclins[32] [*see Figure 9*]. In animal cells, the regulation system is more complex, with different cyclin-dependent kinases and multiple cyclins regulating different cell cycle transitions.

Signals from outside the cell, which involve the interaction of growth factors or other molecules with surface receptors, can regulate progression through the cell cycle. The activation of cell surface receptors leads to the activation of signal transduction pathways that ultimately result in changes in gene expression. The mechanism by which these changes in gene expression lead to re-entry into the cell cycle is not fully understood. Growth factors activate the expression of cyclins that are necessary for the G_1/S transition.[33] In addition, growth factors can regulate the expression of proteins that inhibit the activity of cyclin-dependent kinases. Although the biochemical details of these regulatory mechanisms are not clearly understood, several observations suggest that defects in the cell cycle machinery that responds to external signals may underlie certain types of cancer.[34] For example, cyclins may be overexpressed or structurally altered in some parathyroid adenomas, centrocytic B cell lymphomas, and breast carcinomas. Most recently, investigators have observed that genes encoding proteins that inhibit cyclin-dependent kinases are altered in many human cancers.[34,35]

In addition to being regulated by external signals, the cell cycle clock is regulated by an internal control system. The events of the cell cycle—DNA replication and mitosis—must occur in an orderly succession. The cell therefore needs to determine whether one phase of the cycle is complete before entering the next phase. For example, the cell must monitor whether the S phase is complete before preparing to undergo mitosis. If DNA replication is inhibited, normal cells arrest in the S phase and do not proceed into mitosis. This regulatory mechanism protects the cell from the catastrophic effects of attempting to divide while the chromosomes are not yet replicated. This type of control has been termed *checkpoint control* [26,27] [*see Figure 9*]. Similarly, if cellular DNA is damaged by mutagenic agents (e.g., carcinogens), the cellular division cycle is arrested until DNA damage is repaired; in some cell types, DNA damage results in programmed cell death (apoptosis), which actually destroys the damaged cell.[36] Another checkpoint control mechanism is important in maintaining the fidelity of chromosome transmission at mitosis. Mitosis proceeds to completion only if the chromosome movement machinery (the mitotic spindle) is first correctly assembled; this characteristic again reflects the operation of a checkpoint control mechanism, which monitors assembly of the spindle.[27]

Defects in checkpoint control mechanisms probably have an important role in carcinogenesis. In mammalian cells, the checkpoint control system that monitors DNA damage requires the function of the p53 protein, the product of a tumor suppressor gene that plays a key role in human cancer. This gene, and the effects of deficiency in p53 on the response to DNA damage, are discussed in greater detail in Chapter 6. In addition, some investigators have speculated that the chromosomal instability that is prevalent in human cancer may reflect (at least in part) errors in mitosis resulting from failures in the checkpoint control that monitors spindle assembly.[27]

Finally, tissue homeostasis depends not only on the rate of cell proliferation but also on the rate of cell death. The growth of tumors may depend both on an increase in the fraction of cells that are proceeding through the cell division cycle and on a decrease in the fraction of the cells that undergo programmed cell death. Programmed cell death, or apoptosis, is a physiologic process that involves a series of characteristic, genetically controlled steps, including chromatin condensation and fragmentation and cell shrinkage; it culminates in the engulfment of the cell by neighboring cells, such as macrophages, without a concomitant inflammatory response. In contrast, necrosis(pathological or unprogrammed cell death) results in cell lysis and often provokes an inflammatory response. Apoptosis is essential both to normal development and to tissue homeostasis in the adult.[37] The formation of cavities within the embryo, the removal of nerve cells that have not found the correct connections, the regression of mammary epithelium during the menstrual cycle, the killing of virus-infected cells by cytotoxic T cells, and many other developmental processes all depend on programmed cell death. Apoptosis occurs in simple invertebrates, such as the roundworm *Caenorhabditis* and the fruit fly *Drosophila*, and the genes that regulate programmed cell death in invertebrates are related to those that regulate it in vertebrates.[37] Thus, apoptosis represents an evolutionarily conserved cellular response. Apoptosis also serves as a mechanism for preventing the proliferation of damaged cells: when cells that have sustained DNA damage are stimulated to divide by exposure to growth factors, they may undergo apoptosis, which in this instance represents a form of checkpoint control.[36] The failure of certain tumor cell types to undergo apoptosis appears to be one of the factors underlying the genetic instability of these cell types, their resistance to chemotherapeutic agents, and their increased proliferation.

Disturbances of Differentiation

Benign tumors generally contain well-differentiated cells that retain much of the organization of normal tissue. Malignant tumors, conversely, tend to be less well differentiated: they lose some of the specific features of the normal cells from which they originate. In normal tissues, differentiation may be accompanied by an irreversible commitment to a nonproliferating postmitotic state; when such terminally differentiated cells are produced from a self-renewing stem-cell population, as is the case in the hematopoietic system, a block in maturation results in an increase in proliferation and tumor development [*see Figure 10*]. Classically, the loss of differentiated features is known as *anaplasia,* and the degree of anaplasia is used by pathologists as one criterion in the staging of tumors. In advanced metastatic cancers, the loss of differentiated function may have progressed so far that readily determining the cell of origin may no longer be possible. The tumor cell has thus diverted its biosynthetic capacity from the generation of products that are of functional value to the host organism to the production of macromolecules that are required for cell growth and division.

Studies on the transformation of differentiating cells in culture have suggested that transformation may directly inhibit differentiation. Differentiating muscle cells can be transformed by sarcoma viruses,[38] and differentiating hematopoietic cells can be transformed by acute leukemia viruses.[18,23] Viral transformation frequently results in a suppression of cell differentiation. For example, normal myoblasts (muscle precursor cells) cease DNA replication and fuse to form muscle fibers, which express muscle-specific proteins, whereas virally transformed myoblasts continue to proliferate as single cells and show no signs of muscle-specific differentiation.[38] Similarly, virally transformed erythroid cells proliferate and fail to mature into functional erythrocytes,[20] transformed myeloid cells fail to mature into functional macrophages or granulocytes,[19,21] and transformed lymphoid cells fail to mature into functional lymphocytes.[18] A detailed characterization of

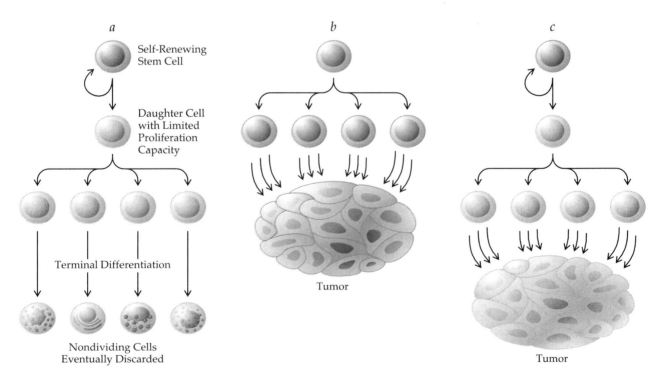

Figure 10 *Normal and deranged control of cell production from stem cells. (a) The normal pathway for producing new differentiated cells. (b) Stem cell fails to produce one non–stem cell daughter in each division and thereby proliferates to form a tumor. (c) Daughter cells fail to differentiate normally and thereby proliferate to form a tumor.*

the proteins expressed in these transformed cells suggests that they are blocked at an early stage in the differentiation process. Similar results have been obtained with human leukemia cells. Moreover, some of these cells can be induced to differentiate by external agents, such as retinoic acid and vitamin A. These observations support the idea that the leukemias represent cells that are arrested within a normal pathway of differentiation.

For an understanding of the basis for this alteration in the differentiation of tumor cells, the process of differentiation must be reviewed. Different cells in the adult express different proteins, according to the functional needs of the tissue. Skeletal muscle cells express a specific form of the protein myosin, which is required for contraction; liver cells synthesize many of the proteins of blood plasma; and erythroblasts synthesize hemoglobin, which is required for oxygen transport. This differential synthesis does not generally reflect changes in the DNA itself. Instead, differential synthesisis achieved primarily through regulation of gene expression: different genes are transcribed (copied into RNA) in different tissues. Thus, the messenger RNA that encodes myosin is expressed only in muscle cells, the messenger RNA that encodes globin is expressed only in developing erythroblasts, and so forth. This differential synthesis is regulated by specific proteins known as *transcription factors*. Transcription, the process by which messenger RNAs are generated, is initiated at a specific site at the end of each gene. Transcription factors function by binding to DNA and promoting (or inhibiting) the initiation of transcription. Different cell types express different transcription factors because the genes that encode transcription factors are themselves under the control of transcription factors expressed at earlier stages of development. Differentiation can therefore be viewed as the execution of a series of transcriptional programs, in which arrays of genes are switched on or off as a result of the expression of specific sets of transcription factors.

Many cells must withdraw from the cell cycle, that is, enter the G_0 state, so that they can differentiate. This phenomenon is most apparent in terminally differentiating cells, which cease dividing and withdraw permanently from the cell cycle when they undergo the final stages of differentiation. Thus, in some instances, differentiation and cell division can be viewed as alternative transcriptional programs. If the cell differentiates, certain genes are turned on, whereas genes involved in cell cycle progression are repressed. Conversely, if the cell proceeds through the cell cycle, the expression of genes required for cell cycle progression (e.g., cyclins, replication proteins) is induced, whereas the expression of genes involved in differentiation is repressed. The switch from one transcriptional program to the other is influenced by growth factors. The activation of growth and the induction of the cell cycle program can therefore lead to the suppression of differentiation. Similarly, in tumor cells, the activation of signaling pathways by mutations may divert the cell from expressing its differentiation program and may prompt it to express the program that leads to cell division. Thus, the abnormalities in cell differentiation that are seen in tumor cells may result directly from the mutations responsible for the activation of autonomous cell growth. However, this model is probably an oversimplification. In particular, the genetic instability that is characteristic of cancer is likely to result in random chromosomal alterations that also contribute to the derangement of cell differentiation.

Clonality of Tumors and Tumor Progression

One of the central concepts of modern tumor biology is that most tumors are monoclonal: all the cells in a tumor descend from a single cell, so that the cells within a given tumor (or within metastases from that tumor) represent a clone.[39,40] Tumors originating from multiple cells—polyclonal tumors—are not unknown. For example, tumors induced by rapidly transforming RNA tumor viruses, which can spread from tumor cells to adjacent uninfected cells, are polyclonal. Other examples exist of tumors appearing to arise from multiple cells, either because of the presence of an infectious agent, or, as in certain hereditary cancer syndromes, because the initiating event is very common. However, most spontaneous tumors are monoclonal and originate from a single cell.

The monoclonal origin of spontaneous tumors has been demonstrated by the use of markers that show clonal heterogeneity in normal tissues. For example, females that are heterozygous for sex-linked markers are mosaic as the result of the process of X-inactivation. This process occurs early in development and results in the random inactivation of one of the two X chromosomes within each cell; the descendants of a cell in which X-inactivation has occurred retain one inactive and one active X chromosome. For example, in a female that is heterozygous for some X-linked gene, whose genotype can be represented A/a, some of her cells are phenotypically A, and others are phenotypically a. Tumors that arise in such heterozygous females are found to be either A or a in phenotype. This finding indicates that the tumors must each have arisen from a single cell. A similar approach can be used for the study of tumors of the immune system. The genes encoding immunoglobulins and the components of the T cell antigen receptor undergo rearrangement during somatic development, so that individual cells express unique products (e.g., a unique immunoglobulin or a unique T cell receptor). Tumors of lymphoid cells generally contain a unique rearrangement of the immunoglobulin or T cell receptor genes. If the tumor cells secrete an immunoglobulin, as occurs in multiple myeloma, the secreted protein invariably has a unique sequence that differs from the sequence of the protein secreted by other tumors of the same type, indicating once again that the tumors are of monoclonal origin.

Even when no markers are available to distinguish between cells in normal tissues, cytologic or genetic analysis can often provide evidence that tumors are of monoclonal origin. The cells of a tumor commonly carry the same chromosomal alteration within an otherwise heterogeneous variety of chromosomal abnormalities, implying that the cells of the tumor have all descended from the cell in which the chromosomal change took place. Similarly, if all of the cells bear a specific mutation in a particular proto-oncogene, it can be concluded that all of the cells of the tumor are derived from the cell in which that mutation occurred.[40]

The finding that tumors generally develop by clonal expansion from a single cell has important theoretical implications. In particular, it implies that

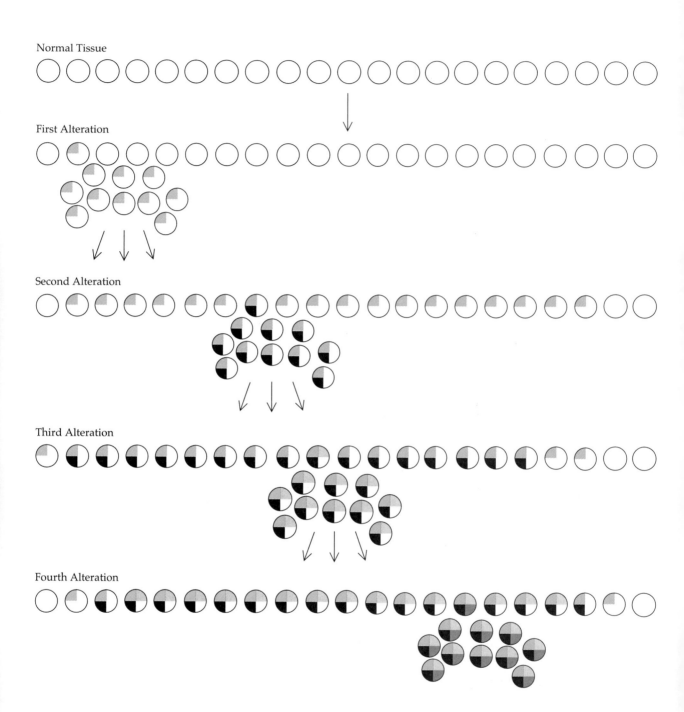

Normal Tissue

First Alteration

Second Alteration

Third Alteration

Fourth Alteration

Figure 11 *A cell clone may sustain successive multiple alterations (mutations) in its genome that allow it to compete with increasing success against cells that lack the full complement of mutations. Tumor progression is shown to equal a series of clonal expansions that are analogous to darwinian evolution in response to natural selection. Growth of most tumors is initiated by an alteration in a single cell. This initial change might lead to partial growth autonomy or a small increase in growth rate, or it might increase the genetic instability of the cell and its descendants. This altered cell divides to give rise to a small clone. One of its descendants subsequently undergoes a second alteration that gives its descendants a selective advantage. Thus, this cell gives rise to a subclone of cells that gradually outgrows the original clone. Another change gives rise to yet another subclone of cells, which has a still greater growth advantage.*

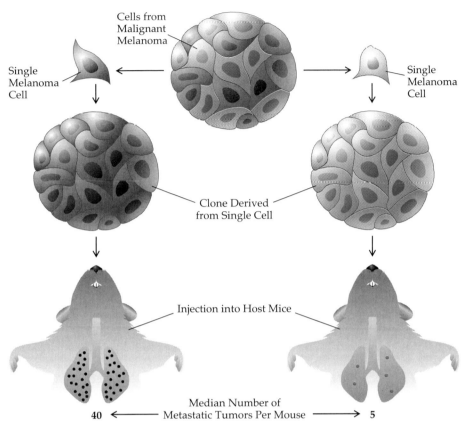

Cells from Malignant Melanoma

Single Melanoma Cell

Single Melanoma Cell

Clone Derived from Single Cell

Injection into Host Mice

Median Number of
40 ← Metastatic Tumors Per Mouse → 5

Figure 12   Experiment showing the clonally heritable differences between the cells of a single tumor with respect to their ability to metastasize. Cells derived from a single cancer cell line are subcloned, and standard aliquots of each subclone are tested by injection into the bloodstream of host mice. The subclones differ markedly in the number of resulting metastases per mouse.

the malignant or tumorigenic state is an intrinsic, clonally inherited property of the tumor cells and that the initiating event is rare. The tumor cells are clearly dependent on the surrounding stroma and on a capillary supply. Nevertheless, the growth of the tumor must result from the autonomous behavior of the tumor cells rather than from a change in the surrounding tissue. The properties of the tumor cells are clonally inherited because they result from genetic alterations within the cell. Stable changes in gene expression ("epigenetic changes") may also underlie some of the changes in malignant cells. However, genetic changes in proto-oncogenes and tumor suppressor genes are primarily responsible for tumor initiation and progression.

Benign tumors frequently evolve into more malignant forms, a phenomenon known as *tumor progression*.[41] This process involves the progressive evolution of the tumor cell population toward more autonomous and more rapidly growing forms. Increased secretion of angiogenic factors allows the growth of the tumor beyond a certain limiting size and can represent a critical step in tumor progression. The malignant cancers that ultimately emerge can invade surrounding normal tissue and, in later stages of the disease, can metastasize to distant sites. Analysis of mutations and chromosomal alterations within tumors at different stages of progression has revealed that tumors evolve as the result of the successive appearance of new clones of more rapidly growing cells within the original tumor cell population [40,41] [*see Figure 11*]. In this way, by progressive selection of more rapidly growing variants, the cell population evolves to a more malignant phenotype. (A similar process of variation and selection accounts for the appearance of drug-resistant variants in patients exposed to chemotherapeutic agents).

The progression ultimately leads to the appearance of invasive or metastatic cancers. Local invasion requires an ability to penetrate and move through the extracellular matrix. For example, a carcinoma invades the underlying connective tissue by penetrating the basement membrane beneath the epithelium in which the tumor arose. Metastasis is an even more complex process. The metastatic cells must penetrate the endothelium surrounding a capillary (or the wall of a lymphatic vessel), and then after transport in the blood, they must adhere to the capillary endothelium at some distant site. Finally, the cells must escape from the capillary and lodge in their new growth environment. Clones derived from a single tumor cell line vary in invasiveness and metastatic potential, indicating that these properties are clonally heritable [*see Figure 12*]. Metastatic potential appears to be correlated with secretion of enzymes, such as metalloproteinases and serine proteases, that degrade the extracellular matrix, and with the altered expression of cell surface molecules involved in cell adhesion and motility.[42] Unfortunately, the molecular basis for the acquisition of malignancy is not yet understood, although it does appear to be based on cumulative mutations that either activate or inactivate genes.

The growth of tumors is thus a darwinian process in which a succession of changes within the tumor cell population leads to the appearance and evolution of progressively more malignant cells.

References

1. Harris H: *The Cells of the Body.* Cold Spring Harbor Press, Cold Spring Harbor, NY, 1995
2. Lin CQ, Bissell MJ: Multi-faceted regulation of cell differentiation by extracellular matrix. *Faseb J* 7:737, 1993
3. Metcalf D: The molecular control of cell division, differentiation commitment and maturation in haemopoietic cells. *Nature* 339:27,1989
4. Cross M, Dexter TM: Growth factors in development, transformation, and tumorigenesis. *Cell* 64:271, 1991
5. Heath JK: *Growth Factors.* IRL Press at Oxford University, Oxford, New York, 1993
6. Clark EA, Brugge JS: Integrins and signal transduction pathways: the road taken. *Science* 268:233, 1995
7. Hayflick L: The limited in vitro lifetime of human diploid cell strains. *Exp Cell Res* 37:614, 1965
8. Chen Q, Fischer A, Reagan JD, et al: Oxidative DNA damage and senescence of human diploid fibroblast cells. *Proc Natl Acad Sci USA* 92:4337, 1995
9. Harley DB, Villeponteau B: Telomeres and telomerase in aging and cancer. *Curr Opin Genet Dev* 5:249, 1995
10. Todaro GJ, Green H: Quantitative studies of the growth of mouse embryo cells in culture and their development into established lines. *J Cell Biol* 17:299, 1963
11. Boone CW: Malignant hemangioendotheliomas produced by subcutaneous inoculation of Balb-3T3 cells attached to glass beads. *Science* 188:68, 1975
12. Shin SI, Freedman VH, Risser R, Pollack R: Tumorigenicity of virus-transformed cells in nude mice is correlated specifically with anchorage independent growth in vitro. *Proc Natl Acad Sci USA* 72:4435, 1975
13. Pollack R, Osborn M, Weber K: Patterns of organization of actin and myosin in normal and transformed cultured cells. *Proc Natl Acad Sci USA* 72:994, 1975
14. Turner CE, Burridge K: Transmembrane molecular assemblies in cell-extracellular matrix interactions. *Curr Opin Cell Biol* 3:849, 1991

15. Hanafusa H: Rapid transformation of cells by Rous sarcoma virus. *Proc Natl Acad Sci USA* 63:318, 1969

16. Temin HM, Rubin H: Characteristics of an assay for Rous sarcoma virus and Rous saroma cells in tissue culture. *Virology* 6:669, 1958

17. Macpherson I, Montagnier L: Agar suspension culture for the selective assay of cells transformed by polyoma virus. *Virology* 23:291, 1964

18. Rosenberg N: Abl-mediated transformation, immunoglobulin gene rearrangements and arrest of B lymphocyte differentiation. *Semin Cancer Biol* 5:95, 1994

19. Beug H, Kirchbach AV, Doderlein G, et al: Chicken hematopoietic cells transformed by seven strains of defective avian leukemia viruses display three distinct phenotypes of differentiation. *Cell* 18:375, 1979

20. Beug H, Mullner EW, Hayman MJ: Insights into erythroid differentiation obtained from studies on avian erythroblastosis virus. *Curr Opin Cell Biol* 6:816, 1994

21. Graf T, Beug H: Avian leukemia viruses: interaction with their target cells in vivo and in vitro. *Biochim Biophys Acta* 516:269, 1978

22. Heidelberger C: Chemical oncogenesis in culture. *Adv Cancer Res* 18:317, 1973

23. Graf T: Leukemia as a multistep process: studies with avian retroviruses containing two oncogenes. *Leukemia* 2:127, 1988

24. Solomon E, Borrow J, Goddard AD: Chromosome aberrations and cancer. *Science* 254:1153, 1991

25. Stark GR: Regulation and mechanisms of mammalian gene amplification. *Adv Cancer Res* 61:87, 1993

26. Hartwell LH, Weinert TA: Checkpoints: controls that ensure the order of cell cycle events. *Science* 246:629, 1989

27. Murray AW: Cell-cycle checkpoints and feedback controls. *Nature* 359:599, 1992

28. Tanaka K, Wood RD: Xeroderma pigmentosum and nucleotide excision repair of DNA. *Trends Biochem Sci* 19:83, 1994

29. Fishel R, Lescoe MK, Rao MR, et al: The human mutator gene homolog MSH2 and its association with hereditary nonpolyposis colon cancer. *Cell* 75:1027, 1993

30. Pastan I, Gottesman MM: Multidrug resistance. *Annu Rev Med* 42:277, 1991

31. Folkman J, Shing Y: Angiogenesis. *J Biol Chem* 267:10931, 1992

32. Murray AW, Hunt T: *The Cell Cycle: An Introduction.* WH Freeman, New York, 1993

33. Sherr CJ, Roberts JM: Inhibitors of mammalian G1 cyclin-dependent kinases. *Genes Dev* 9:1149, 1995

34. Hunter T, Pines J: Cyclins and cancer. II: cyclin D and CDK inhibitors come of age. *Cell* 79:573, 1994

35. Grana X, Reddy EP: Cell cycle control in mammalian cells: role of cyclins, cyclin dependent kinases (CDKs), growth suppressor genes and cyclin-dependent kinase inhibitors (CKIs). *Oncogene* 11:211, 1995

36. Thompson CB: Apoptosis in the pathogenesis and treatment of disease. *Science* 267:1456, 1995

37. Steller H: Mechanisms and genes of cellular suicide. *Science* 267:1445, 1995

38. Alema S, Tato F: Oncogenes and muscle differentiation: multiple mechanisms of interference. *Semin Cancer Biol* 5:147, 1994

39. Fialkow PJ: Clonal origin of human tumors. *Annu Rev Med* 30:135, 1979

40. Fearon ER, Hamilton SR, Vogelstein B: Clonal analysis of human colorectal tumors. *Science* 238:193, 1987

41. Nowell PC: The clonal evolution of tumor cell populations. *Science* 194:23, 1976

42. Stetler-Stevenson WG, Aznavoorian S, Liotta LA: Tumor cell interactions with the extracellular matrix during invasion and metastasis. *Annu Rev Cell Biol* 9:541, 1993

Acknowledgments

Figures 1 and 2   Marcia Kammerer. Adapted from *Molecular Cell Biology*, 3rd ed., by H. Lodish, D. Baltimore, A. Berk, et al., Scientific American Books, New York, 1995.

Figure 3 from *Molecular Cell Biology*, 3rd ed., by H. Lodish, D. Baltimore, A. Berk, et al., Scientific American Books, New York, 1995.

Figure 4   Dimitry Schidlovsky. Adapted from *Genes and the Biology of Cancer*, by H. Varmus and R.A. Weinberg, Scientific American Library, New York, 1993.

Figures 5 and 6 from *Genes and the Biology of Cancer,* H. Varmus and R.A. Weinberg, Scientific American Library, New York, 1993.

Figure 7   Dimitry Schidlovsky. Adapted from *Oncogenes*, 2nd ed., by G. Cooper, Jones and Bartlett, Boston, 1995.

Figure 8   Seward Hung. Adapted from "The Vascularization of Tumors," by J. Folkman, in *Scientific American* 234:58, 1976.

Figure 9   Dimitry Schidlovsky. Adapted from *The Cell Cycle: An Introduction*, by A. W. Murray and T. Hunt, W.H. Freeman, New York, 1993; *Molecular Cell Biology*, 3rd ed., by H. Lodish, D. Baltimore, A. Berk, et al., Scientific American Books, New York, 1995; and *Molecular Biology of the Cell*, 3rd ed., by B. Alberts, D. Bray, J. Lewis, et al., Garland Publishing, New York, 1994.

Figures 10 and 12   Seward Hung. Adapted from *Molecular Biology of the Cell*, 3rd ed., by B. Alberts, D. Bray, J. Lewis, et al., Garland Publishing, New York, 1994.

Figure 11   Marcia Kammerer. Adapted from *Genes and the Biology of Cancer*, by H. Varmus and R.A. Weinberg, Scientific American Library, New York., 1993.

CHAPTER 3

The Causes of Cancer

Douglas R. Lowy, M.D.

The causes of cancer can be categorized in several ways: according to behavior, such as cigarette smoking or dietary habits, that are associated with the development of cancer, or according to the specific physical, chemical, and infectious agents that are etiologically linked to cancer. In addition to these external factors, causal determinants that are intrinsic to the host must be considered. In this context, genetic and nongenetic elements may play a significant role in the manner in which the organism metabolizes a given carcinogen and in the relative susceptibility of the host target tissue to developing particular cancers.

The classification of cancer into multiple clinical types has facilitated etiologic studies because specific causes are usually directly related to only a subset of tumors. However, identifying the origins of one type of cancer may uncover principles that apply to many tumor types. Our notions of the causes of cancer have come from several areas of research, including cancer epidemiology, experimental cancer induced by chemicals and radiation, tumor virology, tumor biology, and study of cancer-prone families.

Extrinsic Origins of Cancer

For centuries, it was unclear whether cancer resulted from endogenous processes or from exposure to external agents. Epidemiologic evidence collected over the past two centuries has clearly established that external factors account for most cancers.[1-4] The incidence of various cancers has been shown to vary enormously among people of similar genetic background, depending on such factors as diet, tobacco exposure, and occupation.

Percivall Pott is usually credited with providing the first clear description of a presumed exposure to an environmental carcinogen. In 1775, he re-

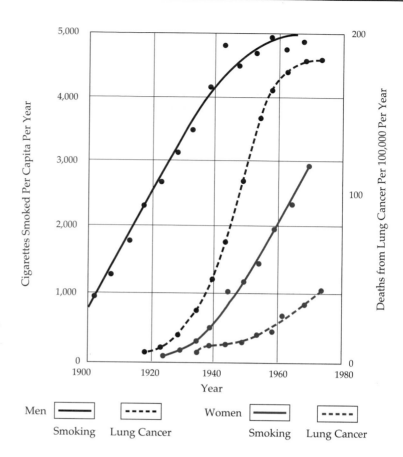

Figure 1 *Correlation between smoking and subsequent rise in the death rate from lung cancer for men and women in England.*

ported a high incidence of scrotal cancer in London men who had been chimney sweeps as boys. Pott's observation linked the development of a particular form of cancer to an occupational exposure, although the nature of the carcinogen remained undefined.

The tracking of cancer incidence in different regions and over time has provided important clues to exogenous causes of cancer. One well-studied example is the relationship between cigarette smoking and lung cancer [*see Figure 1*]. Although lung cancer was relatively uncommon before cigarette smoking became common, this form of cancer is now the most common cause of death from cancer in men and women.[5] The relative risk correlates with the number of cigarettes smoked per day and the length of time a person has been a smoker.[2] The increase in lung cancer incidence started earlier in men than in women, just as widespread smoking in men occurred earlier than it did in women. The striking epidemiological link between cigarette smoking and lung cancer does not, however, rule out the possibility that genetic susceptibility may play a role in determining whether lung cancer develops in a given smoker—indeed, some reports do suggest that the development of lung cancer may be partially determined by genetic characteristics.[6]

Mouse Skin Carcinogenesis

Although epidemiologic studies have supported the conclusion that external factors account for most human cancers and have identified environmental sources that may contribute to the development of cancer, the epidemiologic approach does not lend itself as readily to identifying specific carcinogens within these sources or to determining how carcinogens cause cancer. For example, the studies linking cigarette smoking to lung cancer do not identify the critical carcinogenic components in cigarettes, nor do they elucidate the mechanisms by which cigarette smoking may lead to cancer. Animal models and cell culture systems, which can be readily manipulated and controlled experimentally, are often better suited than epidemiologic studies for identifying the carcinogenic potential of specific agents and revealing how they cause cancer.

Initiators and Promoters

The experimental production of skin cancer in mice is an especially instructive model that has relevance to the pathogenesis of human cancer and the mechanisms by which carcinogenic agents induce tumors. In particular, the studies of Isaac Berenblum, which were begun in the 1940s,[7] were instrumental in establishing certain principles of carcinogenesis. Berenblum identified two types of compounds that had little or no cancer-inducing activity on mouse skin when they were applied individually but cooperated to form cancers at a high rate when an area of mouse skin received both of them [*see Figure 2*]. Furthermore, the compounds could induce cancer efficiently if they were given sequentially, provided that they were administered in a particular order.

The compounds that needed to be given first were designated *initiators*. Initiators included polycyclic aromatic hydrocarbons (PAHs), such as 7,12-dimethylbenz[*a*]anthracene, benzo(*a*)pyrene, and 3-methylcholanthrene, some of which are found in cigarette smoke. Under many circumstances, the skin required only a single application of the initiator. The compounds that were ineffective if given first but led to cancer if given after application of an initiator were called *promoters*. Oil from the *Croton* plant, or its active constituent, 12-*O*-tetradecanoylphorbol-13-acetate (TPA), has been widely used a promoter.[8,9]

In contrast to initiators, promoters needed to be applied repeatedly to the initiated skin. Such treatment of initiated skin with a promoter led to the development of benign skin tumors (papillomas), some of which progressed to carcinomas. Promoter treatment of noninitiated skin did not result in these changes. Although initiated skin appeared to be normal, the initiator had apparently induced an irreversible change in the skin because promoter treatment of initiated skin even one year after the initiator was applied led to cancer formation.

Cancer Is a Multistep Process

This analysis led to the functional classification of some compounds as initiators and others as promoters. Investigators could now ask whether initiators shared fundamental properties and whether promoters shared fundamental properties.

Analysis of PAHs and other initiators indicated that virtually all of them were capable of inducing mutations.[10] Although initiators had other attrib-

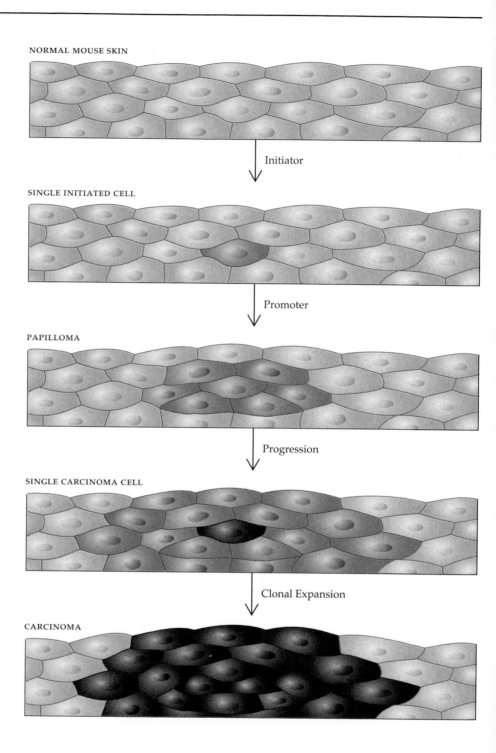

NORMAL MOUSE SKIN

Initiator

SINGLE INITIATED CELL

Promoter

PAPILLOMA

Progression

SINGLE CARCINOMA CELL

Clonal Expansion

CARCINOMA

Figure 2 *Process of tumorigenesis in induced mouse skin tumors.*

utes, the recognition that they were mutagens made it possible that their carcinogenic potential resulted from their activity against DNA. Because the initiated phenotype was long lived, investigators postulated that initiation represented the consequence of generating one or more genetic changes in potential target cells.[11] Promoters, conversely, appeared to stimulate growth of the initiated cells, but they did not seem to be directly mutagenic.[12] Indeed, promotion could be divided into two phases. In the early phase, withdrawal of the promoter led to regression of the papillomas. In the late phase, some papillomas progressed to cancer, whose growth was autonomous and therefore no longer required the promoter. Therefore, continued promoter treatment had led to a second, irreversible change, which led to skin cancer.

These studies and related analyses of chemical carcinogenesis carried out between the 1940s and the 1970s led to several important inferences: (1) cancer arises as a multistep phenomenon that includes initiation, promotion to papilloma formation, and progression to carcinoma, and (2) at least two genetic changes occur during the process (although the precise nature of these alterations was poorly defined). In this model, the initiator induced a genetic change in a small number of skin cells. It was inferred, from the requirement for a promoter, that the genetic alteration in the initiated cell was insufficient by itself to cause abnormal cell growth. Because the promoter did not induce papillomas in noninitiated skin, the initiated cell seemed to contain a genetic abnormality that primed the cell to respond inappropriately to stimulation by the promoter and to give rise to a papilloma via clonal expansion of the initiated cell.

The reversible nature of the early-phase papillomas was interpreted as meaning that the initial promoter treatments had not produced any additional mutations in the initiated cell. By contrast, progression to a cancer whose growth was independent of the promoter implied that at least one additional genetic change had occurred in the cells. Thus, the major role of the promoter, which was not directly mutagenic, was to create conditions that greatly increased the likelihood that the progeny of the initiated cell would sustain a second genetic change that led to cancer.

The promoter presumably created these conditions in at least two ways. First, because the benign papilloma was composed of millions of cells that were derived from a single initiated cell, promoter treatment had led to an enormous increase in the number of initiated cells. The promoter had therefore increased the number of initiated cells that were at risk for undergoing a random genetic alteration that might lead to the development of a skin cancer. Second, treatment with the promoter might have modified the state of the cells in the papilloma so that they were more likely to sustain a mutation. In this regard, studies of cultured cells suggested that mutations were more likely to arise in rapidly growing cells, analogous to those in the papilloma, than in nongrowing cells. The hypothesis that progression from the papilloma stage to cancer represented a separate genetic change was indirectly confirmed by the finding that the progression of first-phase papillomas to carcinomas could occur much more efficiently if the papillomas were treated with an initiator.[13]

The lessons elucidated in the mouse skin model, in which carcinogenesis was induced by mutagenic agents and growth stimulatory promoters, have relevance to human cancer.[3,4] Human carcinogens that are mutagens include x-rays, aflatoxin, and PAHs in tobacco. Conversely, the carcinogenic effects of estrogen in endometrial and breast cancer probably result from its promoter activity on these tissues, and its growth inhibitory activity on ovarian function may account for its anticarcinogenic activity on this organ. Ultraviolet light, which is a potent skin carcinogen, is both mutagenic and growth promoting.[14]

Genetic Factors Can Influence Sensitivity to a Carcinogen

An interesting aspect of the mouse model was that inbred mouse strains varied significantly in their susceptibility to skin cancer induced by PAH initiators. Analysis of this strain-dependent variation led to the recognition that PAHs and many other initiators were actually metabolized inside the cell to a much more chemically reactive form by a cellular enzyme, arylhydrocarbon hydroxylase. When other factors were controlled for, strains whose skin cells possessed high levels of arylhydrocarbon hydroxylase activity in response to PAH initiators were more susceptible to skin cancer induction by PAHs than were strains with low levels of arylhydrocarbon hydroxylase activity.[15]

Two important conclusions followed from this and related observations. First, many carcinogens are taken into the body in the form of a "procarcinogen/promutagen" that becomes highly reactive only after it has been metabolized in the body. Second, genetic differences in metabolism can profoundly influence the rate of mutagenesis and carcinogenesis. Although arylhydrocarbon hydroxylase is an example of an enzyme that activates some carcinogens, other metabolic enzymes exist whose relative activity may influence carcinogenicity by inactivating carcinogens.

Given the many different types of carcinogens and the diverse metabolic systems on which their activation and/or inactivation depend, a given individual might be highly susceptible to one class of carcinogen and relatively resistant to another. In humans, some evidence indicates that an increased risk of bladder cancer exists in individuals whose acetylation of aromatic amines, which are known bladder carcinogens, is genetically determined to be slow. Other investigators have shown that an isoenzyme of cytochrome P_{450}, which can metabolize a wide range of chemicals, may be linked to an increased lung cancer risk.[16,17]

Carcinogens as Mutagens

The recognition that many initiators were mutagens made it important to search for a simple assay for identifying and detecting mutagenic agents and for quantifying their mutagenicity. Because carcinogens had other effects as well, the development of a quantitative assay of mutagenic activity would permit an extensive test of the hypothesis that carcinogens functioned primarily by inducing mutations. The relative mutagenic activity of a compound could then be compared with its in vivo carcinogenicity, which had already been determined for many carcinogens.

The Ames Mutation Test

Because the quantification of mutagenic potency in animal cells was extremely cumbersome, investigators sought simpler methods. One popular assay was developed in the 1970s by Bruce Ames, a microbiologist who worked with bacteria.[18] Ames reasoned that because the DNA of human cells and bacteria was quite similar, the genes of human cells and bacteria might respond similarly to mutagens. If this assumption were correct, bacteria could be used to detect and quantify the response to potentially muta-

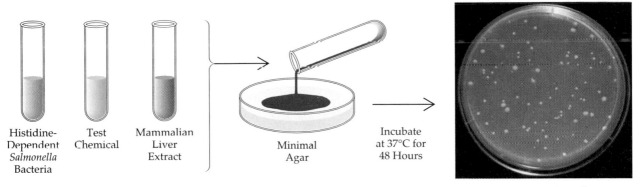

Count Number of
Histidine-Independent Colonies

Figure 3   *The Ames test demonstrates whether a given test chemical, when metabolized by mammalian liver extract, becomes a potent mutagen.*

genic agents because mutations were relatively easy and inexpensive to study in bacteria.

To provide a readily quantitative detection system, Ames exposed the bacteria (a laboratory strain of *Salmonella typhimurium*) to a potential mutagen and then grew them in the absence of an essential nutrient, the amino acid histidine. The starting bacteria needed a high concentration of histidine to be added to their growth medium because their histidine-degrading enzymes were highly active [*see Figure 3*]. Although the starting bacteria did not grow without exogenous histidine, a bacterium with a mutation in an enzyme that degraded histidine had sufficient levels of histidine and therefore was able to grow and form a colony on a Petri dish. By this approach, Ames could expose millions of bacteria to various concentrations of a compound and quantify the compound's mutagenicity simply by counting the number of colonies that formed in the absence of exogenous histidine.

A major obstacle to the widespread application of the Ames assay for testing the mutagenicity of compounds was the fact that, as noted earlier, humans are exposed to many procarcinogens/promutagens whose high mutagenic activity is activated only after being metabolized by the cell. In this respect, it was clear that the bacteria often failed to activate a promutagen because their metabolic systems did not mimic those operating in human cells. To overcome this difficulty, Ames refined the bacterial test by adding extracts of mammalian liver cells to the bacterial plates, a measure that resulted in the metabolic activation of many promutagens.

Analysis of compounds whose carcinogenic activity varied more than one million–fold demonstrated that their relative mutation rates were similar to their carcinogenicity, although also exceptions to this generalization existed. The striking correlation between the mutagenicity of a compound in the Ames assay and its carcinogenic potential in animal tests provided powerful correlative evidence that the mutational activity of many carcinogens accounted for their carcinogenic potential.[18] The Ames assay, or variations of it, is an important, inexpensive technique for screening the mutagenic activity of compounds whose carcinogenic potential is unknown.

Direct versus Indirect Mutagenesis

Most of the environmental factors implicated in human cancer are chemical or physical agents [*see Table 1*].[3,4] Some of these carcinogens, such as x-rays, ultraviolet light, and aflatoxin, appear to function directly as mutagens. However, many carcinogens show negligible mutagenic activity in the Ames assay or in other short-term mutagenesis assays. Rather than concluding that these agents are nonmutagenic, Ames and others have argued that these carcinogens induce mutations indirectly.[18] In this scenario, these carcinogens function as the promoters discussed in the mouse skin carcinogenesis model; they are believed to be mutagenic because they place more cells at risk for mutagenesis by increasing the rate of DNA synthesis, which is error prone, in target cell populations. These carcinogens increase cell growth by diverse mechanisms. Some, such as estrogenic hormones, probably function by directly stimulating DNA synthesis and cell growth. Others, such as alcohol, are believed to act by being cytotoxic, a characteristic that leads to chronic inflammation and reactive proliferation.

Not all mutagens are of exogenous origin. One school of thought argues that oxidants produced by endogenous cellular metabolism may be even more important mutagens than those of exogenous origin.[19] The rate at which these normal metabolic products, which damage DNA and other macromolecules, are formed can be modulated by exogenous agents or inflammation. The high oxidant load of cigarette smoke, in addition to the more classic mutagens found in tobacco, may contribute to the cancer-inducing potential of smoking.

Diet is believed to account for approximately one third of cancers in the United States. However, general dietary factors, rather than specific dietary carcinogens, seem to account for the positive and negative role of diet. Intake of fruits and vegetables is inversely correlated with cancer rates. These foods are high in antioxidants, which may account for their apparent protective effect. Calorie restriction per se, which decreases the mitotic rate in many tissues, has been shown to significantly decrease tumor incidence in animal studies. Thus, diet can influence cancer susceptibility and incidence in at least two ways: by providing antioxidants that counteract the mutagenic products of normal metabolism and by affecting the rate of tissue proliferation.

Table 1   Chemical and Physical Agents Implicated
as Causes of Human Cancer

Agent	Target Organ for Tumors	Probable Mechanism
Sunlight (ultraviolet light)	Skin	Mutagenicity
X-rays	Bone marrow	Mutagenicity
Aflatoxin	Liver	Mutagenicity
Estrogen	Endometrium, breast	Stimulation of cell growth
Tobacco smoke	Lung, esophagus, others	Mutagenicity, oxidant reaction
Asbestos	Lung plura	Cytotoxicity
Alcohol	Liver, esophagus, mouth	Cytotoxicity

Table 2 Viruses Implicated as Causes of Human Cancer

Agent	Target Organ for Tumors
Papillomaviruses	Uterine cervix
Hepatitis B and C viruses	Liver
Epstein-Barr virus	Bone marrow, nasopharynx
Human T cell leukemia virus	Thymus, spleen

Carcinogen-Induced Cancers Are Associated with Changes in Specific Genes

If carcinogens are mutagens, how do the mutations they induce lead to cancer? The mutagenic nature of carcinogens implies the existence of target genes inside normal cells that, once mutated, induce some of the phenotypes of cell transformation. The most effective carcinogenic dosages of initiators are usually relatively low, so that exposed cells sustain only one or a few mutations at most. In the mouse skin cancer model, only a small proportion of the mutated cells carry a genetic alteration that permits them to make a papilloma in response to the promoter.

The process of carcinogenesis as triggered by mutagens is therefore slow and inefficient because the mutagens act randomly, and they usually have adverse effects. Only rarely do mutagens affect a target gene that, once mutated, contributes to the process of tumor formation. The nature of the target genes remained unclear until the 1980s, when investigators recognized that cells contain specific genes that positively and negatively regulate cell growth, and that these genes were commonly altered in tumors.

In summary, investigation of noninfectious carcinogens and of cancer epidemiology provided many insights into the causes of cancer. This body of work indicated that exposure to exogenous chemical and physical agents is the primary cause of human cancer. Some of the major sources of exposure, such as cigarette smoke and diet, have been identified, but the specific carcinogenic agents in most of these sources remain incompletely defined. The mouse skin carcinogenesis model was compatible with the hypothesis that cancer is a multistep phenomenon, in which carcinogens induce tumors by mutating specific target genes in target cells. In humans, the steep rise in the incidence of specific cancers with age and the discrete series of histologic changes associated with the progression to malignancy suggested that human cancer is also a multistep process. Many physical and chemical carcinogens act as direct mutagens, although chemical carcinogens often require metabolic activation. Other carcinogens probably induce mutation indirectly by stimulating an increase in the population of target cells at risk.

Tumor Viruses: Agents of Human Cancer and Models for the Study of Transformation

Although the study of chemical carcinogens revealed cancer to be a multistep phenomenon that included genetic changes, until the 1980s, precisely defining the presumed genetic changes in carcinogen-induced tumors was difficult. The role of specific genes in the development of cancer was able to be tested more directly as a result of the discovery of tumor viruses. These viruses use a small, readily defined repertoire of viral genes to induce cell transformation and thus circumvent the difficulties inherent in searching for a small number of cancer genes residing amid the more than 50,000 other genes in the human genome.[20,21]

Some of these viruses have been revealed to be causative agents for cancer in humans [*see Table 2*]. Tumor viruses have also proved to be extremely useful agents for studying the experimental transformation of cultured cells and the formation of experimental tumors in animals. These viruses are often classified as RNA or DNA viruses, depending on whether the viral genetic information in the virus particles is carried in the form of RNA or DNA molecules. DNA tumor viruses associated with human cancers include human papillomaviruses (associated with cervical cancer), hepatitis B virus (associated with liver cancer), and Epstein-Barr virus (EBV, associated with Burkitt's lymphoma).[22] The human T cell lymphotropic virus type I is an RNA virus that is associated with some lymphoid malignancies.

Tumor Viruses Contain Oncogenes That Can Directly Transform Cells

In addition to causing tumor formation in animals or in people, cancer cells possess abnormal growth properties when they are isolated and cultured in the laboratory, and these altered characteristics are retained indefinitely over many cell divisions. Such observations, as well as the clonal nature of most tumors, imply that the capacity of these cells to form tumors represents a stable, heritable, abnormal trait that is intrinsic to cancer cells. These properties are shared by tumors that are induced by tumor viruses.

An additional feature of some tumor viruses is that they can reproducibly cause the transformation of cultured cells, a property that correlates with their tumorigenic capacity. These observations imply that these tumor viruses bring a small number of viral genes into the infected cell that then transform the growth state of the cell from a normal to a neoplastic configuration. This property of these viruses enabled investigators in the 1960s and 1970s to determine in detail the parts of the virus that were necessary for bringing about these changes.

A major advantage of using a virus to study transformation was that the virus could be readily mutated, the viral gene that carried a mutation could be determined, and the effects of the mutation on cell transformation could be analyzed. Such studies indicated that only a specific subset of the viral genes, usually one or two genes, depending on the virus and the cell system used, are required for inducing the transformation.[20,21] Because these were viral rather than cellular genes, the experiments did not directly address whether cancers that arise independently of tumor viruses result from abnormalities in cellular genes. However, these results established the principle that a small number of specific genes, which were termed *viral oncogenes,* could directly cause cells to become transformed and form tumors in animals.

a   *b*

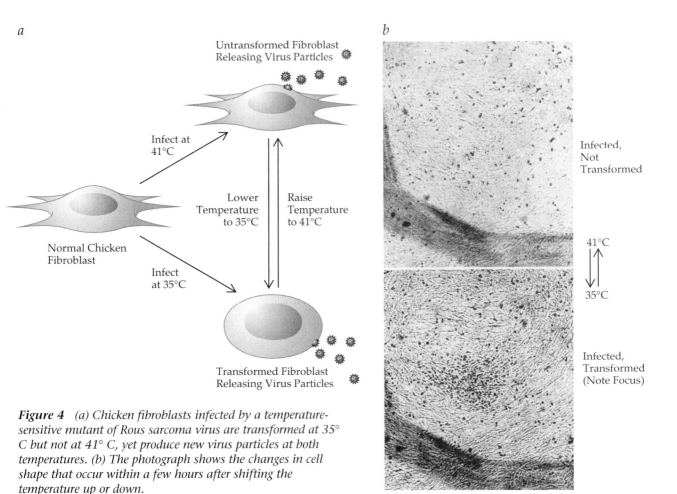

Figure 4 *(a) Chicken fibroblasts infected by a temperature-sensitive mutant of Rous sarcoma virus are transformed at 35° C but not at 41° C, yet produce new virus particles at both temperatures. (b) The photograph shows the changes in cell shape that occur within a few hours after shifting the temperature up or down.*

The initial studies did not determine whether the viral oncogenes were no longer needed once they had induced irreversible cancerous changes in the cell or whether they were required on an ongoing basis because the maintenance of the transformed state depended on the continuous activity of the oncogenes. However, the development of mutant forms of viral oncogenes that were able to function at one temperature but not at another enabled investigators to ascertain that even after a cell had been transformed by a viral oncogene, the continued function of the oncogene was required for the maintenance of the transformed state.[20,23] This conclusion was reached because cells containing a mutant viral oncogene would lose their transformed characteristics when the cells were shifted from a temperature at which the mutant oncogene functioned to one at which it ceased to function [*see Figure 4*].

These results established the paradigm that a small number of genes could reprogram the cell to become cancerous and that the heritable abnormal growth properties of cancer cells required the continued functioning of the genes. Such observations suggest that interfering with the function of those few abnormal genes that are directing the cancer process could, in principle, revert a cancer cell back toward a normal growth state.

Viral Oncoproteins Disturb Normal Growth Control Mechanisms

The studies of such tumor virus genes revealed many important principles, but they did not explain how the viral oncogenes caused the transformation of cells. Because the activities of a gene are carried out through the protein it encodes, a mechanistic understanding of how a gene works is usually obtained through elucidation of the function of the protein encoded by the gene.

Analysis of the oncoproteins encoded by the oncogenes of the RNA viruses known as acute transforming retroviruses revealed one pattern by which tumor viruses transform cells to the neoplastic phenotype.[24] Most of the retroviral oncogenes encode proteins that directly stimulate cell growth. The viral oncogenes of acute transforming retroviruses represent modified versions of normal cellular genes that positively regulate cell growth in many contexts (proto-oncogenes) [see Chapters 4 and 5]. Although proto-oncogenes are subject to stringent control in their normal cellular context, the viral oncogenes cause neoplastic transformation because their proteins are constitutively active.

A different mechanism of transformation emerges from the analysis of oncoproteins encoded by DNA tumor viruses.[24,25] Most viral oncogenes from these viruses encode proteins that transform cells principally by interfering with the function of cellular proteins that negatively regulate cell growth (tumor suppressor genes) [see Chapter 6].

Thus, the oncoproteins of tumor viruses transform cells by disrupting the control mechanisms that normally regulate cell growth. Some induce abnormal growth by mimicking or activating growth stimulatory mechanisms in cells, whereas others do so by inactivating growth inhibitory functions.

Tumor Viruses and Human Cancer

Several tumor viruses have been etiologically linked to the development of human tumors [see Table 2].[22] Although they appear to produce malignant tumors via several mechanisms, these viruses share at least two features. First, most infections with these viruses have a benign outcome. Second, malignant progression is associated with chronic viral infection, with malignancy usually developing only many years after infection. Therefore, other factors in addition to infection are required for malignancy associated with these infectious agents to occur. The best-understood mechanism for tumor progression in association with human tumor viruses involves somatic mutation of cellular target genes in a chronically infected cell. Hence, malignant growth in these situations usually depends on the continued expression of certain viral oncogenes in conjunction with the mutation of cellular genes in the target cell.

Papillomaviruses form a large group of DNA viruses, some of which have been implicated as the causative agents for cervical cancer as well as some less common malignancies.[25] In contrast to these so-called high-risk papillomaviruses, other papillomaviruses, which have been designated low-risk, seem to cause only benign cervical lesions and are not associated with malignant cervical tumors.

As frequently occurs in virally induced cancers, cervical cancers tend to retain and express only those viral genes that continue to be necessary for the maintenance of the carcinogenic state. Although the genomes of papillomaviruses contain about 10 genes, only two of them, *E6* and *E7*, are regularly expressed in cervical cancers. The oncoproteins encoded by these genes in high-risk viruses bind and inactivate the proteins of tumor suppressor genes. E6 inactivates the p53 tumor suppressor protein, and E7 inactivates the Rb protein of the retinoblastoma susceptibility gene [*see Chapter 6*]. In contrast to the oncoproteins specified by the high-risk papillomaviruses, the E6 and E7 proteins of the low-risk papillomaviruses have little or no influence on these tumor suppressor proteins. The differences in the activities of the high-risk and low-risk viruses underline the importance of tumor suppressor protein inactivation in the malignant potential of papillomaviruses associated with cervical cancer.

Several types of viruses other than papillomaviruses are associated with the development of human tumors.[22] Although the oncogenic properties of these viruses are less well understood, they seem to cause tumors by mechanisms that differ from those of the papillomaviruses. EBV is associated with Burkitt's lymphoma in Africa and with nasopharyngeal carcinoma in Asia. The virus encodes several oncoproteins, but none seem to function by mechanisms that are the same as those of papillomavirus oncoproteins. Nevertheless, the EBV viral oncogenes can immortalize cultured lymphocytes that would otherwise have a finite life span. An analogous change in the lymphoid cells of an EBV-infected individual seems to be a prerequisite for the development of Burkitt's lymphoma, but at least one additional somatic alteration in the cell is required. It therefore appears that the virus induces premalignant changes in an infected cell, but that a subsequent somatic mutation in the cell is required to induce malignancy.

Burkitt's lymphoma occurs commonly in children in Central Africa, where it is associated with EBV infection, whereas in other areas of the world, the tumor is uncommon and is not associated with EBV infection. The activation, which occurs via somatic mutation, of a particular cellular proto-oncogene (known as c-*myc*), is characteristic of this tumor in African and non-African cases [*see Chapter 4*]. In the United States, EBV infects an older population than in Africa and is responsible for infectious mononucleosis, which represents a nonmalignant form of lymphocyte proliferation.

Chronic infection with hepatitis B virus and hepatitis C virus is causally linked to the development of liver cancer, which is especially common in some areas of Asia. Some evidence indicates that the hepatitis B virus X protein, which is a transcriptional activator, may contribute directly to growth deregulation.[26] However, it seems more likely that hepatitis B virus (and probably hepatitis C virus as well) promotes the development of malignancy through recurring cycles, over several decades, of virally induced liver damage and the subsequent compensatory regeneration of remaining liver tissue. In these viruses, cell proliferation itself is apparently a carcinogenic influence, likely because cell proliferation tends be mutagenic as a result of errors in DNA replication.

In spite of the large number of retroviruses associated with animal tumors, retroviruses do not seem to be commonly associated with human tumors, although the search for human retroviruses ultimately led to the isolation of human immunodeficiency virus in patients with acquired immunodeficiency syndrome. However, the retrovirus human T cell lymphotropic virus type I is associated with T cell lymphomas. The viral *tax* gene, which is preferentially retained and expressed in T cell lymphomas, appears to be capable of inducing a benign lymphocytic proliferation that may, in a small proportion of chronically infected individuals, progress to lymphoma.

Familial Cancers

Most cancers seem to be induced in ostensibly normal individuals by exposure to exogenous agents. Although cancer-prone families are uncommon, examination of such families has uncovered specific genetic loci that serve as targets of carcinogens. The study of such families has thereby greatly expanded our understanding of human cancer. Analysis of familial cancers in which the abnormalities seemed to involve a single gene has revealed some families in which the susceptibility to cancer appears to be a genetically dominant trait, whereas in other families, the mode of inheritance appears be recessive.[27,28]

The cells of each person contain two copies of each gene, one inherited from the mother and the other from the father. Genetically recessive inheritance means that both copies (or alleles) of a given gene must be abnormal for a particular inherited trait to manifest. An affected individual must therefore receive an abnormal allele from each parent. Unless one of the parents is affected with the condition, this means that each parent carries one normal and one abnormal allele (i.e., they are heterozygous for this gene). Because the chances that any child will receive the abnormal allele of each parent are one in four, approximately 25 percent of the children in the family will have the condition. Conditions with genetically recessive inheritance usually occur in only a single generation because abnormal alleles tend to be uncommon in the general population.

In genetically dominant inheritance, only one allele need be abnormal in order for the trait, such as susceptibility to cancer, to be transmitted [*see Figure 5*]. In dominantly inherited conditions, one of the two alleles in one

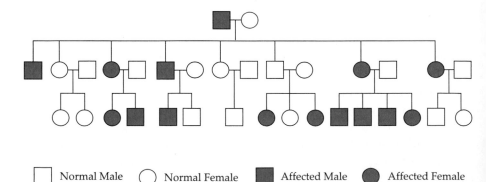

Figure 5 *Three generations of familial retinoblastoma. Blue denotes an affected individual, squares indicate males, and circles indicate females.*

☐ Normal Male   ◯ Normal Female   ■ Affected Male   ● Affected Female

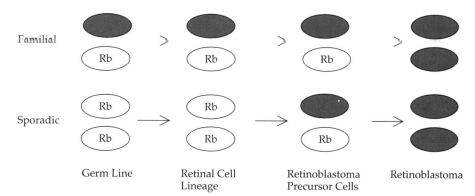

Germaine Line   Retinal Cell   Retinoblastoma   Retinoblastoma
                       Lineage   Precursor Cells

Figure 6 *Similarities and differences between the genetics of familial and sporadic retinoblastoma.*

parent is abnormal, but both alleles of the other parent are normal. Because 50 percent of the children in the family receive the abnormal allele from the affected parent, dominantly inherited diseases tend to occur in about 50 percent of the children in a family with an affected parent. In genetically dominant inheritance, the condition usually manifests over successive generations because, in contrast to recessively inherited conditions, only a single abnormal allele is required.

Retinoblastoma and the Two-Hit Hypothesis

A dominantly inherited tumor that has been examined in detail is the eye cancer retinoblastoma, a tumor that also occurs in some individuals who lack a family history of this cancer. The tumors tend to develop at a younger age in the familial form of the disease than in the sporadic form. In addition, in individuals who have the familial form, multiple independent retinal tumors often develop, whereas in those with the sporadic form, even a second retinal tumor is extremely rare.

Based on these differences between the familial and the sporadic diseases, Alfred Knudson proposed a simple genetic model for the two forms of retinoblastoma [*see Figure 6*]. In a hypothesis known as the "two-hit" theory, Knudson argued that retinoblastoma, whether familial or sporadic, requires two distinct genetic alterations.[29] The first alteration in the familial form would be a mutant gene inherited from a parent. This abnormal gene would be present at conception and would therefore be passed on to all the cells of the body, including those of the retina. The second genetic change would be somatic, occurring in the retinal cells that gave rise to the retinoblastomas. Retinoblastomas that arise as sporadic cases were also proposed to result from two independent mutations, but in this instance, both alterations would arise as a somatic mutation of retinal cells. Because the statistical likelihood of the same retinal cell undergoing the two required mutations is much less than that of the cell undergoing only a single mutation, that requirement would explain the solitary nature and the later age of onset of sporadic retinoblastomas. Conversely, familial retinoblastomas would need only a single somatic mutation in a retinal cell, a requirement that would account for their earlier onset and multiple nature.

In its initial formulation, the two-hit hypothesis did not specify whether the two mutations affected both alleles of the same gene or the alleles of two distinct genes. By the early 1980s, however, progress in our understanding of the genetics of retinoblastoma had made it clear that the two mutations must affect the two alleles of the same gene (designated *Rb*).[30] This conclusion implied that although the familial susceptibility to retinoblastoma displayed a dominant inheritance at the level of the whole organism, development of the tumor cell was a genetically recessive event at the level of the cell because retinoblastoma did not arise until after the second, normal *Rb* allele had been mutated. Mutations that manifest in a genetically recessive manner almost invariably represent alterations in which the normal function of the gene has been lost. It was therefore inferred that the *Rb* gene that was inactivated in retinoblastoma must normally serve to restrict the unrestrained growth of the cell. This type of gene was called a *tumor suppressor gene* because part of its normal function seemed to be to prevent tumor development. The genetics of most familial cancer syndromes are similar to those of retinoblastoma and also represent abnormalities that involve tumor suppressor genes.

Xeroderma Pigmentosum: A Recessively Inherited Cancer Syndrome

In contrast to retinoblastoma and many other familial cancers, xeroderma pigmentosum (XP) is a well studied example of a familial cancer syndrome with a recessive inheritance.[31] Patients with XP usually have a history of severe sunburns, quickly develop extensive sun damage–related skin changes, and form multiple skin cancers of various types on sun-exposed areas at an early age. Thus, sunlight is much more carcinogenic in XP patients than in normal individuals. As in normal individuals, the ultraviolet spectrum in sunlight is responsible for most of the carcinogenicity. The characteristic defect in XP is that the cells from affected individuals are unable to repair ultraviolet light–induced DNA damage. By contrast, most ultraviolet light–induced DNA damage is quickly repaired by cells in normal individuals; this repair is an important, but imperfect, protective mechanism. The XP defect prevents XP cells from carrying out this normal repair process.

Dominantly and Recessively Inherited Cancer Syndromes May Affect Distinct Classes of Genes

The abnormal genes in XP and retinoblastoma are similar in that both predispose affected individuals to the development of cancer. However, the differences in the inheritance pattern of familial retinoblastoma and XP suggest that a fundamental difference may exist between the kinds of genes involved in the two familial cancer syndromes. In other words, why are the parents of patients with XP, who must each be heterozygous for the abnormal *XP* allele, not at greatly increased risk for developing skin cancer, as occurs with retinoblastoma and one abnormal retinoblastoma allele?

One possibility might be that the frequency of mutation of the normal *XP* allele is so low in the cells of the parents that it does not place them at risk. However, it is much more likely that inactivation of the normal *XP* allele occurs with a frequency similar to that of inactivation of the normal retinoblastoma allele. If the risk of mutational inactivation of the *Rb* allelle and the *XP* allele in similar, the likelihood of a cell that has lost the function of the *XP* gene to become malignant must be much lower than that of a cell that has lost the normal retinoblastoma function. The apparent direct involvement of the retinoblastoma allele with growth control means that the loss of its function would lead to a "premalignant" form of inappropriate growth.

By contrast, inactivation of the *XP* gene would not by itself alter the growth of the cell that had lost the function. Because random mutations are more likely to interfere with cell growth rather than to stimulate it, most cells in which the *XP* gene was inactivated would be much more likely to display impaired growth rather than an inappropriately increased growth. Because relatively few cells in XP heterozygotes lose the function of the *XP* allele, these heterozygous individuals are not at greatly increased risk for the development of cancer. However, in patients with XP, the *XP* gene is initially inactive in *all* of their cells. Although the likelihood of ultraviolet light–induced cancerous changes is very small for any one cell, the vast number of abnormal cells at risk leads to the development of the skin cancers.

Unifying Themes in Carcinogenesis

Regardless of the cause of cancer (i.e., environmental exposure to chemical, physical, and viral agents), some common themes emerge. One is that cancer is a multistep, progressive phenomenon that arises because a cell accumulates a series of changes that cause its growth pattern to become progressively more abnormal. Another theme is that a limited number of genetic changes in the cancer cell account for at least some of these alterations, and that more than one genetic modification is required.

Many chemical and physical carcinogens are directly mutagenic, and their carcinogenic potential may correlate with their mutagenic potency. Other carcinogens may induce mutations more indirectly, by directly or indirectly stimulating the growth of potential target cells, thereby placing them at greater risk for mutation. Specific viral genes are responsible for the ability of tumor viruses to directly transform cells. In familial cancers, mutant genes are responsible for the predisposition to the development of cancer.

The importance of promoters, which are not inherently mutagenic, to the development of skin tumors in mice emphasized how factors that are not directly mutagenic can play a significant role in tumor development. Conversely, the ultimate function of a promoter is principally to increase the likelihood that a cell will sustain additional mutations that would push it further toward the cancerous state in which deregulated cell growth is independent of the promoter.

Because most mutations do not increase the growth properties of a cell, the studies discussed in this chapter make it clear that specific genetic changes must underlie the progression to cancer. However, the precise nature of the genes that are being modified in human cancer remained poorly defined before proto-oncogenes and tumor suppressor genes were identified [*see Chapters 4 through 6*].

References

1. Wynder EL, Gori GB: Contribution of the environment to cancer incidence: an epidemiologic exercise. *J Natl Cancer Inst* 58:825, 1977
2. Doll R, Peto R: *The Causes of Cancer.* Oxford University Press, New York, 1981
3. Henderson BE, Ross RK, Pike MC: Toward the primary prevention of cancer. *Science* 254:1131, 1991
4. Ames BN, Gold LS, Willett WC: The causes and prevention of cancer. *Proc Natl Acad Sci USA* 92:5258, 1995
5. Wingo PA, Tong T, Bolden S: Cancer statistics, 1995. *CA Cancer J Clin* 45:8, 1995
6. Tokuhata CK, Lilienfeld AM: Familial aggregations of lung cancer in humans. *J Natl Cancer Inst* 39:289, 1963
7. Berenbrlum I, Shubik P: A new, quantitative approach to the study of the stages of chemical carcinogenesis in the mouse's skin. *Br J Cancer* 1:383, 1947
8. Yuspa SH, Poirer MD: Chemical carcinogenesis: from animal models to molecular models in one decade. *Adv Cancer Res* 50:25, 1988
9. DiGiovanni J: Multistage carcinogenesis in mouse skin. *Pharmacol Ther* 54:63, 1992
10. Miller EC, Miller JA: Mechanisms of chemical carcinogenesis: nature of proximate carcinogens and interactions with macromolecules. *Pharmacol Rev* 18:805, 1966
11. Boutwell RK: Some biological aspects of skin carcinogenesis. *Prog Exp Tumor Res* 4:207, 1964
12. Slaga TJ, Fisher SM, Weeks CE, et al: Cellular and biochemical mechanisms of mouse skin tumor promoters. *Reviews in Biochemical Toxicology* Hodgson E, Bend J, Philpot RM, Eds. Elsevier/North-Holland Press, New York, 1981, p 231
13. Hennings H, Shores R, Weick ML, et al: Malignant conversion of mouse skin tumor is increased by tumor initiators and unaffected by tumor promoters. *Nature* 304:67, 1983
14. Ananthaswamy HN, Pierceall WE: Molecular mechanisms of ultraviolet radiation carcinogenesis. *Photochem Photobiol* 52:1119, 1990
15. Swanson HI, Bradfield CH: The *Ah* receptor: genetics, structure and function. *Pharmacogenetics* 3:213, 1993
16. Cartwright RA, Glashan RW, Rogers HJ, et al: Role of N-acetyltransferase phenotypes in bladder carcinogenesis: a pharmacologic epidemiological approach to bladder cancer. Lancet 2:842, 1982
17. Law MR, Hetzel MR, Idle JR: Debrisoquine metabolism and genetic predisposition to lung cancer. *Br J Cancer* 59:686, 1989
18. McCann J, Choi E, Yamasaki E, et al: Detection of carcinogens as mutagens in the Salmonella/microsome test: assay of 300 chemicals. *Proc Natl Acad Sci USA* 72:5135, 1975
19. Ames BN, Shigenaga MK, Hagen TM: Oxidants, antioxidants, and the degenerative diseases of aging. *Proc Natl Acad Sci USA* 90:7915, 1993
20. Topp WC, Lane D, Pollack R: Transformation by SV40 and polyoma virus. In *DNA Tumor Viruses.* Tooze J, Ed. Cold Spring Harbor Laboratory, New York, 1980, p 205
21. Linial M, Blair D: Genetics of retroviruses. *RNA Tumor Viruses.* Weiss R, Teich N, Varmus H, Coffin J, Eds. Cold Spring Harbor Laboratory, New York, 1984, p 649
22. Howley PM: Principles of carcinogenesis: viral. *Cancer: Principles and Practice of Oncology.* DeVita VT, Hellman S, Rosenberg SA, Eds. JB Lippincott Co, Philadelphia, 1993, p 182
23. Martin GS: Rous sarcoma virus: a function required for the maintenance of the transformed state. *Nature* 227:1021, 1970
24. Bishop JM: Molecular themes in oncogenesis. *Cell* 64:235, 1991
25. Werness BA, Munger K, Howley PM: Role of the human papillomavirus oncoproteins in transformation and carcinogenic progression. *Important Advances in Oncology 1991.* DeVita VT, Hellman S, Rosenberg SA, Eds. JB Lippincott Co, Philadelphia, 1991, p 3
26. Kim C-Y, Koike K, Saito I, et al: HBx gene of hepatitis B virus induces liver cancer in transgenic mice. *Nature* 351:317, 1991
27. German J: Heritable conditions that predispose to cancer. *Genetics in Clinical Oncology.* Chaganti RSK, German J, Eds. Oxford University Press, New York, 1985, p 80
28. Lynch HT, Hirayama T, Eds: *Genetic Epidemiology of Cancer.* CRC Press, Boca Raton, FL, 1990
29. Knudson AG: Mutation and cancer: statistical study of retinoblastoma. *Proc Natl Acad Sci USA* 68:820, 1971

30. Cavenee WK, Dryja TP, Phillips RA, et al: Expression of recessive alleles by chromosomal mechanisms in retinoblastoma. *Nature* 305:779, 1983

31. Clever JE, Kraemer KH: Xeroderma pigmentosum. *The Metabolic Basis of Inherited Disease*. Scriver CR, Beandet AL, Sly WS, Valle D, Eds. McGraw-Hill, New York, 1989, p 2949

Acknowledgments

Figures 1 and 5   Marcia Kammerer. Adapted from *Genes and the Biology of Cancer*, by H. Varmus and R.A. Weinberg, Scientific American Library, New York, 1993.

Figures 2 through 4   Seward Hung. Adapted and modified from *Genes and the Biology of Cancer*, by H. Varmus and R.A. Weinberg, Scientific American Library, New York, 1993.

Figure 6   Marcia Kammerer.

CHAPTER 4

Proto-oncogenes in Normal and Neoplastic Cells

J. Michael Bishop, M.D., Hidesaburo Hanafusa, Ph.D.

The lines of inquiry outlined in the previous chapters converged on the hypothesis that cancer is caused by genetic damage. When this hypothesis first reached maturity, the identification of tumorigenic damage and the genes that it might affect seemed well beyond the reach of contemporary technology. The prospects changed, however, with the discovery that many retroviruses possess oncogenes that have been pirated from host cells during viral replication. The expropriated genes become tumorigenic because of their sustained expression from the viral genome and because of mutations that alter the gene products.

The acquisition of cellular genes by retroviruses has been called *transduction* because it resembles the transfer of host genes from one bacterium to another by bacteriophage, the phenomenon for which the term transduction was first devised. Transduction by retroviruses revealed for the first time the existence of cellular genes whose anomalous activities can contribute to tumorigenesis. These cellular genes have been designated *proto-oncogenes*, in recognition of their role as progenitors of oncogenes.

The discovery of transduction by retroviruses provided the first access to proto-oncogenes. Other means have since been used to uncover these genes, based on direct analysis of the DNA in cancer cells. The number of proto-oncogenes identified now exceeds 100, many of which are thought to be involved in the genesis of human tumors [*see Chapter 7*]. The purpose of this chapter is to describe the rationales and strategies that led to the discovery and elaboration of proto-oncogenes and to explain the fundamental principles that underlie the conversion of these genes to oncogenic forms. The role that proto-oncogenes play in tumorigenesis and the biochemical mechanisms by which they act are described in detail elsewhere in this volume.

Retroviral Oncogenes

At the turn of the twentieth century, Ellerman and Bang, in Denmark, and Peyton Rous, in the United States, reported the discovery of infectious agents that could elicit malignancies in chickens. These reports represented the earliest sightings of what we now call *retroviruses*, which are renowned for their use of reverse transcriptase in replication [*see Chapter 2*]. Retroviruses represent a large and ubiquitous family of viruses that cause diverse kinds of tumors in many species. Paradoxically, retroviruses have been implicated in the causation of only one form of human malignancy (the relatively rare acute T cell leukemia [*see Chapter 2*]). Nonetheless, the study of retroviruses acquired a larger significance by providing experimental access to the genetic underpinnings of all forms of tumorigenesis, regardless of their causes. The first step in gaining that access came with the realization that the tumorigenicity of many retroviruses could be attributed to specific viral oncogenes.

Many tumorigenic retroviruses transform cells in culture to a neoplastic phenotype [*see Chapter 3*]. This property facilitated the genetic analysis of viruses and provided the means for uncovering oncogenes. Studies with the avian sarcoma virus discovered by Peyton Rous (Rous sarcoma virus [RSV]) provided the basis for this area of research. An initial clue was provided by the observation that different strains of RSV induced different changes in cellular shape, a property that bred true as the viral strains were propagated.[1] Thus, the behavior of the transformed cells seemed to be under the direct control of the viral genome. That conclusion was then secured by analysis of two sorts of viral mutants.

One type of mutation was conditional [*see Chapter 3 and Figure 1*]: at 36° C, the mutant virus could transform fibroblasts in culture, but at 41° C, transformation either did not occur or could be reversed, if it had already been established at the lower temperature.[2,3] The temperature sensitivity of transformation presumably reflected some structural abnormality in a protein encoded by the mutant virus. The virus replicated normally at both temperatures, as if the ability to transform cells and the ability to replicate were separable. For geneticists familiar with the properties of conditional mutations, these findings strongly implied that an RSV gene was required for, and also dedicated exclusively to, both the initiation and the maintenance of cellular transformation. It was the first such gene ever identified.

The second type of mutation was nonconditional: it caused a permanent loss of transforming ability but, again, had no effect on viral replication.[4] The loss of transformation was caused by a large deletion that excised what proved to be the viral oncogene. Deletions of this sort had special value because they allowed the oncogene to be mapped to an exact position on the genome of RSV [*see Figure 2*]. The oncogene was soon dubbed v-*src*, for the types of tumors that it induces.

The preceding work was all performed before molecular cloning was invented. However, with the advent of recombinant DNA, it became possible to isolate v-*src* in large quantities and to show that the independent action of this gene could both transform cells in culture and cause tumors in birds and mammals. There was now no doubt that a bona fide cancer gene had been identified. It was equally clear that RSV possesses two types of genes

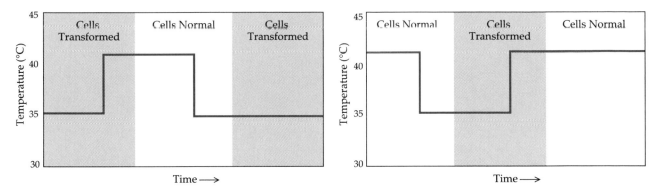

Figure 1 *Conditional mutation of a gene results in the reversible inactivation of the protein it encodes. In the case of a temperature-sensitive mutant of* src, *infected cells are transformed when they are cultured at 35° C but revert to (or remain in) the normal state at 41° C. The discovery of such mutants implies that a viral gene is probably mediated by a protein product and that the sustained action of the gene is necessary for transformation.*

[*see Figure 2*]: those used for the reproduction of the virus, of which there are three; and a fourth gene, v-*src*, whose only function is the transformation of cells to neoplastic growth.

The discovery of v-*src* brought clarity to what had been a muddled business. Earlier research had indicated that the elemental secrets of cancer might be hidden among the genes of the cancer cell, but in the oncogene of RSV, scientists found an explicit example of a gene that could switch a cell's growth from normal to cancerous. Additional examples of the gene were soon found. We now know of more than 30 distinctive retroviral oncogenes that are capable of causing many different forms of cancer [*see Table 1*]. It was immediately clear that the study of these oncogenes would provide valuable insight into the biochemical mechanisms of neoplastic growth [*see Chapter 5*], but the significance of retroviral oncogenes grew even larger with the discovery that these genes are manifestations of a genetic repertoire that might underlie all forms of tumorigenesis, even those that do not involve retroviruses.

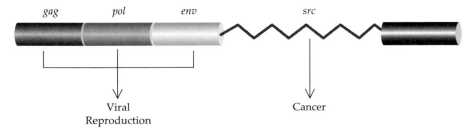

Figure 2 *The genes of Rous sarcoma virus. The single-stranded RNA genome of Rous sarcoma virus carries four genes. Three are devoted to replication, encoding the capsid proteins of the virus (gag), the enzymes for reverse transcription and integration of proviral DNA (pol), and the surface glycoprotein of the viral envelope (env). The fourth gene (src) plays no role in viral replication but elicits neoplastic transformation of cells and causes sarcomas in birds and mammals.*

Table 1   Retroviral Oncogenes

Oncogene	Prototype Virus	Major Disease	Species of Origin
src	Rous sarcoma	Sarcoma	Chicken
yes	Y73 avian sarcoma	Sarcoma	Chicken
fps	Fujinami avian sarcoma	Sarcoma	Chicken
ros	UR2 avian sarcoma	Sarcoma	Chicken
crk	CT10 avian sarcoma	Sarcoma	Chicken
jun	Avian sarcoma 17	Sarcoma	Chicken
eyk	RPL30 avian sarcoma	Sarcoma	Chicken
maf	AS42 avian sarcoma	Sarcoma	Chicken
qin	Avian sarcoma 31	Sarcoma	Chicken
mil	Mill Hill-2	Carcinoma and myeloid leukemia	Chicken
myc	MC29 avian myelocytomatosis	Carcinoma and myeloid leukemia	Chicken
sea	S13 avian erythroblastosis	Erythroleukemia	Chicken
myb	Avian myeloblastosis	Myeloid leukemia	Chicken
erb-B	Avian erythroblastosis	Erythroleukemia and sarcoma	Chicken
erb-A	Avian erythroblastosis	Erythroleukemia	Chicken
ets	E26 avian erythroblastosis	Erythroleukemia	Chicken
ski	Avian SK77	Carcinoma	Chicken
rel	Avian reticuloendotheliosis	Reticuloendotheliosis	Turkey
abl	Abelson murine leukemia	Pre–B cell lymphoma	Mouse
mos	Moloney murine sarcoma	Sarcoma	Mouse
raf	3611 murine sarcoma	Sarcoma	Mouse
fos	FBJ murine osteosarcoma	Osteosarcoma	Mouse
cbl	Cas NS-1	Pre–B cell lymphoma	Mouse
akt	AKT8	T cell lymphoma	Mouse
H-*ras*	Harvey murine sarcoma	Sarcoma	Rat
K-*ras*	Kirsten murine sarcoma	Sarcoma	Rat
fes	ST and GA feline sarcoma	Sarcoma	Cat
fms	SM feline sarcoma	Sarcoma	Cat
fgr	GR feline sarcoma	Sarcoma	Cat
kit	HZ4 feline sarcoma	Sarcoma	Cat
sis	Simian sarcoma	Sarcoma	Monkey

The Discovery of Proto-oncogenes

The larger significance of retroviral oncogenes was realized as a result of two considerations. The first was an evolutionary puzzle. Genetic analysis had made it clear that retroviral oncogenes are not essential for the replication of the viruses. Why then are these genes present in retroviruses, and from whence did they come? Might they have arisen by genetic recombination with the genome of the host cell, an event that is central to the life cycle of retroviruses [*see Chapter 2*]? The second consideration was the oncogene hypothesis, which proposed that all tumorigenic agents act by inducing the expression of otherwise cryptic retroviral genes already resident in the germ lines of vertebrates as a result of infection at some early point during the evolution of metazoan species.[5] Both arguments inspired investigators to search for evidence indicating that retroviral oncogenes might also be present in vertebrate DNA.

Once again, research on RSV provided the first insights. The results were unexpected but clear: chicken DNA contains a very close relative of v-*src*, and more divergent versions of the same gene were also found in the DNA of other vertebrates.[6,7] Eventually, it became clear that the cellular version of *src* was an authentic vertebrate gene rather than a retroviral oncogene.[8] Thus, the allele of *src* found in RSV had been acquired ("transduced") from the chicken genome. As a result of this transduction, the normal *src* proto-oncogene was converted to a tumorigenic oncogene, which was now carried in the genome of a retrovirus [*see Figure 3*].

The findings with *src* were soon generalized to other retroviral oncogenes, each derived from a distinct cellular proto-oncogene. More than 30 examples are now on record [*see Table 1*]. The discovery of transduction inverted the original oncogene hypothesis. It was not retroviruses that had conferred cancer genes on cells, but rather cells that had served as the source of retroviral oncogenes. Nevertheless, the inversion retained one of the original thoughts of the oncogene hypothesis: proto-oncogenes might represent a final common pathway of tumorigenesis and may be targets for carcinogens of various sorts [*see Figure 3*]. It was a thought that would bear abundant fruit.

Despite the number and diversity of retroviral oncogenes, transduction of proto-oncogenes is actually rare in both natural and experimental settings.

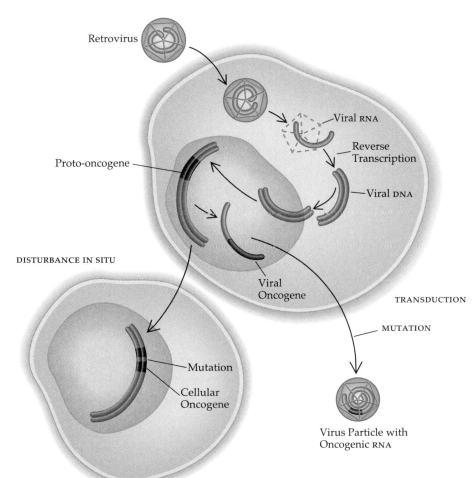

Figure 3 *Proto-oncogenes as precursors of cancer genes. Proto-oncogenes can become oncogenes either by transduction into retroviruses or by disturbance at their sites of residence in chromosomes. In either event, the consequence is an abnormal gain of function in the form of either unleashed expression of the gene or deregulation of the protein product.*

There is no reason to believe that transduction by retroviruses is limited to proto-oncogenes, but transduction of other sorts of genes would be easily overlooked because the phenomenon is not likely to give a phenotype that can be easily perceived.

Expanding the Inventory of Proto-oncogenes

Soon after retroviral transduction was discovered, it became apparent that other genetic mechanisms could also convert proto-oncogenes to tumorigenic forms. The study of these mechanisms provided a way of further expanding the inventory of proto-oncogenes. In the process, evidence was obtained that indicated a role for proto-oncogenes in the genesis of human cancer [*see Chapter 7*].

Insertional Mutagenesis

Although it was the study of oncogenes that first brought attention to retroviruses in cancer research, most retroviruses cause tumors without the benefit of an oncogene in their genome. Instead, such retroviruses directly affect proto-oncogenes at their sites of residence in cellular DNA by a process known as *insertional mutagenesis*. As part of their normal replicative cycle, retroviruses insert a DNA copy of their RNA genome (a "provirus") into the chromosomal DNA of host cells [*see Chapter 2*]. Occasionally, this insertion occurs in the vicinity of a proto-oncogene. The insertion converts the nearby proto-oncogene to an active oncogene.

The discovery of insertional mutagenesis was made by study of B cell tumors that had been induced in chickens by a retrovirus that carries no oncogene.[9,10] Although integration of retroviral DNA is thought to occur virtually at random throughout the cellular genome, most of the chicken B cell tumors were found to contain a provirus that had been inserted in the same limited region of chromosomal DNA. This finding suggested that a biologic selection might exist for cells with those particular integrations and prompted the notion that the presence of a provirus might induce tumors by disturbing the function of a nearby proto-oncogene. The notion was soon confirmed by the finding that the allegedly pathogenic proviruses were integrated in the vicinity of a previously identified proto-oncogene known as *myc* and were indeed disturbing its function [*see Figures 4 and 5*].[11,12] This finding was especially fortunate because *myc* had already been established as a proto-oncogene by transduction into retroviruses; thus, its pathogenic potential in the context of insertional mutagenesis was relatively easy to imagine.

Further study of insertional mutagenesis revealed examples that did not involve previously identified proto-oncogenes. In such settings, experimentalists were able to exploit the fact that insertion of proviral DNA provides a molecular tag for adjacent cellular DNA. When that DNA was examined, it was found to contain proto-oncogenes that were previously unknown. By this means, more than a dozen proto-oncogenes have been added to the list compiled through the study of transduction.[13]

To the best of our knowledge, insertional mutagenesis by retroviruses

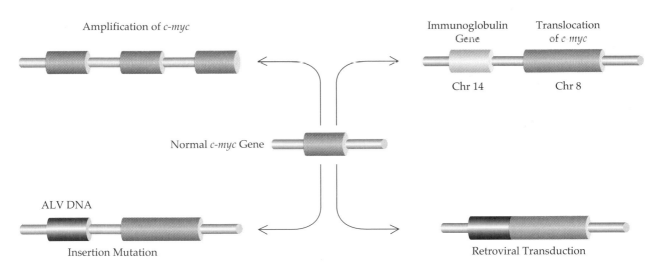

Figure 4 *Ways in which a proto-oncogene can be converted to an oncogene are illustrated with the c-myc gene, which has been found to be activated by gene amplification, chromosomal translocation, retroviral transduction (forming a viral oncogene), and proviral insertion mutations. ALV; avian leukemia virus.*

plays no role in the genesis of any human cancer (although insertions of mobile DNA from within the human genome can sometimes cause disease [*see Chapter 7*]). Nevertheless, the phenomenon was important to the genetic paradigm of cancer in two ways. First, by expanding the inventory of proto-oncogenes, it enlarged our view of the genetic keyboard on which tumorigenic agents might play. Second, it provided the first indication that proto-oncogenes can participate in tumorigenesis while still residing within the chromosomes of cells and, thus, are authentic candidates for progenitors of cancer genes, regardless of the nature of the tumorigenic agent.

Chromosomal Translocations

The consistent appearance of chromosomal abnormalities in many sorts of tumors provided an early hint that genetic damage might be the fundamental ailment in cancer cells [*see Chapters 2 and 3*]. Prominent among these abnormalities are translocations between two chromosomes and inversions within single chromosomes. Translocations and inversions create new molecular joints within chromosomes, at positions known as *breakpoints*. The DNA adjacent to breakpoints is of great interest because it may harbor genes that, when damaged, can contribute to tumorigenesis.

How the DNA at breakpoints might be isolated was not initially clear. The discovery of transduced proto-oncogenes provided unexpected access to the problem because a few of these genes were found to be located in the vicinity of known breakpoints on human chromosomes. The earliest examples again involved the *myc* proto-oncogene and were found in human and mouse B cell tumors (Burkitt's lymphoma and plasmacytomas, respectively), which contain consistent chromosomal translocations [*see Chapter 7*]. The breakpoints in these translocations were adjoined on one side by an immunoglobulin gene, which is contributed by one of the participating chromosomes, and by the *myc* gene on the other side, which is contributed by the second chromosome.[14-16] By isolating single fragments of DNA that bore both of these genes from tumor cells, investigators were able to isolate the actual point of fusion created by the translocations [*see Figure 4*]. It then became possible to examine the molecular consequences of the translocations in detail.

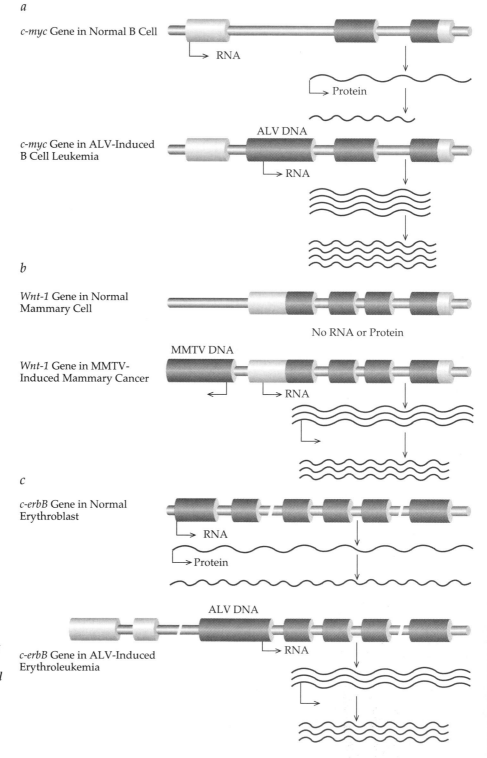

Figure 5 *Insertions of retroviral DNA can increase the production of RNA and protein by a proto-oncogene (a), turn on a previously silent proto-oncogene (b), or cause the production of an abnormal (e.g., truncated) protein (c). ALV; avian leukemia virus. MMTV; mouse mammary tumor virus*

Another early example deserves mention because it provided a molecular description of the Philadelphia chromosome in chronic myelogenous leukemia, the discovery of which in 1960 launched the modern cytogenetic analysis of cancer cells.[17] The Philadelphia chromosome is formed by a reciprocal translocation—a regional exchange of chromosomal arms—between chromosomes 9 and 22 [*see Chapter 7*]. After the discovery of transduced proto-oncogenes, it was noted that one of these (*abl*) is situated at the breakpoint on chromosome 9 in the Philadelphia chromosome. The *abl* proto-oncogene provided a molecular marker by which the point of fusion in the translocation could be isolated. Moreover, *abl* itself proved to be fractured by the translocation.[18,19]

Most of the numerous translocations associated with human tumors do not involve previously identified proto-oncogenes. The molecular characterization of these translocations was achieved by use of genetic markers other than proto-oncogenes. The strategy succeeded first with genes for immunoglobulins, which are found at or near the breakpoints of translocations involved in various B cell tumors (including translocations that affect *myc*). Use of the immunoglobulin genes as entry points for the molecular cloning of DNA adjoining the breakpoints enabled additional proto-oncogenes to be discovered in the vicinity of breakpoints.[20,21] Another highly productive source was translocations in T cell leukemias, the breakpoints of which are adjoined by genes for the antigen receptor of T cells. These genes, like the immunoglobulin genes, served as guideposts for the cloning of previously unrecognized proto-oncogenes.[20,21]

As the science of human genomics progressed, physical markers for many positions on human chromosomes were identified, some of which are fortuitously located in the vicinity of translocation breakpoints. These markers permitted the molecular dissection of previously inaccessible breakpoints, each revealing an additional proto-oncogene. The number of proto-oncogenes uncovered in this manner now exceeds 50 and could eventually reach 100 or more because the variety of translocations and inversions associated with particular human tumors is at least that numerous [*see Chapter 7*].[21] To date, most molecular characterizations of translocations have been performed with the DNA of human leukemias and lymphomas, a bias arising from the fact that cytogenetic analysis of solid tumors has lagged well behind cytogenetic analysis of hematologic malignancies.

Amplified DNA

Many tumor cells contain regions of chromosomes in which the DNA has been abnormally reduplicated, sometimes in excess of 100- or even 1,000-fold. The reduplicated DNA is said to have been "amplified." Amplification of DNA in turn gives rise to cytogenetic abnormalities known as homogeneously staining regions and double-minute chromosomes [*see Chapter 3*]. The first examples of abnormally amplified DNA in vertebrates were provided by human tumor cells that had become resistant to cytotoxic drugs. At that time, amplification of DNA was considered to be exclusively a consequence of therapy. It is now apparent, however, that amplified DNA is a common feature of tumors before therapy is initiated and that the amplification sometimes affects previously identified proto-oncogenes.[22] The first

Human Tumor Cells or Chemically
Transformed Rodent Cells

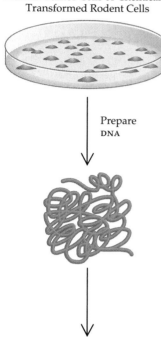

Prepare
DNA

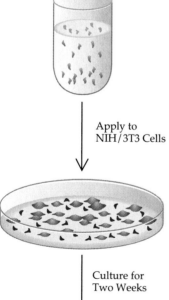

Precipitate DNA in Calcium
Phosphate Crystals

Apply to
NIH/3T3 Cells

Culture for
Two Weeks

Focus of Transformed
NIH/3T3 Cells Growing among
Untransformed Cells

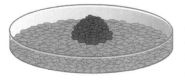

examples of amplification in human tumor cells were again provided by *myc* [*see Figure 4*], echoing the experience with insertional mutagenesis and chromosomal translocation. Several previously identified proto-oncogenes have since been shown to be amplified consistently in one form of human tumor or another.

Because many instances of amplification do not involve a previously identified proto-oncogene, probing the amplified DNA for additional candidates has been necessary. Two approaches have been successful. The first was inadvertent but productive: testing amplified DNA for the presence of a known proto-oncogene occasionally uncovered a related gene instead. This strategy led to the discovery of the proto-oncogene N-*myc*, which is closely related to *myc* and is commonly amplified in human neuroblastomas.[23,24] Another member of this kindred, known as L-*myc*, has been found in the amplified DNA of human small cell carcinoma of the lung.[25]

The second strategy was to first purify the amplified DNA and then to scan this DNA for candidate proto-oncogenes. The yield to date from this strategy has been limited but significant. For example, dissection of amplified DNA in a mouse cell line uncovered the *mdm*2 gene,[26,27] which is now recognized as an important component of the machinery that regulates the cell division cycle and is amplified in several forms of human tumors [*see Chapter 7*]. Another proto-oncogene, designated as *gli*, was first identified in the amplified DNA of human gliomas and has since been implicated in the pathogenesis of these and other human tumors [*see Chapter 7*].[28]

Gene Transfer by Transfection

The example of viral oncogenes also inspired a more direct tactic for the detection of cancer genes: the search for biologically active oncogenes in the DNA of human tumors. The tactic uncovered a mutant proto-oncogene that has since proved to be among the most prevalent genetic anomalies in cancer cells.

Much of the progress in the study of viral oncogenes has been based on their ability to transform cells in culture to a neoplastic phenotype. Assays for transformation originally used infectious viruses, but eventually, techniques were developed that allowed the transformation of cells by isolated DNA that carries viral oncogenes, in a procedure known as *transfection* [*see Figure 6*]. The first successful transfections were performed with purified viral DNA,[29] but investigators were also able to transform cells by use of DNA from cells transformed by RSV; in this instance the retroviral provirus and its oncogene were diluted by vast amounts of cellular DNA.[30]

The availability of transfection and the precedent provided by viral oncogenes inspired the belief that malignant cells might also contain genes that could be detected by transformation in cell culture. The first success with this strategy occurred with DNA extracted from mouse cells that had been

Figure 6   *The presence of an oncogene in chemically transformed mouse cells or human tumor cells could be demonstrated by preparing tumor cell DNA, transfecting it into NIH3T3 cells, and scanning for the appearance of transformed cells several weeks later.*

transformed by a chemical carcinogen.[31] The procedure was then applied to various cell lines from human tumors and numerous specimens taken directly from tumors. Transforming activity has now been detected with DNA representing a large variety of human malignancies.[32,33] Some types of tumors rarely, if ever, contain detectable transforming genes, whereas others do so with consistency [*see Chapter 7*]. At least some of the variation may be the result of difficulties with the biological assay, which is relatively insensitive and technically demanding. Once the nature of the transforming genes had been established, however, it became possible to develop molecular tests for these abnormal genes that supplanted transfection and could be used in clinical applications [*see Chapter 7*].

The transforming activity found in the DNA of human tumors provided an assay by which the responsible genes could be isolated and authenticated. The first success was achieved with a cell line that was derived from a bladder carcinoma[34-36] and has been repeated numerous times with many types of tumors. This work was initiated with the expectation that it would lead to a new genre of cancer gene, but most transforming genes isolated from human tumors proved to be members of a previously identified family of proto-oncogenes known by the general term *ras*.[34-36] Two of these genes (H-*ras* and K-*ras*) were first encountered as transduced oncogenes in retroviruses and serve as prototypes for the gene family; the third (N-*ras*) came to view through the use of transfection with tumor DNA.

Transfection has produced only a few other examples of biologically active proto-oncogenes from human tumors, and none of these has a prevalence that approximates that of active *ras* genes [*see Chapter 7*]. Whether the predominance of *ras* genes in the harvest from transfection represents a biologic reality or limitations inherent to the assay is not yet clear. One additional example, *ret*, deserves mention because it is the only proto-oncogene that has been implicated in heritable cancer.[37] Mutant alleles of *ret* are apparently responsible for several congenital syndromes that feature inherited predispositions to tumors of endocrine tissues, particularly the thyroid, parathyroid, and adrenal medulla; these syndromes include multiple endocrine neoplasia types IIA and IIB and familial medullary thyroid carcinoma [*see Chapter 7*].

Families of Proto-oncogenes

Many proto-oncogenes are members of gene families that have been generated by repeated duplication and subsequent diversification of a progenitor gene during the course of evolution. Once one member of a gene family has been isolated, the other members can be identified by virtue of their cross-reaction in molecular hybridization with the original isolate. For example, the gene family originally defined by *src* is now known to contain at least nine members, all of which have properties of proto-oncogenes. Many of the proto-oncogenes uncovered in this manner have been poorly studied, and it remains to be seen how many of these play a role in the genesis of human cancer. Nonetheless, the pursuit of proto-oncogene families has greatly enlarged our catalogue of functions involved in the regulation of normal cells.

Authenticating Proto-oncogenes

Proto-oncogenes were first encountered as progenitors for the oncogenes of retroviruses. Accordingly, the definition of these genes rests mainly on the fact that they can be converted into oncogenes by genetic damage (or "activated" as this event is often called). The transforming alleles of *ras* genes isolated from human tumors already possess the activity of oncogenes, so they inherently obey the definition. In other contexts, candidate proto-oncogenes are at first defined only by circumstantial evidence, such as the consistency with which particular genes are found in association with insertional mutagenesis, translocation, or amplification in tumor cells.

For a proto-oncogene to be properly authenticated, however, it is necessary to demonstrate that the gene can be converted to an oncogene and have the consequent ability to transform cells to neoplastic growth. Many activated proto-oncogenes can transform fibroblasts, but the more selective tissue specificity of some genes necessitates the use of specialized cell cultures.

N-*myc* provides an example of how a proto-oncogene can be authenticated. This gene was found amid a large domain of amplified DNA, in the company of other genes whose number and nature are undetermined. For what reasons is N-*myc* regarded as an authentic proto-oncogene? At least two indirect indications exist. First, N-*myc* is a close relative of *myc*, an archetypal proto-oncogene.[38] Second, amplification of N-*myc* in neuroblastomas is limited to the more aggressive stages of the disease; amplification in this situation provides a prognostic indicator of grave outcome and suggests that the amplification may be partly responsible for the behavior of the tumor [*see Chapter 7*].[39-41] More direct experimental tests provided an even stronger case: N-*myc* can transform cells in culture when the gene is expressed from the context of a retroviral vector.[42-44] When it is inserted as a transgene in mice, N-*myc* elicits tumors.[45,46]

General Considerations

The number of authenticated and candidate proto-oncogenes now exceeds 100, and the number will likely continue to grow. For example, dozens of chromosomal translocations exist for which the affected proto-oncogenes have yet to be identified. Only a few of the proto-oncogenes first uncovered by retroviral transduction or insertional mutagenesis have been implicated in human tumors. However, some of these same genes have had a great impact on the course of discovery. Consider *myc*, which has been a great provider of information [*see Figure 4*]. First discovered as a transduced oncogene in a leukemia/carcinoma virus of chickens, *myc* eventually proved to be crucial in the discovery of insertional mutagenesis, the molecular nature of chromosomal translocation and the genes that it affects, and the potential role of amplification in tumorigenesis.

Most proto-oncogenes are conserved across vast reaches of phylogenic time. For example, the prototypic *src* has been found in all metazoan organisms that have been examined, ranging from echinoderms to mammals, and the same is true of many other proto-oncogenes. Conservation of this magnitude suggests that the course of evolution has selected proto-onco-

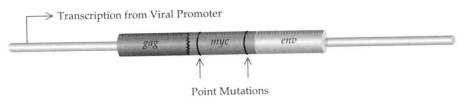

Transcription from Viral Promoter

gag   myc   env

Point Mutations

Figure 7   *Activation of* myc *by transduction.*

genes for vital purposes. Pursuit of those purposes has greatly illuminated the mechanisms by which cells govern themselves and how that governance goes awry in cancer [*see Chapter 5*].

Conversion of Proto-oncogenes to Oncogenes

What is the nature of the genetic damage that is responsible for converting proto-oncogenes to oncogenes? The answer to this question varies with the biologic context and is best considered by use of specific examples.

Activation by Retroviral Transduction and Insertional Mutagenesis

Although retroviral oncogenes have not figured in the genesis of human tumors, the means by which they are activated have helped illuminate the genetic origins of tumorigenesis. Transduction can convert proto-oncogenes to oncogenes in at least three ways [*see Figure 7*]: (1) by placing expression of the gene under the control of the viral genome; (2) by fusing part or all of the proto-oncogene to a structural gene of the virus, creating a hybrid gene and protein product; and (3) by inflicting more focal damage, such as point mutations and small deletions, on the coding domain of the proto-oncogene.

The first two phenomena are consequences of the initial recombination that implants a proto-oncogene into a retroviral genome. The third arises both from changes inflicted by the process of transduction itself and from mutagenesis that occurs during subsequent viral propagation. As dramatized by the timely example of human immunodeficiency virus, the replication of retroviral genomes is exceedingly prone to error, giving rise to a high rate of mutagenesis within many portions of the viral genome—including any transduced proto-oncogene.

Insertional mutagenesis activates proto-oncogenes to oncogenes principally by commandeering control of their expression. The retroviral provirus is equipped with powerful devices for the vigorous expression of viral genes; these same devices can co-opt the expression of proto-oncogenes that lie in the vicinity of the integrated provirus. The result can be either activation of a previously silent gene or sustained and augmented expression of a previously active gene [*see Figure 5*]. In some instances, however, integration of proviral DNA also disturbs the coding domain of the affected proto-oncogene, giving rise to an anomalous gene product [*see Figure 5*].

The transduced version of *myc* provides an illustration of the various mechanisms by which proto-oncogenes are converted to oncogenes [*see Figure 7*]. The transduced gene has been brought under the influence of viral transcriptional controls, has been fused to a viral structural gene to create a hybrid protein, and has sustained point mutations in focal regions of the coding domain. Each of these changes contributes to the potency of tumorigenesis by transduced *myc*, and in combination, they anticipate the activation of proto-oncogenes to oncogenes in human tumors.

Activation by Chromosomal Translocations

Translocations can affect proto-oncogenes in either of two ways. First, they can relocate the gene into the vicinity of strong transcriptional controls that will commandeer expression of the proto-oncogene. The prototype is the translocation of *myc* found in Burkitt's lymphoma, which typically brings the proto-oncogene under the influence of the transcriptional controls for an immunoglobulin gene.[47] In the most prevalent example, the transcriptional unit for the immunoglobulin gene is embedded within that of *myc* and becomes the controlling factor for the expression of the proto-oncogene [*see Figure 8; see also Chapter 7*]. Other configurations are observed less frequently, but the functional consequences are generally similar. It has recently become apparent, however, that many of the translocated alleles of *myc* have also sustained point mutations in a focal domain of the encoded protein, much as is found in transduced alleles of *myc*.[48] Based on the example of transduced *myc*, these mutations may also contribute to the activation of translocated *myc*, but this interpretation remains speculative.

The second form of damage inflicted by translocations on proto-oncogenes results when the breakpoints of the translocations fuse portions of two genes together in a manner that creates a hybrid protein that is composed of domains derived from both genes. The configuration resembles that found in transduced proto-oncogenes that have been fused with viral structural genes [*see Figure 7*]. The first example was provided by the Philadelphia chromosome, which joins the previously identified proto-oncogene *abl* with a gene known as *bcr*.[18,19] Many of the other translocations described in human leukemias fuse portions of two transcription factors together [*see Chapter 7*].[21] In principle, both of the genes involved in such fusions could be considered to be proto-oncogenes. In some instances, however, it may be necessary for only one of the genes to contribute a biochemical activity to the hybrid protein. The contribution from the other gene may be passive, such as disruption or replacement of a regulatory domain [*see Chapter 7*].

Activation by Gene Amplification

Amplification of a proto-oncogene increases the amount of template available for transcription of messenger RNA from the gene and, thus, increases the amount of gene product produced in the cell. Because the extent of the amplification can be 100-fold or more, the increase in gene product can also be immense. In addition, some amplified alleles of proto-oncogenes sustain mutations within their protein-coding domains before the amplification.[22] A reasonable interpretation of these successive changes is that the mutation of the gene's coding domain conferred some selective advantage on the cell.

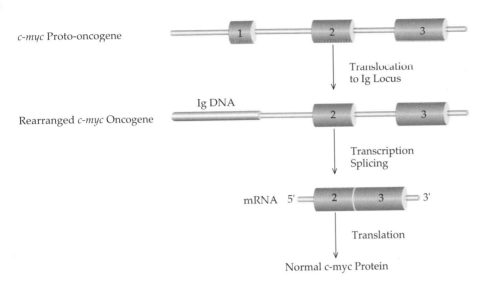

c-myc Proto-oncogene

Rearranged *c-myc* Oncogene

Translocation
to Ig Locus

Ig DNA

Transcription
Splicing

mRNA   5'   2   3   3'

Translation

Normal c-myc Protein

Figure 8 *Activation of* c-myc *by translocation in mouse plasmacytomas.*

Amplification of the mutant gene then enhanced the advantage. At present, it appears that amplification of an otherwise normal proto-oncogene is the usual finding in human tumors.

Activation by Point Mutations

Many human tumors contain alleles of *ras* genes that readily transform cells in culture, whereas the normal counterparts of these genes do not.[32,49] The transforming alleles all contain point mutations that change a single amino acid residue in the gene product, usually at residue 12, 13, or 61 [*see Figure 9*].[32,49] Suitable testing quickly showed that these mutations are responsible for the transforming activity. As with other proto-oncogenes, even wild-type alleles of *ras* genes can transform cells when expressed in sufficient abundance.[49] The point mutations appear to enhance transforming activity at least 100-fold. Similar point mutations at codon 12 also activate the transduced alleles of *ras* present in retroviral genomes.

Activated alleles of *ras* genes are exceedingly common in human tumors. They occur only sporadically (or not at all) in some forms of cancer, and with reasonable or great consistency in others [*see Chapter 7*]. These findings advanced our understanding of human cancer by providing a clear example of how mutation of a human gene could directly cause transforming activity. Because such mutations were found to be prevalent in many different sorts of human tumors, they gave further credence to the genetic paradigm for cancer.

Activated alleles of the *ret* proto-oncogene are far less common in human tumors than are those of *ras* proto-oncogenes. However, the mutant alleles of *ret* are more varied than those of *ras* proto-oncogenes and, thus, provide a broader sampling of the mechanisms by which human proto-oncogenes can be activated. The *ret* proto-oncogene was discovered through the use of transfection. The biologic activity in the first instance was caused by a genetic rearrangement that apparently occurred as an artifact during transfection.[37] The rearrangement fused *ret* to a portion of another gene and, in the process, replaced an amino-terminal domain of the Ret protein—a malfor-

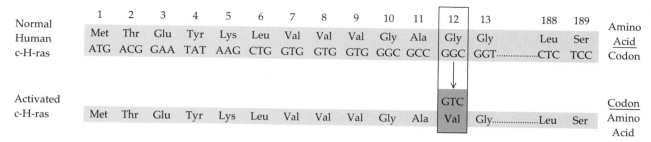

	1	2	3	4	5	6	7	8	9	10	11	12	13		188	189	
Normal Human c-H-ras	Met	Thr	Glu	Tyr	Lys	Leu	Val	Val	Val	Gly	Ala	Gly	Gly		Leu	Ser	Amino Acid
	ATG	ACG	GAA	TAT	AAG	CTG	GTG	GTG	GTG	GGC	GCC	GGC	GGT..............CTC		TCC		Codon
Activated c-H-ras												GTC					Codon
	Met	Thr	Glu	Tyr	Lys	Leu	Val	Val	Val	Gly	Ala	Val	Gly..............Leu		Ser		Amino Acid

Figure 9 *The active H-ras oncogene often differs from the H-ras proto-oncogene by a single nucleotide change in the 12th codon, causing an important alteration in the amino acid sequence of ras protein.*

mation reminiscent of the gene fusions seen in some proto-oncogenes activated by transduction, insertional mutagenesis, or translocation. Fortuitously, similar rearrangements activate *ret* in many papillary carcinomas of the thyroid.[37] In contrast, the alleles of *ret* that are responsible for the aforementioned inherited endocrine tumors contain point mutations in either of two portions of the coding domain. These mutations also activate the transforming potential of the gene.

Mechanisms Responsible for Damage to Proto-oncogenes

The mechanisms responsible for the genetic damage displayed by proto-oncogenes in tumor cells are poorly understood. Chromosomal translocations are common in leukemias and lymphomas of both B and T cells. In B cell tumors, the translocations typically involve an immunoglobulin gene, whereas in T cell tumors, they involve one of the genes for the cell-surface antigen receptor. These findings have prompted the notion that the translocations might arise from misbegotten actions of the enzymatic mechanisms that normally rearrange and fuse DNA segments in order to assemble functional genes that encode immunoglobulins and T cell receptors. Circumstantial evidence supports this view, but no decisive proof exists. The translocations found in nonlymphoid tumors remain unexplained. The only hint of an explanation for these last cases is the possibility that the translocations arise from errant versions of homologous recombination, which normally facilitates meiotic crossing over between chromosomes. Whatever the mechanisms by which translocations occur, a provoking cause for these aberrations has not been identified.

The causes and mechanisms of gene amplification are also obscure.[50] One venerable hypothesis holds that the first step in amplification is the occurrence of repetitive initiations within one replicon of DNA during a single S phase of the cell cycle. A more recent view is that the initial event is breakage of DNA, but the events that follow remain a matter of controversy. Whatever the mechanism of amplification might be, no exogenous cause of the abnormality has been found. It does appear that amplification is rarely, if ever, the initial event in tumorigenesis. Instead, it occurs later, as the emerging tumor cell progresses toward full malignancy [*see Chapter 7*].

The sorts of point mutations found in the *ras* genes of human tumors are familiar to students of mutagenesis. Nevertheless, the mechanisms that create these mutant alleles remain elusive. The best clue comes from certain tumors that have been induced in rodents by use of chemical or physical carcinogens.[51] These tumors carry mutant alleles of *ras* that are similar to those found in human tumors, and the nature of the mutations is consistent with what is known about the responsible carcinogens' chemical reactivity with DNA. Thus, it appears that the mutations were elicited directly by the exogenous carcinogens, and the naturally occurring mutations of *ras* genes in human tumors may have arisen in a similar way (although the nature of the carcinogens responsible for the human tumors is generally not known). However, a portion of the mutations arising in human *ras* genes may be caused by spontaneous errors in DNA replication that are unprovoked by any external agent.[52]

Point mutations are also prevalent in several domains of translocated *myc* genes.[48] Because the translocations in question have occurred in B cells, the point mutations have been ascribed to the mechanisms that normally diversify immunoglobulin genes by somatic mutation. Accordingly, the activation of *myc* in malignant B cells may derive from the ensemble of enzymatic mechanisms that are normally devoted to the genesis of mature immunoglobulin genes, including the mechanisms responsible for assembling the genes through genetic rearrangement and the mechanisms responsible for final diversification of the genes through somatic mutation. The derangement of *myc* by these mechanisms is likely to be a rare and nonspecific anomaly, but the functional consequences of the derangement provide a strong selective advantage for those rare cells in which the anomaly happens to occur.

The causes and mechanisms of genetic damage in the proto-oncogenes of human tumors are not abstruse issues. It may eventually be possible to deduce the causes of cancers from the nature of the genetic damage found in the cancers, thereby joining molecular biology with epidemiology in the search for the causes of human cancer [*see Chapter 7*].

Pathophysiology of Proto-oncogenes

A diversity of genetic mechanisms can damage proto-oncogenes and activate them to become oncogenes. How might the damage affect the function of the genes? Two answers have been proposed to this question: a quantitative model, in which pathogenesis is caused merely by the sustained and perhaps excessive activity of the gene or its protein product, and a qualitative model, which posits a change in either the specificity or the actual function of the gene product.[53] Although this contrast may be too starkly drawn, it has framed the experimental data in a useful manner. Most adequately studied examples conform to the quantitative model. The various forms of genetic damage that have been chronicled for proto-oncogenes in tumor cells generally represent "gain-of-function" mutations that confer constitutive or even excessive activity on the genes and/or their products, whose functions otherwise remain normal. The genesis of this unwanted activity takes several forms.

Gain of Function Through Altered Gene Expression

Several forms of the genetic damage that afflict proto-oncogenes in tumor cells alter expression of the genes. Transduction and insertional mutagenesis by retroviruses place the affected genes under the influence of viral elements for the control of transcription. Similarly, chromosomal translocations reconfigure the transcriptional control of proto-oncogenes. In all these instances, expression of the gene may be augmented. However, it may be equally (or even more) important that expression of the proto-oncogene has become constitutive rather than regulated by physiologic circumstances. As a result, forces that might otherwise inhibit expression of the gene can no longer do so.

A similar situation arises from gene amplification, which can vastly increase expression of the affected genes. In principle, the amplified DNA might remain susceptible to normal controls that are imposed on transcription. In practice, the amplification is likely to overwhelm these controls. The end result is equivalent to a gain-of-function mutation, viz, constitutive and vastly augmented expression.

Often, the increased expression of a proto-oncogene cannot be ascribed to any obvious mechanism. The proto-oncogene *myc* is the most prevalent example. In these instances, overexpression of the gene is assumed to result from subtle genetic disturbances of the transcriptional apparatus that are more difficult to detect than are translocation and amplification. Because the degradation of messenger RNA is also subject to specific control, disturbance of this control could likewise enhance gene expression. These possibilities have yet to be explored in detail.

In summary, a variety of genetic damage can lead to the constitutive expression of proto-oncogenes. In these instances, the inability of the cell to silence the gene presumably leads to pathogenesis: the cell falls prey to inappropriately sustained activity of an otherwise normal gene. However, several forms of genetic damage can also cause a large increase in gene expression; this increase appears to be essential to transformation in some settings. The impact of this overexpression is not well understood and may require relatively subtle explanations. For example, the sheer quantity of gene product may overwhelm various cellular controls, including normal thresholds in biochemical pathways, the degradative machinery that normally disposes of proteins, or other quantitative controls. Alternatively, large concentrations of gene product may drive signaling by means of mass action. One proven example of this is the transmembrane receptors that are protein-tyrosine kinases [*see Chapter 5*]. Signaling from these receptors is triggered by dimerization of the receptor proteins in the plane of the plasma membrane, a process that is normally mediated by binding of ligand but might also be driven by inordinately large quantities of receptor monomer.

Gain of Function Through Disturbance of Protein Structure

Several forms of genetic damage affect the coding domains of proto-oncogenes in human tumors, including point mutations, deletions, and fusions with other genes. These changes have a common result: the mutant proteins are unleashed from controls that normally constrain their activity. The functional consequence is the same as that produced by deregulation of gene expression: constitutive and perhaps augmented activity that cannot be bridled by physiologic signals but is otherwise normal.

The activated alleles of *ras* proto-oncogenes illustrate this point clearly. The proteins encoded by *ras* genes are signaling devices that are triggered by the binding of guanosine triphosphate (GTP) and then proceed to turn themselves off by hydrolyzing the bound GTP to guanosine diphosphate [*see Chapter 5*]. The hydrolysis is designed to limit the duration of signaling by the Ras protein. Another protein, known as GAP (for GTPase-activating protein), interacts directly with the Ras protein to enhance the hydrolysis of GTP many fold; indeed, without the action of GAP, spontaneous hydrolysis of GTP by Ras proteins is inconsequential. The mutations that convert *ras* proto-oncogenes to oncogenes cripple the ability of the gene products to hydrolyze GTP, mainly by impeding the response to GAP. As a consequence, the mutant ras proteins signal constitutively—a quantitative gain-of-function mutation that acts directly through the gene product rather than through gene expression.

The *ret* proto-oncogene provides another example of how point mutations activate oncogenes. *Ret* encodes a cell surface receptor with a cytoplasmic protein-tyrosine kinase that is activated by binding of ligand to the extracellular domain of the receptor.[37] All of the *ret* mutations associated with inherited endocrine tumors apparently bestow constitutive activity on the gene product, eliminating the requirement for ligand binding.[37] However, some of these mutations may also alter the substrate specificity of the kinase. If so, they could represent an example of the qualitative model for pathogenesis by activated oncogenes.

Even the more drastic disturbances of proto-oncogene structure may engender constitutive activity of otherwise normal functions. For example, some genetic rearrangements delete or replace regulatory domains of proteins, giving rise to constitutive activity (e.g., *ret*, in the form of the rearrangements found in many papillary carcinomas of the thyroid[37]). These rearrangements replace part of the ligand-binding domain of the Ret protein with a domain derived from another gene. As a result, the protein-tyrosine kinase encoded by *ret* becomes constitutively active. Similar anomalies have been described in other proto-oncogenes that encode protein kinases. Prominent examples include *erb*-B1 (whose product is the receptor for epidermal growth factor, which can be activated by deletion of its ligand-binding domain), *abl* (whose fusion with *bcr* in the Philadelphia chromosome is thought to constitutively activate the protein-tyrosine kinase encoded by *abl*), and *raf* (whose product is a cytoplasmic serine-threonine protein kinase, which can be activated by deletion or replacement of a regulatory domain within the protein) [*see Chapter 5*].

Many of the translocations in human leukemias create hybrids between two transcription factors.[21] In such situations, a qualitative change in function may occur, such as action on a novel spectrum of genes or alteration of tissue specificity [*see Chapter 7*]. The matter requires further study.

Pathogenesis by Gain-of-Function Mutations in Proto-oncogenes

The great diversity of proto-oncogenes confounded early efforts to explain why activated versions of all these genes have the same biologic effects: cellular transformation and tumorigenesis. The first hint of a solution to this puzzle came with the discoveries that two proto-oncogenes (*sis* and *erb*-B1) encode well-recognized elements in the signaling pathways that are used to excite and sustain cellular proliferation—the B-subunit of platelet-derived growth factor and the cellular receptor for epidermal growth factor, respectively. As prefigured by these discoveries, it is now apparent that proto-oncogenes encode many switching points in the elaborate biochemical circuitry that is used to elicit cellular proliferation in response to physiologic signals [*see Chapter 5*]. The diversity of proto-oncogenes and their products reflects the complexity of this circuitry and offers exceptional experimental access to the circuitry. Indeed, many of the known proto-oncogenes define signaling functions that might otherwise remain undetected.

The elucidation of how proto-oncogenes serve normal cells provided an explanation for the transformational and tumorigenic potential of these genes. Each gain-of-function mutation in a proto-oncogene represents a short-circuit in the signal transduction that leads to cellular proliferation. Thus, the constitutive and even augmented activity of a proto-oncogene or its protein product can free cells from their usual requirement for external signals to excite and sustain proliferation. This freedom is one of the most fundamental properties of neoplastic cells.

Conclusion

Uncovering the multitude of proto-oncogenes has paid rich dividends. Pursuit of these genes has provided initial access to several of the genetic maladies in human cancers, unveiled diverse forms of genetic damage that can contribute to tumorigenesis, revealed a general scheme by which cancer cells can acquire their proliferative prowess, and helped to illuminate the elaborate biochemical circuitry that governs the behavior of both normal and neoplastic cells.

Transduced proto-oncogenes are uncommonly potent, perhaps because they have been subjected to prolonged biologic selection for tumorigenicity. More often than not, only a single retroviral oncogene is required for tumorigenesis. In contrast, most, if not all, human tumors arise from a combination of genetic lesions [*see Chapters 7 and 8*]. The multistep nature of tumorigenesis can sometimes be embodied in single proto-oncogenes: for full tumorigenic potential to be realized, deregulated expression can combine with activating mutations within coding domains. Typically, however, the genesis of human tumors involves not only multiple genetic lesions but also multiple genes. In particular, proto-oncogenes inevitably share the stage with another genre of gene (tumor suppressor genes) in tumorigenesis [*see Chapters 6, 7, and 8*].

Transduction by retroviruses has been eclipsed as a source of discovery in our assault on the genome of the cancer cell, but its energizing influence remains apparent. It was transduction by retroviruses that first gave physical reality to the belief that the vertebrate genome harbors potential cancer genes. With the discovery of transduction, the genetic paradigm became the prevailing force in cancer research. The remainder of this book shows how far that force has now taken us toward a unified understanding of tumorigenesis.

References

1. Temin HM: The control of cellular morphology on embryonic cells infected with Rous sarcoma virus in vitro. *Virology* 10:182, 1960

2. Martin GS: Rous sarcoma virus: a function required for the maintenance of the transformed state. *Nature* 227:1021, 1970

3. Kawai S, Hanafusa H: The effects of reciprocal changes in temperature on the transformed state of cells infected with a Rous sarcoma virus mutant. *Virology* 46:470, 1971

4. Vogt PK: Spontaneous segregation of nontransforming viruses from cloned sarcoma viruses. *Virology* 46:939, 1971

5. Huebner RJ, Todaro GJ: Oncogenes of RNA tumor viruses as determinants of cancer. *Proc Natl Acad Sci USA* 64:1087, 1969

6. Stehelin D, Varmus HE, Bishop JM, et al: DNA related to the transforming gene(s) of avian sarcoma viruses is present in normal avian DNA. *Nature* 260:170, 1976

7. Spector DH, Varmus HE, Bishop JM: Nucleotide sequences related to the transforming gene of avian sarcoma virus are present in DNA of uninfected vertebrates. *Proc Natl Acad Sci USA* 75:4102, 1978

8. Bishop JM: Cellular oncogenes and retroviruses. *Annu Rev Biochem* 52:301, 1983

9. Neel BG, Hayward WS, Robinson HL, et al: Avian leukosis virus-induced tumors have common proviral integration sites and synthesize discrete new RNAs: oncogenesis by promoter insertion. *Cell* 23:323, 1981

10. Payne GS, Courtneidge SA, Crittenden LB, et al: Analysis of avian leukosis virus DNA and RNA in bursal tumors: viral gene expression is not required for maintenance of the tumor state. *Cell* 23:311, 1981

11. Hayward WS, Neel BG, Astrin SM: Activation of a cellular *onc* gene by promoter insertion in ALV-induced lymphoid leukosis. *Nature* 290:475, 1981

12. Payne GS, Bishop JM, Varmus HE: Multiple arrangements of virus DNA and an activated host oncogene in bursal lymphomas. *Nature* 295:209, 1982

13. Varmus H: An historical overview of oncogenes. *Oncogenes and the Molecular Origins of Cancer.* Weinberg RA, Ed. Cold Spring Harbor Laboratory Press, Cold Spring Harbor, NY, 1989, p.3

14. Taub R, Kirsch I, Morton C, et al: Translocation of the c-*myc* gene into the immunoglobulin heavy chain locus in human Burkitt lymphoma and murine plasmacytoma cells. *Proc Natl Acad Sci USA* 79:7837, 1982

15. Dalla-Favera R, Bregni M, Erickson J, et al: Human c-*myc onc* gene is located on the region of chromosome 8 that is translocated in Burkitt lymphoma cells. *Proc Natl Acad Sci USA* 79:7824, 1982

16. Leder PJ, Battey G, Lenoir C, et al: Translocations among antibody genes in human cancer. *Science* 222:765, 1984

17. Nowell PC, Hungerford DA: A minute chromosome in human chronic granulocytic leukemia. *Science* 132:1497, 1960

18. Groffen J, Stephenson JR, Heisterkamp N, et al: Philadelphia chromosomal breakpoints are clustered within a limited region, *bcr*, on chromosome 22. *Cell* 36:93, 1984

19. Shtivelman E, Lifshitz B, Gale RP, et al: Fused transcript of *abl* and *bcr* genes in chronic myelogenous leukaemia. *Nature* 315:550, 1985

20. Haluska FG, Tsujimoto Y, Croce CM: Oncogene activation by chromosome translocation in human malignancy. *Annu Rev Genet* 21:321, 1987

21. Rabbitts TH: Chromosomal translocations in human cancer. *Nature* 372:143, 1994

22. Alitalo K, Schwab M: Oncogene amplification in tumor cells. *Adv Cancer Res* 47:235, 1986

23. Schwab M, Alitalo K, Klempnauer KH, et al: Amplified DNA with limited homology to *myc* cellular oncogene is shared by human neuroblastoma cell lines and a neuroblastoma tumour. *Nature* 305:245, 1983

24. Kohl NE, Kanda N, Schreck RR, et al: Transposition and amplification of oncogene-related sequences in human neuroblastomas. *Cell* 35:359, 1983

25. Nau MM, Brooks BJ, Battey J, et al: L-*myc*, a new *myc*-related gene amplified and ex-

pressed in human small cell lung cancer. *Nature* 318:69, 1985

26. Fakharzadeh SS, Trusko SP, George DL: Tumorigenic potential associated with enhanced expression of a gene that is amplified in a mouse tumor cell line. *EMBO J* 10:1565, 1991

27. Momand J, Zambetti GP, Olson DC, et al: The *mdm*-2 oncogene product forms a complex with the p53 protein and inhibits p53-mediated transactivation. *Cell* 69:1237, 1992

28. Kinzler KW, Bigner SH, Bigner DD, et al: Identification of an amplified, highly expressed gene in a human glioma. *Science* 236:70, 1987

29. Graham FL, van der Eb AJ: A new technique for the assay of infectivity of human adenovirus 5 DNA. *Virology* 52:456, 1973

30. Hill M, Hillova J: Recovery of the temperature-sensitive mutant of Rous sarcoma virus from chicken cells exposed to DNA extracted from hamster cells transformed by the mutant. *Virology* 49:309, 1972

31. Shih C, Shilo B-Z, Goldfarb MP, et al: Passage of phenotypes of chemically transformed cells via transfection of DNA and chromatin. *Proc Natl Acad Sci USA* 76:5714, 1979

32. Weinberg RA: Oncogenes of spontaneous and chemically induced tumors. *Adv Cancer Res* 36:149, 1982

33. Varmus HE: The molecular genetics of cellular oncogenes. *Annu Rev Genet* 18:553, 1984

34. Parada LF, Tabin CJ, Shih C, et al: Human EJ bladder carcinoma oncogene is homologue of Harvey sarcoma virus *ras* gene. *Nature* 297:474, 1982

35. Der CJ, Krontiris TG, Cooper GM: Transforming genes of human bladder and lung carcinoma cell lines are homologues to the *ras* genes of Harvey and Kirsten sarcoma viruses. *Proc Natl Acad Sci USA* 79:3637, 1982

36. Santos E, Tronick SR, Aaronson SA, et al: T24 human bladder carcinoma oncogene is an activated form of the normal human homologue of BALB- and Harvey-MSV transforming genes. *Nature* 298:343, 1982

37. van Heyningen V: One gene: four syndromes. *Nature* 367:319, 1994

38. Stanton LW, Schwab M, Bishop JM: Nucleotide sequence of the human N-*myc* gene. *Proc Natl Acad Sci USA* 83:1772, 1986

39. Seeger RC, Brodeur GM, Sather H, et al: Association of multiple copies of the N-*myc* oncogene with rapid progression of neuroblastomas. *N Engl J Med* 313:1111, 1985

40. Brodeur GM, Hayes FA, Green AA, et al: Consistent N-*myc* copy number in simultaneous or consecutive neuroblastoma samples from sixty individual patients. *Cancer Res* 47:4248, 1987

41. Schwab M, Ellison J, Busch M, et al: Enhanced expression of the human gene N-*myc* consequent to amplification of DNA may contribute to malignant progression of neuroblastoma. *Proc Natl Acad Sci USA* 81:4940, 1984

42. Schwab M, Varmus HE, Bishop JM: Human N-*myc* gene contributes to neoplastic transformation of mammalian cells in culture. *Nature* 316:160,1985

43. Yancopoulos GD, Nisen PD, Tesfaye A, et al: N-*myc* can cooperate with *ras* to transform normal cells in culture. *Proc Natl Acad Sci USA* 82:5455, 1985

44. Small MB, Hay N, Schwab M, et al: Neoplastic transformation by the human gene N-*myc*. *Mol Cell Biol* 7:1638, 1987

45. Rosenbaum H, Webb E, Adams JM, et al: N-*myc* transgene promotes B lymphoid proliferation, elicits lymphomas and reveals cross-regulation with c-*myc*. *EMBO J* 8:749, 1989

46. Dildrop R, Ma A, Zimmerman K, et al: IgH enhancer-mediated deregulation of N-*myc* gene expression in transgenic mice: generation of lymphoid neoplasias that lack c-*myc* expression. *EMBO J* 8:1121, 1989

47. Cory S: Activation of cellular oncogenes in hemopoietic cells by chromosome translocation. *Adv Cancer Res* 47:189,1986

48. Bhatia KK, Huppi G, Spangler D, et al: Point mutations in the c-myc transactivation domain are common in Burkitt's lymphoma and mouse plasmacytoma. *Nat Genet* 5:56, 1993

49. Barbacid M: *Ras* genes. *Annu Rev Biochem* 56:779, 1987

50. Stark GR, Wahl GM: Gene amplification. *Annu Rev Biochem* 53:447, 1984

51. Sukumar S: *Ras* oncogenes in chemical carcinogenesis. *Curr Top Microbiol Immunol* 148:93, 1989

52. Meuth M: The structure of mutation in mammalian cells. *Biochim Biophys Acta* 1032:1, 1990

53. Bishop JM: Molecular themes in oncogenesis. *Cell* 64:235, 1991

Acknowledgments

Figure 1   Marcia Kammerer. Adapted from "Oncogenes," by J.M. Bishop, in *Scientific American* 246·80, 1982.

Figures 2 and 8   Talar Agasyan.

Figure 3   Dimitry Schidlovsky.

Figures 4, 5, and 7   Talar Agasyan. Adapted from *Genes and the Biology of Cancer*, by H. Varmus and R.A. Weinberg, Scientific American Library, New York, 1993.

Figure 6   Dimitry Schidlovsky. Adapted from *Genes and the Biology of Cancer*, by H. Varmus and R.A. Weinberg, Scientific American Library, New York, 1993.

Figure 9   Marcia Kammerer. Adapted from *Genes and the Biology of Cancer*, by H. Varmus and R.A. Weinberg, Scientific American Library, New York, 1993.

CHAPTER 5

The Biochemical Mechanisms of Oncogene Action

Tony Pawson, Ph.D.

Mammalian cells are generally functionally inert until they receive an extracellular signal that modifies their behavior in some specific way. Hence, the growth, the differentiation, and frequently the survival of normal cells are dependent on such external signals. The process of cellular communication is initiated when one cell produces a signaling molecule, often in the form of a soluble hormone, which then binds tightly to a receptor on a target cell.

Transmission of Signals Between Cells

Because the ability of a hormone to induce a cellular response is entirely dependent on its association with a specific receptor displayed on the surface of the target cell, a hormone has no biologic impact on a cell that lacks the relevant receptor. In addition, cells that do not normally react to a hormone because they do not synthesize the appropriate receptor can be rendered responsive by the artificial expression of the receptor.

   Binding of a hormone generally converts its receptor from a dormant to an active state by stimulating some intrinsic biochemical function of the receptor. The activated receptor then modifies intracellular signaling pathways that control gene expression, progression through the cell cycle, cell metabolism, cytoskeletal architecture, and cell adhesion or migration. Signaling hormones can regulate all aspects of cellular behavior. For example, platelet-derived growth factor (PDGF) and epidermal growth factor (EGF) can act as mitogens to stimulate cell proliferation, and hormones such as nerve growth factor and macrophage colony-stimulating factor promote cell differentiation and are required for the survival of their neuronal or hematopoietic targets.[1] These latter factors therefore promote the progression of undifferentiated stem cells to more mature cell types. The actions of these and many other hormones are largely responsible for the orderly development and specialization of cells and tissues in the embryo. In the adult, they are essential for metabolic control, acute responses to infection and wounding, and ongoing production and differentiation of hematopoietic cells.

Examples of Signaling Molecules and Receptors

Most hormones, including all of the polypeptide hormones, are unable to penetrate the cell's plasma membrane. For this reason, their receptors are displayed on the cell surface and, in their simplest form, possess an extracellular domain that binds a specific ligand, a transmembrane region, and a cytoplasmic domain that couples to internal biochemical pathways.[2,3] Many hormones with diverse signaling properties bind transmembrane receptors that possess cytoplasmic protein-tyrosine kinase (PTK) domains. On activation, these receptors phosphorylate both themselves and other intracellular proteins on the amino acid tyrosine [see Figure 1]. Although hormones that bind to PTK receptors can influence differentiation and metabolism, they are also frequently involved in the control of cell growth and are therefore commonly referred to as *growth factors*. Apparently for this reason, the genes encoding both PTK receptors and the intracellular proteins that mediate their effects on cell proliferation are frequently altered by oncogenic mutations and, as a consequence, can contribute to the formation of a wide range of human and animal cancers.

Cells can deliver growth factors to PTK receptors in several ways. The hormone-producing cell can be distant from its target, as occurs in endocrine stimulation by a hormone such as insulin, or nearby, as observed in paracrine stimulation.[4] Moreover, rather than being secreted as freely diffusible soluble hormones, growth and differentiation factors are sometimes tethered to the membrane of the producing cell and can bind to receptors only on neighboring cells. A nice example is provided by Steel factor (also known as mast cell growth factor and stem cell factor), which controls various facets of hematopoiesis, melanogenesis, and gametogenesis by binding to a PTK receptor, termed Kit.[5,6] Steel factor is produced as a transmembrane protein, a fraction of which is subsequently cleaved to yield a soluble form. A mutation in the mouse *Steel* gene that specifically interferes with the transmembrane form of Steel factor but allows the production of the soluble hormone results in a mutant phenotype, indicating that the membrane-associated form of the factor is biologically important.[7] Another common class of cell-surface receptors spans the membrane seven times [see Figure 1] and signals through its ability to regulate heterotrimeric guanine nucleotide-binding proteins (so-called large G proteins).[8] These G proteins can also be subverted as oncoproteins in some cell types.

Steroid hormones and related hydrophobic compounds, such as thyroid hormone and retinoic acid, are able to passively diffuse across the plasma membrane, and their receptors are therefore located within the cell in the cytoplasm or nucleus.[9] These receptors act as transcription factors, whose ability to directly modify gene expression is controlled by hormone bind-

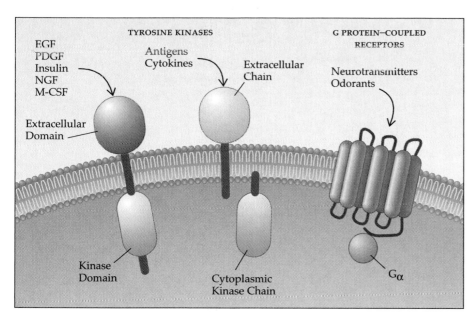

Figure 1   *Cell surface receptors. Receptors for growth factors (e.g., epidermal growth factor [EGF] and platelet-derived growth factor [PDGF]), for insulin, and for differentiation and survival factors (e.g., nerve growth factor [NGF] or macrophage colony-stimulatory factor [M-CSF]) are transmembrane proteins with cytoplasmic protein-tyrosine kinase (PTK) domains. Receptors for antigens and cytokines have a binary structure, with one or more chains involved in binding to the extracellular signaling molecules, and an associated intracellular PTK chain. G protein–coupled receptors span the membrane seven times and associate directly with heterotrimeric large G proteins.*

ing. Such nuclear receptors are potentially involved in human malignancies, as is the case with retinoic acid receptor-α, which is altered by a 15;17 chromosome translocation that is characteristic of acute promyelocytic leukemia.[10,11]

Signaling from the Cell Surface to the Nucleus

Receptor Activation and Autophosphorylation

Many of the factors that stimulate cell growth bind to receptor PTKs at the cell surface.[3] How does this interaction stimulate the intrinsic tyrosine kinase activity of the receptor, and how does the activated receptor elicit changes in gene expression, cell morphology, and metabolism? Most receptor PTKs are monomeric in unstimulated cells and are induced to dimerize by the bound growth factor. This phenomenon is most simply understood for hormones such as PDGF and macrophage colony-stimulating factor, which are dimers. Hence, a single molecule of mature PDGF contains two chains, which are covalently linked by disulfide bonds and each of which can bind the extracellular domain of a single receptor subunit. This has the effect of clustering the receptor into dimers [*see Figure 2*].[2,12] The binding of EGF to the EGF receptor has a similar capacity to induce receptor dimerization, although because EGF is itself a monomer,

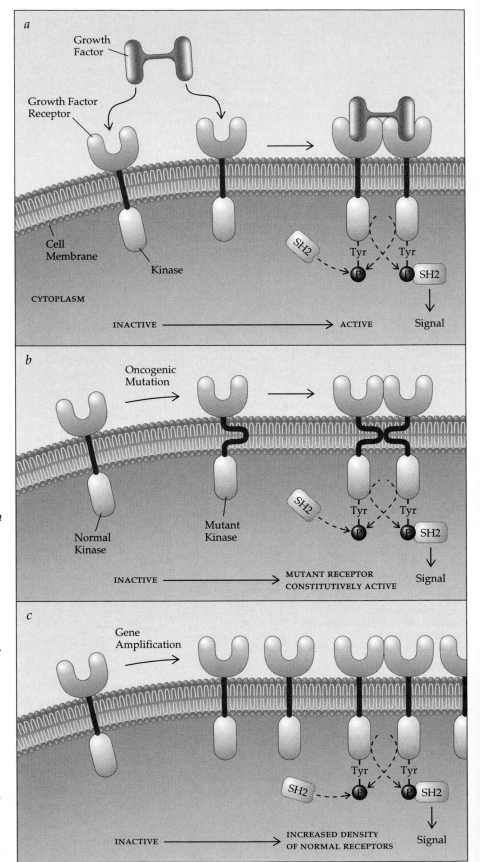

Figure 2 *Activation of growth factor receptors. (a) In the unstimulated cell, receptors exist in an inactive monomeric state. Binding of the growth factor induces receptor dimerization, resulting in activation of the kinase domain and cross-phosphorylation of the paired receptor chains. Receptor autophosphorylation recruits cytoplasmic proteins with SH2 domains to the activated receptor and stimulates a signal output. (b) Oncogenic mutations in the genes for receptor PTKs produce structurally altered receptors that are locked in the activated state. Such variant receptors can form dimers in the absence of the appropriate growth factor. (c) A similar effect is achieved by gene amplification and consequent overexpression of the normal receptor. Owing to their increased density in the plasma membrane, these receptors can cluster and self-activate in the absence of an extracellular ligand.*

this effect may be achieved by the ability of a single EGF molecule to bind simultaneously to two receptors.[13]

The initial consequence of receptor dimerization is to induce the cytoplasmic PTK domains of the two receptor chains to phosphorylate one another on tyrosine. Recent structural analysis suggests that the inactive receptor has a tyrosine residue located within its catalytic domain that sits in the active site and thereby represses enzymatic activity.[14] Autophosphorylation of this tyrosine by the neighboring chain of the dimerized receptor releases this inhibition and stimulates tyrosine kinase activity. The activated receptor then liberally autophosphorylates additional tyrosines that are positioned in noncatalytic regions of the cytoplasmic part of the receptor. These latter autophosphorylation sites serve to recruit cytoplasmic targets of the receptor that have in common a polypeptide sequence module termed the Src homology 2 (SH2) domain. SH2 domains bind with high affinity to specific phosphotyrosine sites that are present on activated receptors and are created by the action of their kinase domains [*see Figure 2a*].[15-17]

PTK Receptors Are Coupled to Ras

The mitogenic signaling pathway activated by PTK receptors is now well established in outline [*see Figure 3*]. One of the proteins attracted to autophosphorylated receptors via an SH2 domain is Grb2. In addition to an SH2 domain, Grb2 also possesses two SH3 domains[18]; SH3 domains are distinct modules that bind proline-rich motifs.[16,17,19,20] In the case of Grb2, the SH3 domains bind to one of two closely related proteins, termed Sos, which function as guanine nucleotide exchange factors for the small (21 kilodaltons; 189 amino acids) membrane-associated Ras proteins.[21-25] This phenomenon, in turn, activates the Ras proteins. The Ras polypeptides are anchored at the cytoplasmic face of the plasma membrane and are biologically inactive when bound to guanosine diphosphate (GDP).[20,26] The affinity of Ras for GDP is very high, and hence the inactive form of Ras is rather stable. The Sos protein induces Ras to release GDP and to bind guanosine triphosphate (GTP), which is present at a much higher concentration than GDP within the cell. The association of the Grb2-Sos complex with the receptor may activate Sos, which consequently converts Ras from the inactive GDP-bound state to the active GTP-bound form.

On exchanging GDP for GTP, Ras undergoes a conformational change [*see Figure 4*] that involves an effector loop between residues 32 and 40, which is relatively inaccessible when Ras is bound to GDP but becomes exposed and positioned for interactions with other proteins in the GTP-bound state.[26-28] In its activated form, Ras can potentially interact with its immediate downstream targets, one of which is the soluble cytosolic protein kinase Raf; this protein kinase in turn, phosphorylates serine and threonine residues on downstream substrates.[29-32] The Raf protein possesses an N-terminal region, which associates with GTP-bound Ras, and a C-terminal protein kinase domain. One function of the interaction between Ras and Raf may be to recruit Raf to the plasma membrane, because Raf can be artificially activated as an oncogene by incorporation of a membrane-targeting se-

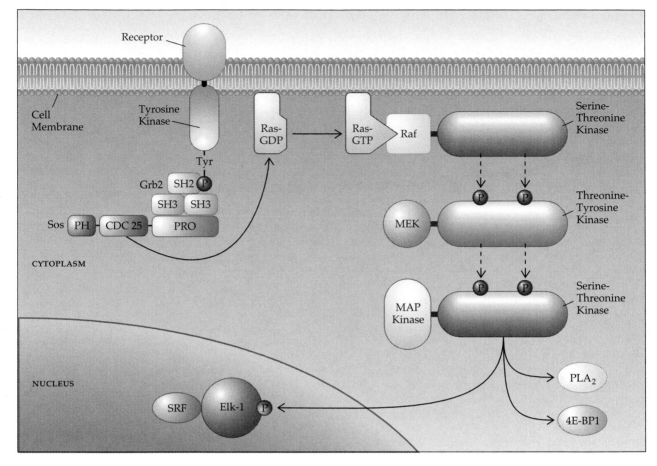

Figure 3 *A signaling pathway from tyrosine kinases to the nucleus. An activated receptor PTK induces Ras activation, leading to a protein kinase cascade that ultimately impinges on Map kinase. The Map kinase phosphorylates and regulates a variety of critical proteins, including transcription factors (e.g., Elk-1), regulators of protein synthesis (e.g., 4E-BP1), and enzymes (e.g., phospholipase A_2 [PLA_2]) that control phospholipid metabolism. GDP, guanosine diphosphate; GTP, guanosine triphosphate.*

quence into the Raf protein that results in its permanent association with the plasma membrane.[33,34] GTP-bound Ras likely has additional targets, which may be involved in modifying the cytoskeletal architecture and cell morphology.[30,35]

A Protein Kinase Cascade Leads to the Nucleus

A cascade of signaling proteins conveys growth factor–initiated signals to the Raf protein. This protein in turn phosphorylates the Mek protein kinase on serine and thereby catalytically activates it.[32,36] The Mek protein kinase has the unusual property of phosphorylating another protein kinase (Map kinase) on both threonine and tyrosine residues, thereby stimulating Map kinase activity. Unlike Raf and Mek, which are rather specific for their protein kinase substrates, Map kinase phosphorylates a wide range of proteins, including transcription factors and regulators of protein synthesis.[32,36,37] Both Raf and Mek can be activated as oncogenes by structural alterations that lock these protein kinases they encode in a permanently active state, an observation that is consistent with the idea that these proteins normally lie on the Ras mitogenic signaling pathway. However, neither *raf* nor *mek* is commonly found as an oncogene in human tumors.

The Map kinase appears to be a key target of this mitogenic pathway, which directly influences gene expression and cell growth. The importance of the various members of this elaborate pathway has been tested by inhibition of their activity in cultured cells. Blocking the pathway at any level generally inhibits the induction of DNA synthesis and cell proliferation. The large number of steps involved in joining the receptor PTK to nuclear events likely allows for amplification of the signal and also provides for the possibility of cross-communication with other signaling pathways. For example, cyclic adenosine monophosphate (cAMP), which is a growth inhibitor in many cell types, acts through cAMP-dependent protein kinase to block the association of active GTP-bound Ras with Raf.[29]

Among the substrates of Map kinase are nuclear transcription factors, which either directly or through their ability to stimulate the expression of additional transcriptional regulators are apparently important for cell proliferation. As anticipated from the fact that they lie at the end of the PTK/Ras/Map kinase mitogenic signaling pathway, several of these transcription factors, such as Fos, Jun, and Ets, are themselves oncogenic when they are overexpressed and indeed were first identified as retroviral oncogene products.

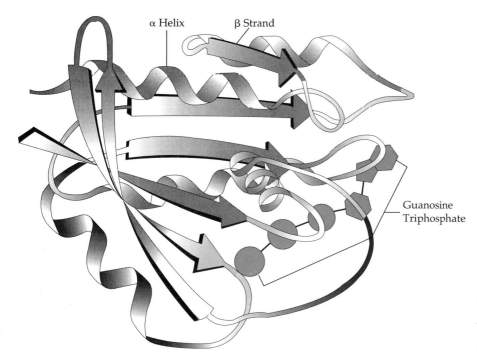

α Helix   β Strand

Guanosine
Triphosphate

Figure 4 *Structure of the Ras protein in the GTP-bound form. The effector loop is shown in dark blue.*

Growth Factor Signaling and Oncogenes

Oncogenic Mutations Affect the Structure and Activity of Mitogenic Signaling Proteins

Many oncogenes encode aberrant forms of the proteins involved in this mitogenic signaling process. A central feature of the PTK/Ras/Map kinase mitogenic signaling pathway, leading from the extracellular growth factor to the nucleus, involves its transient activation and tight regulation in normal cells. Oncogenic mutations frequently involve genes that encode growth factors, growth factor receptors, and intracellular signaling proteins that lie downstream of these receptors. With the exception of the growth factor itself, these signaling proteins can all exist in an inactive and an active state. In each case, the active form is rapidly removed, by dephosphorylation in the case of protein kinases and their immediate targets, or by the hydrolysis of GTP to GDP on Ras. Oncogenic mutations change the coding potential of the relevant genes, such that their protein products are subtly altered and become locked in an activated state.

The expression of a constitutively activated signaling protein, such as that encoded by an oncogene, is interpreted by the cell as a continuous and unrestricted growth-inducing signal. Oncogenes, therefore, have a dominant, positive effect on cell growth by mimicking a normal mitogenic signal. The conversion of a proto-oncogene to an oncogene requires only a single mutation because only one of the two normal alleles needs to be altered.

Oncogenic Mutations Can Affect Growth Factor Expression

The preceding sections introduced the general theme that the constitutive activation of a mitogenic pathway leads to the deregulated growth of cells, and thus to their transformation. The ensuing sections analyze this picture in more detail, by addressing each of the steps in mitogenic signaling by growth factors and the mechanisms by which growth factors contribute to the process of cell transformation.

In normal tissue, the amount of any growth-stimulatory factor available to the cell is controlled by its neighbors or by distant cells that produce and release this factor. This situation ensures normal levels of proliferation and thus tissue homeostasis. However, what happens if a cell makes a growth factor to which it can itself respond? In other words, what would be the consequence of an individual cell expressing both a growth factor and the receptor that confers responsiveness to this factor? This situation (termed *autocrine stimulation* or *self-stimulation*) can result in aberrant cell proliferation.

Once released from the cell, growth factors can be considered to be in an active state because their subsequent binding to a receptor stimulates a cellular response. Growth factor activity is primarily controlled at the level of gene expression, especially by a block to growth factor synthesis in cells that express the cognate receptor. This feature is important because a cell that expresses both a growth factor and its receptor can grow unchecked through autocrine stimulation.[38,39] Thus, the normal regulatory events that prevent prolonged interaction of a growth factor and its receptor are bypassed when both molecules are synthesized in the same cell, contributing to cellular transformation.

Autocrine Stimulation in Tumorigenesis

A strong clue that aberrant expression of growth factors might stimulate cancerous growth came from an analysis of the v-*sis* oncogene, which was discovered as the transforming component of simian sarcoma virus and was shown to encode a variant form of the PDGF-B chain.[40] The functional PDGF hormone is composed of two PDGF chains, which are covalently linked to one another by disulfide bonds. Two closely related PDGF polypeptides have been identified, PDGF-A and PDGF-B. These can associate to form homodimers (AA or BB) or heterodimers (AB). Similarly, two very similar PTK receptors exist for these dimeric growth factors, the α-PDGF and β-PDGF receptors.[41] Cells transformed by the v-*sis* oncogene express a dimeric growth factor that is both structurally and functionally similar to the naturally occurring BB form of PDGF. In particular, the v-Sis dimer binds to and activates PDGF receptors expressed by these same cells. These results have suggested that the v-*sis* oncogene transforms cells in culture and induces tumors in animals through the autocrine stimulation of PDGF receptors [*see Figure 5*]. This model predicts that the ability of v-*sis* to transform cells should be entirely dependent on their expression of PDGF receptors. Indeed, cells that fail to synthesize PDGF receptors are resistant to transformation by v-*sis* but can be rendered susceptible to v-*sis* transforming activity by introduction of a recombinant expression vector for PDGF receptors, a situation that induces ectopic PDGF-receptor synthesis.[4,42]

The role of PDGF in the induction of cellular transformation has also been addressed by use of inhibitory PDGF mutants, designed to inactivate normal PDGF chains by driving the formation of nonfunctional PDGF heterodimers.[43] Overexpression of PDGF-A or PDGF-B in mouse fibroblasts expressing the α-PDGF and β-PDGF receptors leads to autocrine transformation, but this can be blocked by coexpression of inhibitory PDGF mutants. Such inhibitory mutants have been used to probe the involvement of autocrine PDGF stimulation in human tumors.

Astrocytomas that are pathologically similar to those occurring naturally in humans develop in primates injected intracranially with simian sarcoma virus.[44] Interestingly, most established human malignant astrocytoma cell lines and operative specimens express combinations of PDGF and PDGF receptors that would potentially establish an autocrine stimulatory loop and thereby play a role in glial cell transformation.[45] Consistent with this possibility, expression of inhibitory PDGF mutants in human malignant astrocytoma cell lines results in their reversion toward a nontransformed phenotype, as measured both by growth in culture and tumor formation in nude mice.[43] These results suggest not only that PDGF dimers and their receptors are highly expressed in astrocytomas but also that this expression contributes to their malignant growth through the prolonged stimulation of mitogenic signaling pathways downstream of the PDGF receptor.

This tendency of tumor cells to secrete growth factors may have other consequences for a tumor beyond that of directly affecting the growth of the cancer cell itself. The provision of the tumor with a vascular network is a critical event as a tumor increases in size; this event requires the formation of new blood vessels, a process known as neovascularization. Without this process, the tumor cells become starved of nutrients and oxygen and be-

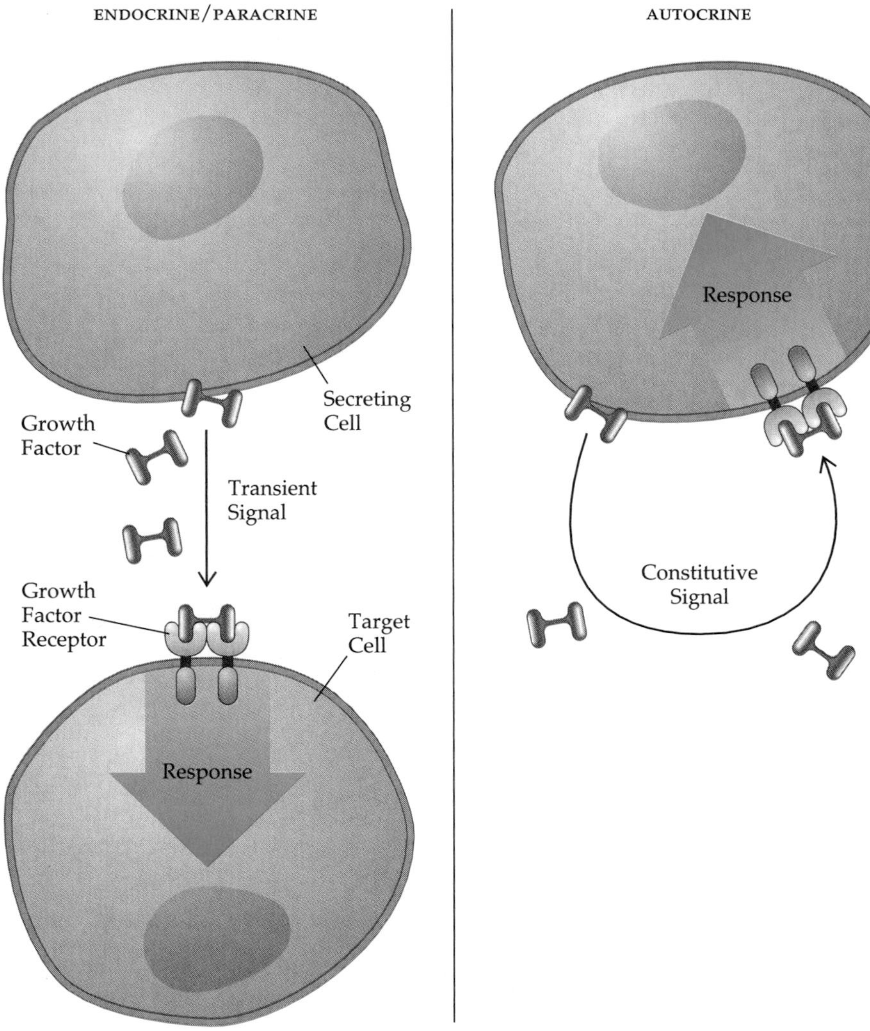

Figure 5 *Autocrine growth. In endocrine and paracrine stimulation, growth factor is produced by one cell type and binds to a receptor on a second distinct cell. The cells that make the growth factor and the cells that respond to its action are therefore physically separated. In autocrine cell growth, the growth factor is produced by a cell that also possesses receptors and is therefore responsive to the growth factor's activity. This establishes a constitutive stimulatory loop that can result in malignant cell growth.*

come necrotic. In glial tumors, abnormal growth factor expression may be important not only in direct transformation of glial cells but also in neovascularization of the resulting tumors. Angiogenic growth factors, such as vascular endothelial growth factor (VEGF), likely play an important role in normal angiogenesis, through paracrine effects on the endothelium. VEGF is structurally related to PDGF and exerts its biologic effects through two PTK receptors, Flt-1 and Flk-1. Although not normally expressed by white matter, VEGF messenger RNA expression is up-regulated in malignant astrocytoma cells around zones of necrosis.[46,47] Endothelial cells expressing Flt-1 proliferate in response to VEGF released from the astrocytoma cells, leading to areas of endothelial hyperproliferation, which is a characteristic feature of malignant astrocytomas.

The likely relevance of VEGF-mediated neovascularization to the growth of malignant astrocytomas has been demonstrated by blocking of the function of either VEGF or its receptor in vivo.[48] Both of these interventions compromise the growth of human astrocytoma cells in mice. Hence, astrocytomas provide a good example of a tumor whose growth is dependent on autocrine stimulation by one growth factor (PDGF) and on paracrine stimulation of angiogenesis by another growth factor (VEGF).

Activation of Growth Factor Receptors

Oncogenic Mutations in Receptors Mimic Growth Factor Stimulation

The next downstream step that might be deregulated involves growth factor receptors. PTK receptors are normally activated by clustering, which is induced by binding of a ligand to the extracellular domain. A structural alteration in a receptor that duplicates the effects of ligand binding might be expected to result in constitutive activation of the receptor, and hence continuous stimulation of the Ras-Map kinase mitogenic pathway described earlier. Indeed, a substantial number of retroviral and cellular oncogenes encode mutant forms of growth factor receptors. Transforming variants of growth factor receptor genes can arise by retroviral capture, by point mutations or deletions within cellular genes, by chromosome rearrangements, or by gene amplification. These genetic events can all convert a previously docile receptor into an unrestrained oncoprotein.

In the early days of research on retroviral oncogenes, it was realized that transforming genes such as v-*erb*-B, v-*fms,* and v-*kit* encode truncated forms of the receptors for EGF, macrophage colony-stimulating factor, and Steel factor, respectively.[5,49,50] These mutant receptors contain various deletions at their N-terminal or C-terminal regions, as well as several amino acid substitutions, but retain in each case an intact PTK domain that is constitutively active. Further experimental mutagenesis of these oncogenes that alters residues known to be critical for tyrosine kinase activity also abolishes their transforming activity. These results led to the idea that mutant receptors with a permanently activated PTK domain can induce a spectrum of neoplasia in vivo and can transform cells in culture in a fashion that is dependent on the function of their kinase domains. Significantly, the transforming activity of these mutant receptors is not dependent on their normal growth factor ligands.

Subsequent analysis of animal and human tumors and transformed cell lines has revealed several examples of cellular oncogenes whose products are variant PTK receptors. For example, altered forms of the c-*erb*-B gene, which contain internal deletions that result in the production of an EGF receptor that lacks part of the extracellular domain (and in this regard resembles the v-*erb*-B retroviral oncogene product), are found in glial tumors, notably grade III (anaplastic astrocytoma) and grade IV (glioblastoma multiforme).[51,52] Experimental evidence suggests that these mutant EGF receptors, whose tyrosine kinase domain fires regardless of the presence of EGF, convert glioblastomas to a more malignant state.[53]

The *neu* oncogene (also known as *erb*-B2 or HER-2) was originally identified in rat neuroblastomas induced by the chemical carcinogen ethylnitrosourea. In its normal form, the *neu* oncogene specifies a transmembrane PTK that is closely related to the EGF receptor. The oncogene isolated from the neuroblastoma has a single point mutation that converts a valine residue in the transmembrane domain to glutamic acid.[54] Many data have suggested that this substitution induces dimerization of the oncogenic Neu protein in the plasma membrane, akin to that normally observed when a growth factor binds its receptor [*see Figure 2b*].[55] As a consequence, the mutant Neu PTK is activated even though no extracellular stimulus is present.

The *neu* gene is frequently amplified and overexpressed in human mammary carcinomas and in ovarian cancers.[56,57] Although the amplified gene appears to encode a structurally normal protein, the Neu receptor in these tumors is autophosphorylated on tyrosine and is in a constitutively active state. This phenomenon may be explained by the simple observation that a substantial increase in the density of receptors in the membrane inevitably favors receptor clustering and activation [*see Figure 2c*]. Amplification of the c-*erb*-B gene and overexpression of the EGF receptor are commonly seen in carcinomas of the breast, ovary, cervix, kidney, and squamous cells.

PTK receptor genes are frequently rearranged with other sequences in human tumors, leading to the production of chimeric proteins in which variable amounts of N-terminal receptor sequence are replaced by foreign polypeptides. A striking example identified in a human osteosarcoma cell line involves the rearrangement of the *met* gene, which encodes the receptor for hepatocyte growth factor (HGF), with a gene termed *tpr*.[58,59] The resulting Tpr-Met fusion protein, which is highly transforming, lacks the entire extracellular and transmembrane regions of Met. The Tpr sequence that replaces them has an element known as a leucine zipper, which forms an amphipathic α helix and consequently associates with itself. The association of the leucine zippers of two distinct Tpr-Met molecules results in their dimerization in the cytoplasm, a situation that mirrors the dimerization of the normal met receptor induced by the binding of its ligand, HGF.[59, 60] The dimeric Tpr-Met PTK is then activated by cross-phosphorylation, resulting in its association with downstream SH2-containing targets and activation of mitogenic signaling pathways.[61]

In summary, receptor PTKs can apparently be activated by various mutations, whose effect is to promote receptor aggregation and thereby emulate the state of the receptor as it exists when it is bound to its physiologic ligand.

An Inherited Receptor PTK Oncogene

In papillary thyroid carcinomas, the *ret* and, to a lesser extent, *trk* genes are commonly rearranged with genes such as *tpr*.[59,62] The *ret* gene encodes a PTK receptor whose normal ligand has not been identified, whereas *trk* encodes the high-affinity receptor for nerve growth factor. These genetic rearrangements frequently produce chimeric genes and proteins, with novel N-terminal elements fused to receptor sequences, a situation that results in constitutive receptor dimerization. The *ret* gene is of particular interest because it corresponds to the gene mutated in the inherited cancer syndromes multiple endocrine neoplasia (MEN) types IIA and IIB.[63,64]

In general, dominantly acting oncogenes are not inherited, presumably because their presence is incompatible with normal embryonic development. The mutant forms of *ret* associated with MEN types IIA and IIB seem to be an exception, in that they function as dominant transforming genes.[65] The mutations observed in MEN type IIA affect the extracellular domain of the receptor; typically, they alter cysteine residues that are expected to participate in the formation of intramolecular disulfide bonds. These substitutions likely promote receptor dimerization by inducing the formation of intermolecular disulfide bonds that would bridge receptor chains. The *ret* mutation observed in the other variant form of this inherited syndrome, MEN IIB, is more subtle. It induces a substitution of a methionine in the kinase domain with a threonine, which likely alters the substrate specificity of the receptor's tyrosine kinase domain to resemble that of intracellular tyrosine kinases. Why this latter mutation renders the Ret protein oncogenic remains to be clarified.

Cytoplasmic Tyrosine Kinases

PTKs can be divided into two broad groups: the transmembrane receptors and the intracellular kinases that apparently form signaling subunits for more complex multichain receptors, such as those for cytokines and antigens [*see Figure 1*].[66,67] Several of these intracellular PTKs, including Src, Abl, and Fps, were originally identified as the products of retroviral oncogenes. Such transforming PTKs have sustained structural alterations that result in their constitutive activation. As an example, the kinase activity of the normal c-Src PTK is repressed by phosphorylation on a tyrosine residue within the short C-terminal tail. This situation apparently leads to an intramolecular interaction with the c-Src SH2 domain, resulting in inhibition of the enzymatic domain.[68] Variants of Src in which the C-terminal tail is deleted or in which its tyrosine phosphorylation site is converted to phenylalanine are transforming because the resulting mutant protein can no longer be kept in an inactive state.[69]

Another intracellular kinase, that encoded by the *abl* gene, is implicated in the cause of Philadelphia chromosome–positive leukemias. During the pathogenesis of these tumors, the *abl* gene, which normally resides on chromosome 9, becomes juxtaposed with the *bcr* gene on chromosome 22 as a result of a reciprocal chromosome translocation t(9;22)(q34.1; q11.1) that is typical of Philadelphia chromosome–positive chronic myelogenous leukemia and acute lymphocytic leukemia.[70,71,72] The *bcr* and *abl* genes are both broken and then joined in such as fashion as to encode one of two Bcr-Abl fusion proteins (P210[bcr-abl] and P185[bcr-abl]) that differ solely in the extent of their N-terminal Bcr sequence.[73,74] In both of these fusion proteins, Bcr sequences replace the N-terminal region of c-Abl [*see Figure 6*]. The P185[bcr-abl] isoform appears to be the more highly transforming, although the reason for this has not been firmly established, and this isoform is more commonly found in acute leukemias.

The joining of Bcr to Abl has several consequences. One consequence is that Bcr promotes oligomerization of the Bcr-Abl fusion protein and subsequent activation of the Abl tyrosine kinase domain by autophosphorylation, much as the autophosphorylation described earlier for oncogenic variants of membrane-spanning receptors.[75] As a consequence of autophosphorylation, the Bcr-Abl oncoprotein associates with SH2 signaling proteins, such as Grb2, and may thereby activate pathways that promote cell survival and proliferation.[76,77] Hence, the fusion of *bcr* and *abl* genes in-

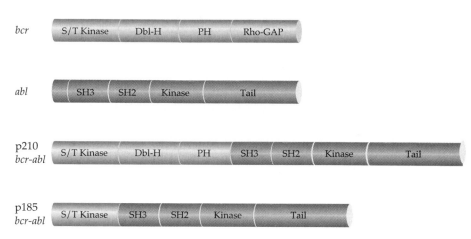

Figure 6 *The Bcr-Abl onco-protein. The normal* bcr *gene encodes a protein with an unusual serine/threonine–specific protein kinase domain, a dbl-homology domain, a PH domain, and a domain that functions as a GAP for Rho proteins (similar in structure to Ras). The Abl protein has SH2, SH3 and PTK domains. The rearrangement of* bcr *and* abl *produces one of two hybrid Bcr-Abl oncoproteins, with constitutive PTK activity.*

duced by the 9;22 chromosome translocation activates the Abl kinase and induces its association with downstream targets.

Intracellular Signal Transducers

Guanine Nucleotide-Binding Proteins

Ras Proteins

The principal mitogenic signaling pathway in many cell types involves the activation of Ras. PTKs are coupled to Ras through the SH2/SH3 adaptor protein Grb2, which is in turn linked to Sos proteins that directly activate ras by inducing the exchange of GDP for GTP [*see Figures 1 and 7*]. Three distinct *ras* genes have been identified, H-*ras*, K-*ras*, and N-*ras*, but in biochemical terms, their products are remarkably similar, and all can be converted to an oncogenic form.[20] The Ras proteins are members of a very large family of small guanine nucleotide-binding proteins, which control such cellular events as formation of the actin cytoskeleton, membrane ruffling, and transport of vesicles between distinct cellular compartments.[78] However, it is the *ras* genes and their product that have the primary role in human cancer, presumably because they play a key role in controlling the mitogenic pathway from cell-surface receptors.

Normal Ras proteins are primarily regulated by two distinct classes of proteins. Guanine nucleotide exchange factors, such as Sos, can activate Ras by promoting the formation of the GTP-bound state. However, GTP-bound Ras is rapidly inactivated in growth factor–stimulated cells by the hydrolysis of its associated GTP to GDP [*see Figure 7*]. This conversion restores Ras to an inactive form, which is unable to interact with downstream effectors, such as the Raf protein kinase [*see Figure 3*].

Although Ras has an intrinsic GTPase activity, this activity is very weak and by itself is insufficient to account for the rapid inactivation of GTP-bound Ras observed in normal cells. The GTPase activity of Ras is tremendously increased, however, by its interaction with proteins known as GTPase-activating proteins (GAPs), which specifically recognize Ras in the

GTP-bound form and cooperate with the intrinsic Ras GTPase activity to hydrolyze bound GTP to GDP. Three ras-GAP proteins have been identified in mammalian cells, p120-GAP, neurofibromin, and GAP-1ᵐ, all of which can function as negative regulators of Ras.[78]

Three distinct mechanisms can therefore be envisaged through which Ras proteins might be constitutively locked in the active GTP-bound form, in which state they can deliver a prolonged mitogenic signal that is capable of eliciting cellular transformation. First, unremitting activation of Sos proteins, as occurs in cells expressing oncogenic tyrosine kinases, elevates the rate of guanine nucleotide exchange, and hence the fraction of Ras in the active GTP-bound state. The same net effect can be achieved by a reduction in cellular GAP activity, which should reduce the rate at which active GTP-bound Ras is converted to GDP-Ras, and indeed one of the GAP proteins (neurofibromin) is either reduced or absent in several human malignancies. Neurofibromin is the product of the *NF*-1 tumor suppressor gene, which is responsible for von Recklinghausen's neurofibromatosis.[79] Loss of both alleles of *NF*-1 has also been observed in juvenile myeloid leukemias. Reduction in the level of neurofibromin might be expected to increase the fraction of GTP-bound Ras, and this effect has been seen in some cells with *NF*-1 mutations, although whether this is the only biochemical consequence of removing neurofibromin remains unclear.[80,81]

By far, the most common mechanism of Ras activation involves mutations within the *ras* genes themselves, which represent one of the most common genetic alterations found in human cancers. These mutations all have a common effect: they induce substitutions that leave intact the ability of Ras proteins to bind GTP and to interact with downstream targets, such as Raf, but block the capacity of Ras to induce GTP hydrolysis, even in the presence of a GAP protein. These oncogenic Ras variants can therefore be activated and can transmit a mitogenic signal but are unable to shut

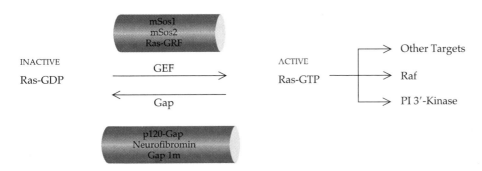

Figure 7 *Regulation of ras proteins. The Ras proteins exist in an inactive GDP-bound state and are stimulated by exchange of GDP for GTP under the control of guanine nucleotide exchange factors, such as Sos. Once in the active GTP-bound state, Ras can interact with its downstream targets, which include the Raf protein kinase and phosphatidylinositol (PI) 3'-kinase and likely additional proteins. Inactivation of Ras is greatly accelerated by GAPs (e.g., p120-GAP, neurofibromin, and GAP-1ᵐ), which stimulate hydrolysis of GTP on Ras to GDP. Oncogenic Ras variants have substitutions that render them resistant to GAP activity, and, as a consequence, they accumulate in the active GTP-bound state.*

themselves off. Activating point mutations in *ras* genes generally affect codons for the glycine residues at positions 12 or 13, or for the glutamine residue at position 61.[20] Gly 12 and Gly 13 are contained within a loop that contacts the α-phosphate and β-phosphate of GTP or GDP [*see Figure 4*]. The Gly 12 codon is a particularly common site of oncogenic mutations; indeed, Ras proteins can be activated by substitution of this residue with any amino acid other than proline. Gln 61 is in a flexible region of the protein implicated in the GTPase reaction. The replacement of the native residues found at these sites most likely excludes a water molecule, which normally serves as the nucleophile that cleaves the γ-phosphate from GTP to yield GDP.[27]

The Ras proteins can also be oncogenically activated by mutations made by site-directed mutagenesis in vitro that have not been observed in human cancers, most likely because two mutations are required for induction of the desired amino acid substitution.[26] For example, substitutions that lower the affinity of Ras proteins for guanine nucleotides increase the rate at which GDP is exchanged for GTP, thereby increasing the amount of Ras bound to GTP.

LARGE G PROTEINS

The Ras proteins are pared down versions of so-called large G proteins that mediate signaling by seven membrane–spanning receptors.[8,26] These large G proteins are composed of three subunits: G_α proteins, which bind guanine nucleotides in a fashion similar to Ras, to which they are related in sequence, and G_β and G_γ, which are permanently complexed with one another. The prototypic α subunit is $G_{s\alpha}$, which is activated by the β-adrenergic receptor, which it couples to the downstream effector adenylate cyclase. This latter enzyme catalyzes the conversion of adenosine triphosphate to cAMP. cAMP in turn stimulates the cAMP-dependent protein kinase, which has among its many substrates the transcription factor CREB (cAMP response element binding factor), whose ability to stimulate gene expression is induced by its phosphorylation.[37] In unstimulated cells, $G_{s\alpha}$ is bound to GDP and is physically associated with the β and γ subunits. Binding of an agonist to the receptor induces a conformational change in the receptor's cytoplasmic region, allowing the receptor itself to serve as a guanine nucleotide exchange factor and to convert $G_{s\alpha}$ to a GTP-bound form, which then dissociates from β/γ and interacts with its target, adenylate cyclase. Unlike Ras, $G_{s\alpha}$ has an intrinsically high rate of GTPase activity, but in essence the regulatory cycle of $G_{s\alpha}$ and the many related large G proteins is similar to that of Ras proteins. In principle, then, G_α proteins could be locked in an active GTP-bound state by mutations, similar to those found in Ras proteins, which destroy their intrinsic GTPase activity and result in the permanent activation of downstream targets, such as adenylate cyclase.

In most cells, the product of adenylate cyclase, cAMP, is actually growth inhibitory. In pituitary somatotrophs, however, growth hormone–releasing hormone acts through a seven membrane–spanning receptor to stimulate $G_{s\alpha}$ and elevate cAMP levels, which in turn elicits cellular proliferation and secretion of growth hormone [*see Figure 8*]. One might therefore anticipate that in this cell type, mutations that activated $G_{s\alpha}$ would stimulate cell growth. Indeed, in a subset of pituitary tumors that secrete high levels of

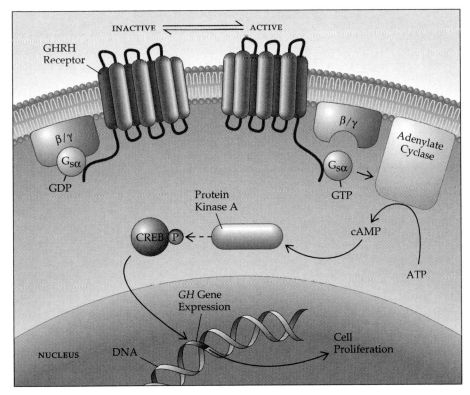

Figure 8 *A mitogenic pathway involving $G_{s\alpha}$. The binding of growth hormone–releasing hormone (GHRH) to its receptor activates $G_{s\alpha}$ by inducing its dissociation from the β/γ subunits and exchange of GDP for GTP. GTP-bound $G_{s\alpha}$ stimulates adenylate cyclase activity, resulting in the production of cyclic adenosine monophosphate (AMP), the activation of cAMP-dependent protein kinase, and the phosphorylation of the transcription factor CREB (cAMP response element binding factor). CREB stimulates transcription of the growth hormone (GH) gene and induces proliferation. Oncogenic variants of $G_{s\alpha}$ lack intrinsic GAP activity and are locked in the active GTP-bound state.*

growth hormone and have constitutively elevated levels of cAMP, mutations have been found in the gene for $G_{s\alpha}$.[82] These mutations induce substitutions that block $G_{s\alpha}$ GTPase activity. Hence, $G_{s\alpha}$ is left in the active GTP-bound state, inducing high levels of cAMP, and presumably contributing to tumorigenesis. These oncogenic $G_{s\alpha}$ alleles (referred to as *gsp*) would only have transforming activity in cells that have a proliferative response to cAMP. These results show how the susceptibility of a particular cell to transformation by a specific oncogene depends on its internal biochemical signaling pathways. The spectrum of cells transformed by an oncogene such as *gsp* is very narrow, whereas oncogenes such as *ras* have a much broader transforming potential. In addition to the α subunit of G_s, activating point mutations have been found in the α subunit of another large G protein, G_{i2}, in ovarian and adrenal tumors,[83] whereas other activated α subunits can transform specific cells in culture.

Transcription Factors as Oncogenes

The final targets of mitogenic signal transduction pathways are transcription factors, which function within the nucleus to drive the expression of specific genes, that most likely encode proteins involved in passage through the cell cycle. Such transcription factors are normally regulated in two ways. First, the ability of preexisting factors to activate transcription can be stimulated by their phosphorylation. Second, their own expression is tightly controlled and can be greatly enhanced by mitogenic signals. Several of these transcription factors can themselves function as oncoproteins. The three archetypes of these oncogenic transcription factors are *fos*, *jun*, and *myc*, of which *myc* is an important contributor to human tumorigenesis.

The Fos and Jun proteins associate with one another through a leucine zipper motif to form a transcription factor termed AP-1. These proteins are normally regulated at the level of expression and by phosphorylation on serine and threonine residues.[84,85] *fos* and *jun* were both originally identified as retroviral oncogenes, indicating that their aberrant expression can contribute to cellular transformation.[86]

myc Genes

Growth factor stimulation leads to the rapid accumulation of the Myc nuclear proteins.[87] Under normal circumstances, *myc* gene expression is tightly controlled by cytoplasmic mitogen-activated signaling pathways. However, in tumors, its expression can become uncoupled from normal mitogenic regulators, leading to constitutively high levels of the Myc protein. *myc* was originally found as a retroviral oncogene, in which the principal effect of retroviral capture is to drive high levels of Myc protein expression. Amplification of *myc*, or its close relatives N-*myc* and L-*myc*, is a frequent event in some cancers and leads to overproduction of Myc proteins. Chromosome translocations that bring the *myc* gene under the control of strong promoters or enhancers, as observed in Burkitt's lymphoma, can have the same effect of increasing *myc* transcription and accumulation of the Myc protein.

The nuclear location of the Myc protein suggested that it might be a transcriptional regulator that was capable of inducing the expression of genes involved in cell cycle control. Recent evidence has confirmed this early suggestion and has indicated how Myc might participate in transcriptional regulation. The Myc protein has a lengthy N-terminal region, followed by a basic DNA-binding region. At its C-terminal, Myc has a helix-loop-helix motif and a leucine zipper region, both of which are implicated in protein dimerization. Despite this array of interesting elements, Myc alone has no independent DNA-binding activity. However, Myc is able to form heterodimers with another nuclear factor, Max, and in this state can bind to CACGTG enhancer elements and stimulate gene expression [*see Figure 9*].[88] The Max nuclear factor itself is able to form homodimers and can also associate with the related Mad protein. The Max-Max or Mad-Max dimers are both able to bind DNA at CACGTG sites but have the opposite effect of Myc-Max heterodimers in the sense that they repress gene expression. These results have suggested a scheme in which Max stimulates the expression of genes required for DNA synthesis when complexed with Myc but blocks transcription when bound to Mad [*see Figure 9*].[89] The effect of elevated Myc synthesis on growth factor stimulation is then to drive Max into a partnership with Myc and activate gene expression. The level of Myc protein therefore appears to be crucial for the control of growth of normal cells. Indeed, the cessation of proliferation that accompanies cell differentiation is commonly accompanied by a decline in c-*myc* expression and a loss of the stimulatory Myc-Max heterodimers, which are replaced by inhibitory Mad-Max complexes.

As might be anticipated from this scheme, the level of Myc protein is reg-

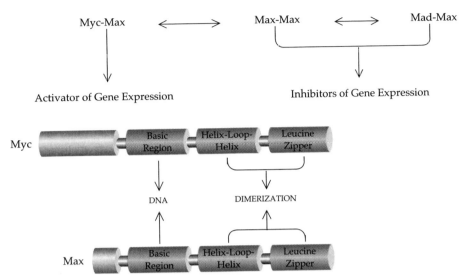

Figure 9 *The c-Myc transcription factor activates gene expression when dimerized with Max and promotes proliferation. In contrast, when associated with itself or with Mad, Max is a transcriptional repressor and is likely an inhibitor of the cell cycle. Overexpression of Myc disturbs this equilibrium by increasing the concentration of Myc-Max and contributes to aberrant cell proliferation. The structures of the Myc and Max proteins and the domains involved in DNA binding and the formation of heterodimers are shown.*

ulated in many ways. First, the Myc protein is very rapidly degraded within the cell, in contrast to Max, which is rather stable. In addition, transcription of the *myc* gene is controlled at the level of transcriptional initiation and elongation. Consistent with the view that the level of Myc protein, and hence of the Myc-Max heterodimers, is of crucial importance, c-*myc* is activated as an oncogene by genetic rearrangements that induce its overexpression. Unlike many other oncogenes, mutations that affect the structure of the protein seem less important. Overexpression of *myc* therefore disturbs the fine balance of transcriptional regulators by elevating the relative concentration of activating Myc-Max heterodimers and consequently drives continued rounds of cell proliferation.

Oncoproteins in Control of the Cell Cycle

The mammalian cell cycle is largely regulated during the G_1 phase [*see Chapter 1*]. External signals, such as those provided by growth factors, are required for cells to move from a quiescent state (G_0) and pass through G_1 into the S phase, where DNA synthesis takes place. The passage through G_1 requires the sequential actions of cyclin-dependent kinases and the inhibition of the Rb protein through phosphorylation. The cycling cell must activate a series of positive factors and repress the functions of inhibitors. It can then be envisaged that genetic events that lock in place the activators of the G_1 phase of the cell cycle might create dominantly acting oncogenes, whereas loss-of-function mutations in inhibitory cell cycle genes would inactivate tumor suppressors.

Several lines of evidence point to cyclin D as a dominantly acting oncoprotein that can contribute to tumorigenesis.[90] First, cyclin D isoforms, through their association with cyclin-dependent kinases (Cdk4 and Cdk6), are apparently required for the phosphorylation of Rb, and therefore for passage through G_1. Growth factors, such as macrophage colony-stimulating factor, induce cyclin D expression when these factors are applied to quiescent cells. Aberrantly high expression of cyclin D might therefore be expected to derange the cell cycle clock, by promoting passage through G_1. Indeed, chromosome rearrangements seen in several tumors appear to act by elevating transcription of the gene for cyclin D1. In parathyroid adenoma, an intrachromosomal inversion affecting chromosome 11 places the 5' promoter of the parathyroid hormone gene upstream of the gene for cyclin D1, at 11q13. This result suggests that cyclin D1 would be abnormally expressed in these cells, under the influence of the parathyroid hormone regulatory sequences, and might thereby contribute to tumorigenesis. Chromosome translocations involving 11q13 have also been seen in numerous tumors, including some chronic B cell neoplasms and breast cancers, suggesting the existence of an oncogene (originally termed bcl-1) at this site. Although the breakpoints map about 110 kb upstream of the gene for cyclin D1, they nonetheless lead to up-regulation of cyclin D1 expression.

Consistent with the view that overexpression of cyclin D1 might stimulate aberrant cell proliferation, artificially high expression of D-type cyclins shortens the G_1 phase of rodent fibroblasts, although it does not induce overt morphological transformation.[91] These results suggest that elevated levels of D-type cyclins may provide cells with a growth advantage, thereby contributing to tumorigenesis.

Therapeutic Implications

Tyrosine Kinase Inhibitors

The aforementioned data suggest that growth factors, their receptors, and the cytoplasmic targets of the activated receptors are of fundamental importance for the development of many human cancers. Molecules that specifically antagonize these oncogene products are potentially useful from a therapeutic point of view. One possible mode of intervention is to block of the association of growth factors with their receptors in tumors that are subject to autocrine stimulation. The potential value of this approach has been demonstrated by the use of dominant-negative variants of PDGF-A, which halt the growth of some astrocytoma cell lines in culture.

Perhaps the greatest effort to date has been put into the development of specific tyrosine kinase inhibitors.[92] Such compounds are small-molecule drugs that must penetrate into the cell, show selectivity for the tyrosine kinase responsible for the growth of a specific tumor, and not have toxic side effects. Many protein kinase inhibitors have been isolated that generally block kinase activity through competition with adenosine triphosphate. Rather remarkably, these compounds can be engineered to be quite selective. Compounds such as 4,5-dianilinophthalimide (DHAP-1) and the quinazoline PD 153035 are specific for inhibition of the EGF-receptor. The latter compound blocks EGF-receptor kinase activity with a Ki of 5 pM and inhibits the EGF-receptor in EGF-stimulated cells with an IC50 of 15 nM. DHAP-1 has been shown in nude mice to block the growth of tumors that are dependent on an activated EGF-receptor for malignancy but to have no effect on tumors that are dependent on the PDGF-receptor. These results lead to considerable hope that tyrosine kinase inhibitors might be valuable in the treatment of some cancers. These compounds may well arrest the growth of tumor cells, although they are less likely to induce their destruction.

The process of signaling downstream of PTK receptors involves a series of protein-protein interactions involving protein modules, such as the SH2 and SH3 domains. Both of these domains recognize short peptide motifs of five to 10 amino acids, which might be mimicked by small molecules. If such compounds can be rendered selective for particular signaling pathways, they could be used to block mitogenic signaling in tumors that depend on tyrosine kinases for their growth. A great deal of work is presently in progress to pursue this possibility.

Ras Inhibitors

In principle, drugs can be designed to interfere with those parts of Ras that are essential for interactions with targets such as Raf.[92] Of particular interest in this regard, Ras proteins must become attached to the inner face of the plasma membrane so that they can send a mitogenic signal. This fact highlights the common observation that the proper subcellular localization of intracellular signaling proteins is crucial for their activity. This presumably reflects the fact that many signaling proteins exert their effects through precise interactions with downstream proteins; therefore, the signaling protein and its target must meet at the same place in the cell for a productive outcome. The association of Ras proteins with the plasma membrane is mediated by the very C-terminal region of the protein, which contains a cysteine at residue 186, three amino acids from the end of the polypeptide. During posttranslational processing of Ras proteins, this cysteine becomes covalently attached to a hydrophobic 15-carbon isoprenyl group (a farnesyl moiety) that inserts into the membrane.[93] If oncogenic Ras proteins are altered by the substitution of this cysteine with another amino acid, they no longer become modified by the farnesyl group, fail to stably associate with the membrane, and lose their transforming ability. A potential means of inhibiting oncogenic Ras proteins would be to block their farnesylation in vivo. Analogues of the Ras C-terminal sequence have been developed that act as competitive inhibitors of the enzyme that farnesylates Ras proteins. These inhibitors can revert the phenotype of cells transformed by *ras* oncogenes, but surprisingly, they appear to be relatively nontoxic. These compounds serve as prototypes for antitumor drugs that might block the malignant growth of tumors carrying activated *ras* oncogenes.[94]

The transforming activity of oncogenic Ras proteins is also abolished by substitutions in the effector loop that also prevent the association of activated Ras with the N-terminal region of Raf. This finding highlights the importance of Raf as a downstream target of Ras and raises the possibility that compounds that interfere with the Ras-Raf interaction might also block mitogenic signaling downstream of Ras and, hence, inhibit Ras-dependent transformation.

Summary

A complex signal-transducing circuitry exists that reaches from the extracellular space through the cytoplasm to the cell cycle clock in the nucleus, the central regulator of cell proliferation. Mutations in the genes whose products control many of the growth-promoting steps in this signaling cascade can convert these proteins into potent oncoproteins that drive cell growth, even in the absence of externally applied mitogens. Such autonomous growth is essential for the deregulated cell proliferation that is the essence of neoplasia. Drugs specifically designed to inhibit these oncoproteins have been identified and are presently being tested in vivo. These compounds offer considerable hope for a new range of antineoplastic agents.

References

1. Pawson T, Bernstein A: Receptor tyrosine kinases: genetic evidence for their role in *Drosophila* and mouse development. *Trends Genet* 6:350, 1990
2. Ullrich A, Schlessinger J: Signal transduction by receptors with tyrosine kinase activity. *Cell* 61:203, 1990
3. van der Geer P, Hunter T: Receptor protein-tyrosine kinases and their signal transduction pathways. *Annu Rev Cell Biol* 10:251, 1994
4. Leal P, Williams LT, Robbins KC, Aaronson SA:Evidence that the v-sis gene product transforms by interaction with the receptor for platelet-derived growth factor. *Science* 230:327, 1985
5. Chabot B, Stephenson DA, Chapman VM, et al: The proto-oncogene c-*kit* encoding a transmembrane tyrosine kinase receptor maps to the mouse W locus. *Nature* 335:88, 1988
6. Geissler EN, Ryan MA, Housman DE: The dominant-white spotting (W) locus of the mouse encodes the c-*kit* proto-oncogene. *Cell* 55:185, 1988
7. Anderson DM, Lyman SD, Baird A, et al: Molecular cloning of mast cell growth factor, a hematopoietin that is active in both membrane bound and soluble forms. *Cell* 63:235, 1990
8. Neer EJ: Heterotrimeric G proteins: organizers of transmembrane signals. *Cell* 80:249, 1995
9. Evans RM: The steroid and thyroid hormone receptor superfamily. *Science* 240:889, 1988
10. de The H, Chomienne C, Lanotte M, et al: The t(15;17) translocation of acute promyelocytic leukemia fuses the retinoic acid receptor a gene to a novel transcribed locus. *Nature* 347:558, 1990
11. Borrow J, Goddard AD, Sheer D, Solomon E: Molecular analysis of acute promyelocytic leukemia breakpoint cluster region on chromosome 17. *Science* 249:1577, 1990
12. Heldin CH: Dimerization of cell surface receptors in signal transduction. *Cell* 80:213, 1995
13. Lemmon MA, Schlessinger J: Regulation of signal transduction and signal diversity by receptor oligomerizaton. *Trends Biochem Sci* 19:459, 1994
14. Hubbard SR, Wei L, Ellis L, Hendrickson WA: Crystal structure of the tyrosine kinase domain of the human insulin receptor. *Nature* 372:746, 1994
15. Pawson T, Schlessinger J: SH2 and SH3 domains. *Curr Biol* 3:434, 1993
16. Pawson T: Protein modules and signaling networks. *Nature* 373:573, 1995
17. Cohen GB, Ren R, Baltimore D: Modular binding domains in signal transduction proteins. *Cell* 80:237, 1995
18. Lowenstein EJ, Daly RJ, Batzer AG, et al: The SH2 and SH3 domain-containing protein-Grb2 links receptor tyrosine kinases to Ras signaling. *Cell* 70:431, 1992
19. Ren R, Mayer BJ, Cicchetti P, Baltimore D: Identification of a ten-amino acid proline-rich SH3 binding site. *Science* 259:1157, 1993
20. Barbacid MA: *ras* genes. *Annu Rev Biochem* 56:779, 1987
21. Egan SE, Giddings BW, Brooks MW, et al: Association of Sos Ras exchange protein with Grb2 is implicated in tyrosine kinase signal transduction and transformation. *Nature* 363:45, 1993
22. Rozakis-Adcock M, Fernley R, Wade J, et al: The SH2 and SH3 domains of mammalian Grb2 couple the EGF-receptor to mSos1, an activator of Ras. *Nature* 363:83, 1993
23. Gale WN, Kaplan D, Lowenstein EJ, et al: Grb2 mediates the EGF-dependent activation

of guanine nucleotide exchange on Ras. *Nature* 363:88, 1993

24. Li N, Batzer A, Daly R, et al: Guanine nucleotide releasing factor hSos1 binds to Grb2 and links receptor tyrosine kinases to ras signaling. *Nature* 363:85, 1993

25. Buday L, Downward J: Epidermal growth factor regulates p21ras through the formation of a complex of receptor, Grb2 adaptor protein, and Sos nucleotide exchange factor. *Cell* 73:611, 1993

26. Bourne HR, Sanders DA, McCormick F: The GTPase superfamily: conserved structure and molecular mechanism. *Nature* 349:117, 1991

27. Pai EF, Krengel U, Petsko GA, et al: Refined crystal structure of the triphosphate conformation of H-ras p21 at 1.35 Å resolution: implications for the mechanism of GTP hydrolysis. *EMBO J* 9:2351, 1990

28. Pai EF, Kabsch W, Krengel V, et al: Structure of the guanine nucleotide-binding domain of the Ha-*ras* oncogene product in the thiophosphate conformation. *Nature* 341:209, 1989

29. McCormick F: Activators and effectors of ras p21 proteins. *Curr Opin Genet Dev* 4:71, 1994

30. Vojtek AB, Hollenberg SM, Cooper JA: Mammalian Ras interacts directly with the serine/threonine kinase Raf. *Cell* 74:205, 1993

31. Warne PH, Viciana PR, Downward J: Direct interaction of ras and the amino-terminal region of Raf-1 in vitro. *Nature* 364:352, 1993

32. Marshall CJ: Map kinase kinase kinase, MAP kinase kinase and MAP kinase. *Curr Opin Genet Dev* 4:82, 1994

33. Stokoe D, Macdonald SG, Cadwallader K, et al: Activation of Raf as a result of recruitment to the plasma membrane. *Science* 264:1463, 1994

34. Hall A: A biochemical function of ras—at last. *Science* 264:1413, 1994

35. Rodriguez-Viciana P, Warne PH, Dhand R, et al: Phosphatidylinositol-3-OH kinase acts as a direct target of Ras. *Nature* 370:527, 1994

36. Marshall CJ: Specificity of receptor tyrosine kinase signaling: transient versus sustained extracellular signal-regulated kinase activation. *Cell* 80:179, 1995

37. Hill CS, Treisman R: Transcriptional regulation by extracellular signals: mechanisms and specificity. *Cell* 80:199,1995

38. Sporn MB, Todaro GJ: Autocrine secretion and malignant transformation of cells. *N Engl J Med* 878:30, 1980

39. Aaronson SA: Growth factors and cancer. *Science* 254:1146, 1991

40. Deuel TF: Polypeptide growth factors: roles in normal and abnormal cell growth. *Annu Rev Cell Biol* 3:443, 1987

41. Claesson-Welsh L: Platelet-derived growth factor receptor signals. *J Biol Chem* 269:32023, 1994

42. Garrett JS, Coughlin SR, Niman HL, et al: Blockade of autocrine stimulation in simian sarcoma virus-transformed cells reverses down-regulation of platelet-derived growth factor receptors. *Proc Natl Acad Sci USA* 81:7466, 1984

43. Shamah S, Stiles C, Guha A: Dominant-negative mutants of platelet-derived growth factor (PDGF) revert the transformed phenotype of human astrocytoma cells. *Mol Cell Biol* 13:7203, 1993

44. Deinhardt F: Biology of primate retroviruses. *Viral Oncology*. Klein, G, Ed. Raven Press, New York, 1980, p. 357

45. Nistér M, Claesson-Welsh L, Eriksson A, et al: Differential expression of platelet derived growth factor receptors in human malignant glioma cell lines. *J Biol Chem* 266:16755, 1991

46. Plate KH, Breier G, Weich HA, Risau W: Vascular endothelial growth factor is a potential tumor angiogenesis factor in human gliomas. *Nature* 359:845, 1992

47. Kim KJ, Li B, Armanini M, et al: Inhibition of vascular endothelial growth factor-induced angiogenesis suppresses tumor growth in vivo. *Nature* 362:841, 1993

48. Millauer B, Shawver LK, Plate KH, et al: Glioblastoma growth inhibited in vivo by a dominant-negative Flk-1 mutant. *Nature* 367:576, 1994

49. Downward J, Yarden Y, Mayers E, et al: Close similarity of the epidermal growth factor-receptor and v-*erb*B oncogene protein sequences. *Nature* 307:521, 1984

50. Sherr CJ, Rettenmeier CW, Sacca R, et al: The c-*fms* proto-oncogene product is related to the receptor for the mononuclear phagocyte growth factor, CSF-1. *Cell* 41:665, 1985

51. Ekstrand AJ, Sugawa N, James CD, Collins VP: Amplified and rearranged epidermal growth factor receptor genes in human glioblastomas reveal deletions of sequences en-

coding portions of the N- and /or C-terminal tails. *Proc Natl Acad Sci USA* 89:4309, 1992

52. Ekstrand AJ, Longo N, Hamid ML, et al: Functional characterization of an EGF receptor with a truncated extracellular domain expressed in glioblastoma with EGFR gene amplification. *Oncogene* 9:2313, 1994

53. Nishikawa R, Ji X-D, Harmon RC, et al: A mutant epidermal growth factor receptor common in human glioma confers enhanced tumorigenicity. *Proc Natl Acad Sci USA* 91:7727, 1994

54. Bargmann CI, Hung M-C, Weinberg RA: Multiple independent activations of the *neu* oncogene by a point mutation altering the transmembrane domain of p185. *Cell* 45:649, 1986

55. Weiner DB, Liu J, Cohen JA, et al: A point mutation in the *neu* oncogene mimics ligand induction of receptor aggregation. *Nature* 339:230, 1989

56. Slamon DJ, Clark GM, Wong SG, et al: Human breast cancer: correlation of relapse and survival with amplification of the HER-2/*neu* oncogene. *Science* 235:177, 1987

57. Slamon DJ, Godolphin W, Jones LA, et al: Studies of the HER-2/*neu* proto-oncogene in human breast and ovarian cancer. *Science* 244:707, 1989

58. Park M, Dean M, Cooper CS, et al: Mechanism of *met* oncogene activation. *Cell* 45:895, 1986

59. Rodrigues GA, Park M: Oncogenic activation of tyrosine kinases. *Curr Opin Genet Dev* 4:15, 1994

60. Rodrigues G, Park M: Dimerization mediated by a leucine zipper oncogenically activates the *met* receptor tyrosine kinase. *Mol Cell Biol* 13:6711, 1993

61. Ponzetto C, Bardelli A, Zhen Z, et al: A multifunctional docking site mediates signaling and transformation by the hepatocyte growth factor/scatter factor receptor family. *Cell* 77:261, 1994

62. Grieco M, Santoro M, Berlingieri MT, et al: PTC is a novel rearranged form of the *ret* proto-oncogene and is frequently detected in vivo in human thyroid papillary carcinomas. *Cell* 60:557, 1990

63. Mulligan LM, Kwok JBJ, Healey CS, et al: Germ-line mutations of the *ret* proto-oncogene in multiple endocrine neoplasia type 2A. *Nature* 363:458, 1993

64. Hofstra RM, Landsvater RM, Ceccherini I, et al: A mutation in the *ret* proto-oncogene associated with multiple endocrine neoplasia type 2B and sporadic medullary thyroid carcinoma. *Nature* 367:375, 1994

65. Santoro M, Carlomagno F, Romano A, et al: Activation of *ret* as a dominant transforming gene by germline mutations of MEN2A and MEN2B. *Science* 267:381, 1995

66. Stahl N, Yancopoulos GD: The alphas, betas, and kinases of cytokine receptor complexes. *Cell* 74:587, 1993

67. Weiss A: T cell antigen receptor signal transduction: a tale of tails and cytoplasmic protein-tyrosine kinases. *Cell* 73:209, 1993

68. Superti-Furga G, Fumagalli S, Koegl M, et al: Csk inhibition of c-*src* activity requires both the SH2 and SH3 domains of Src. *EMBO J* 12:2625, 1993

69. Parsons JT, Weber MJ: Genetics of *src*: structure and functional organization of a protein tyrosine kinase. *Curr Top Microbiol Immunol* 147:79, 1989

70. Nowell PC, Hungerford DA: Minute chromosome in human chronic granulocytic leukemia. *Science* 132:1497, 1960

71. Daley R, Ben-Neriah Y: Implicating the *bcr/abl* gene in the pathogenesis of Philadelphia chromosome-positive human leukemia. *Adv Cancer Res* 57:151, 1991

72. Heisterkamp N, Stam K, Groffen J: Structural organization of the *bcr* gene and its role in the Ph' translocation. *Nature* 315:758, 1985

73. Konopka JB, Watanabe SM, Witte ON: An alteration of the human c-abl protein in K562 leukemia cells unmasks associated tyrosine kinase activity. *Cell* 37:1035, 1984

74. Clark SS, McLaughlin J, Crist WM, et al: Unique forms of the abl tyrosine kinase distinguish Ph1-positive CML from Ph1-positive ALL. *Science* 235:85, 1987

75. McWhirter JR, Wang JYJ: An actin-binding function contributes to transformation by the *bcr-abl* oncoprotein of Philadelphia chromosome-positive human leukemias. *EMBO J* 12:1533, 1993

76. Pendergast AM, Quilliam LA, Cripe LD: BCR-ABL-induced oncogenesis is mediated by direct interaction with the SH2 domain of the GRB-2 adaptor protein. *Cell* 75:175, 1993

77. Puil L, Liu X, Gish G, et al: BCR-ABL oncoproteins bind directly to activators of the Ras signaling pathway. *EMBO J* 13:764, 1994

78. Boguski MS, McCormick F: Proteins regulating Ras and its relatives. *Nature* 366:643, 1994

79. Xu G, O'Connell P, Viskochil D, et al: The neurofibromatosis type 1 gene encodes a protein related to GAP. *Cell* 62:599, 1990

80. Basu TN, Gutmann DH, Fletcher JA, et al: Aberrant regulation of Ras proteins in malignant tumour cells from type 1 neurofibromatosis patients. *Nature* 356:713, 1992

81. DeClue JE, Papageorge AG, Fletcher JA, et al: Abnormal regulation of mammalian p21ras contributes to malignant tumor growth in von Recklinghausen (type 1) neurofibromatosis. *Cell* 69:265, 1992

82. Landis CA, Masters SB, Spada A, et al: GTPase inhibitory mutations activate the α chain of Gs and stimulate adenylyl cyclase in human pituitary tumors. *Nature* 340:692, 1989

83. Lyons J, Landis CA, Harsh G, et al: Two G protein oncogenes in human endocrine tumors. *Science* 249:655, 1990

84. Treisman R: Ternary complex factors: growth factor regulated transcriptional activators. *Curr Opin Genet Dev* 4:96, 1994

85. Hunter T, Karin M: The regulation of transcription by phosphorylation. *Cell* 70:375, 1992

86. Vogt PK, Boss TJ: jun: oncogene and transcription factor. *Adv Cancer Res* 55:1, 1990

87. Marcu KB, Bossone SA, Patel AJ: Myc function and regulation. *Annu Rev Biochem* 61:809, 1992

88. Blackwood EM, Eisenman RN: Max: a helix-loop-helix zipper protein that forms asequence-specific DNA-binding complex with myc. *Science* 251:1211, 1991

89. Amati B, Land H: Myc-max-mad: a transcription factor network controlling cell cycle progression, differentiation and death. *Curr Opin Genet Dev* 4:102, 1994

90. Sherr CJ: Mammalian G1 cyclins. *Cell* 73:1059, 1993

91. Quelle DE, Ashmun RA, Shurtlett SA, et al: Overexpression of mouse D-type cyclins accelerates G1 phase in rodent fibroblasts. *Genes Dev* 7:1559, 1993

92. Gibbs JB, Oliff A: Pharmaceutical research in molecular oncology. *Cell* 79:193, 1994

93. Gibbs JB: Ras C-terminal processing enzymes: new drug targets? *Cell* 65:1, 1991

94. Gibbs JB, Oliff A, Kohl NE: Farnesyltransferase inhibitors: ras research yields a potentialcancer therapeutic. *Cell* 77:175, 1994

Acknowledgments

Figures 1, 2, 3, 5, and 8   Seward Hung.

Figures 4, 6, 7, 9   Talar Agasyan.

CHAPTER 6

The Tumor Suppressor Genes and Their Mechanisms of Action

José F. Leis, M.D., Ph.D., David M. Livingston, M.D.

Tumor formation results, at least partly, from mutations in two classes of cellular genes, proto-oncogenes and tumor suppressor genes. Proto-oncogenes are genes whose protein products deliver signals leading to cell proliferation [*see Chapters 4 and 5*]. Proto-oncogene products participate in all levels of the signaling pathways that fuel cell growth and can usually be categorized into four types: growth factors, growth factor receptors, intracellular signal transducers, and transcription factors. Mutations in proto-oncogenes often result in a gain of function that manifests itself in the unceasing stimulation of cell growth. Typically, such mutated proto-oncogenes, now referred to as *oncogenes*, functionally dominate the wild-type allele at the molecular level. More than 50 proto-oncogenes have been described to date. Almost invariably, these genes become involved in cancer pathogenesis through somatic mutations that strike cells within target tissues. Only one example of a mutant proto-oncogene inherited through the germ line currently exists.[1]

The products of tumor suppressor genes, in contrast, generally provide signals that constrain cell proliferation. These genes are involved in tumorigenesis when they sustain loss-of-function mutations. Mutations in prototypical tumor suppressor genes generally behave in a recessive manner at the molecular level. Hence, only when both copies of the gene are inactivated does an abnormal phenotype become manifest in a cell. Because of this recessive genetic behavior, a single mutant allele of such a gene can be passed through the germ line. Such a mutant allele is often tolerated during embryogenesis because its presence is revealed in a tissue only when the remaining wild-type allele is lost. This loss may occur many years after birth. In this way, such an inherited tumor suppressor allele may serve as a predisposing determinant to cancer.[2] Features of proto-oncogenes and tumor suppressor genes are presented in Table 1.

Research on tumor suppressor genes has lagged 10 years behind research on oncogenes, mainly because of the technical difficulties encountered in the study of genes that become apparent only when their function is lost. However, knowledge in this area has exploded during the past decade. Almost a dozen genes of this type have now been isolated as molecular clones. The emphasis of this chapter is on the general principles involved in the identification and authentication of tumor suppressor genes, with the retinoblastoma susceptibility locus serving as a prototype. Several excellent reviews of these genes now exist.[3-7]

The Evidence for Tumor Suppressor Genes

Evidence for the existence of tumor suppressor genes has come from three major lines of research: somatic cell hybrid experiments, studies of familial cancers, and detection of loss of heterozygosity (LOH) in tumors. These lines of inquiry have converged during the past decade to support the notion that loss-of-function mutations in tumor suppressor genes are linked to tumorigenesis.

Somatic Cell Hybridization

The earliest evidence that tumors could be suppressed and that cancer may be recessive at the cellular level dates back nearly a quarter of a century.[8,9] Experiments in this area focused on the study of somatic cell hybrids formed by the experimental fusion of tumor cells with normal cells. These hybrid cells contain genomic information provided by both parental cell lines. The underlying question was whether the resulting hybrid cell was malignant or normal. If the malignant phenotype were dominant, as one might have predicted based on the characteristics of proto-oncogenes, these hybrids should have been tumorigenic. On the other hand, if the loss of an important regulatory gene contributed to the neoplastic transformation of the parental tumor cell line, then acquisition of a normal copy of this gene

Table 1 Properties of Tumor Suppressor Genes
and Proto-oncogenes

Property	*Tumor Suppressor Genes*	*Proto-oncogenes*
Alleles mutated in cancer	Both alleles	One allele
Germ line transmission of mutant allele	Frequently seen	Rare*
Somatic mutation involved in tumor formation	Yes	Yes
Function of mutant allele(s)	Loss of function (recessive allele)	Gain of function (dominant allele)
Effects on cell growth	Inhibit cell growth	Promote cell growth
Cancer predisposition as a result of mutational event	Specific cancer type	Many types of cancer

*Only one example known at this time.

from the normal cell fusion partner should result in a reversion of the neo-plastic phenotype.

The cell hybrids resulting from these fusions were usually found to be nontumorigenic, although they still exhibited many features of trans formed cells. Moreover, suppression of the tumorigenic phenotype was observed regardless of whether the cells used for the generation of the hybrid cells were derived from chemically, virally, or spontaneously induced tumors. These results indicated that the normal cell used in the fusion contributed genes to the malignant cell that normalized its growth and implied strongly that recessive alleles present in tumor cell genomes play an important role in tumorigenesis. This work also provided the first indication that tumor cells lack critical growth-regulating genetic information that is present in normal cells.[10]

Although the cell hybrids were initially nontumorigenic, propagation of hybrid cell clones in culture often led to reversion to a tumorigenic phenotype. An explanation for this phenomenon came from the observation that these hybrids often exhibited karyotypic instability and would preferentially lose chromosomes that were contributed by one or the other parent cell. In certain cases, loss of a single, specific chromosome originally contributed by the normal parent was linked to reversion to a tumorigenic phenotype. The fact that reversion could result from the loss of a single chromosome suggested that a single gene or a small number of genes on that chromosome were active in tumor suppression.

Interestingly, the results of hybridization experiments that used a wide variety of tumor cell lines fused to normal cells revealed that putative tumor suppressor genes exist on multiple chromosomes. For example, loss of chromosome 11 from the normal parent of HeLa cervical carcinoma cell X normal fibroblast hybrids resulted in reversion to tumorigenicity, whereas loss of the normal copy of chromosome 1 from fibrosarcoma cell fusions was correlated with this outcome.[11,12] This finding was the first suggestion that multiple, distinct tumor suppressor genes exist and that loss of function of at least one such gene is a characteristic of many tumor cells.

The technique of microcell-mediated chromosome transfer (microcell fusion) further refined our understanding of the process of tumor suppression.[13,14] Microcell fusion allows investigators to transfer a single tagged chromosome from a normal cell to a tumor cell by membrane fusion. The transferred chromosome is then passed on to successive progeny cells. By use of this technique on a wide variety of tumor cell lines, a single copy of a given normal chromosome was found to be sufficient to suppress the tumorigenic phenotype of certain tumor cells. Furthermore, transfer of other chromosomes had no such effect. The results of microcell fusion experiments reinforced the conclusions of earlier somatic cell hybrid studies that multiple tumor suppressor genes exist.

Studies of Familial Cancers

The study of familial cancers provided a second line of evidence for the existence of tumor suppressor genes.[15] Pioneering research on familial retinoblastoma and Wilms' tumor revealed that the genes that conferred inherited tumor susceptibility behaved as mendelian dominants. The penetrance of the mutant gene or genes appeared to vary and was often incomplete. Furthermore, in most affected families (e.g., families with hereditary retinoblastoma), the predisposition was limited to a single or to few types of cancer and not to cancer in general.

CYTOGENETIC STUDIES OF HERITABLE TUMORS

In a small number of cases, the genetic basis of these inborn susceptibilities became apparent through karyotypic analysis of a patient's leukocytes, which revealed a recurrent chromosomal deletion in one member of a chromosomal pair. For example, the otherwise normal leukocyte karyotype of approximately five percent of patients with hereditary retinoblastoma revealed a gross deletion of part or all of the long arm of one copy of chromosome 13. Although the extent of the deletions and their end points were variable, loss of band q14 on chromosome 13 was common to all deletions.[16] In addition, with improvements in cytogenetic techniques, deletions in this region of chromosome 13 were also detected in the tumors. In some patients with nonhereditary retinoblastoma, deletions in 13q were detected in the tumor cells of the patient but not in the cells of other tissues, indicating somatic loss of this chromosomal region.[17]

Analogous leukocyte karyotype analysis performed on patients with Wilms' tumor, an embryonic kidney tumor, revealed deletions within the short arm of chromosome 11, particularly involving 11p13, implying that a Wilms' tumor suppressor gene exists in that chromosomal segment. Recurrent chromosomal deletions have now been demonstrated in several heritable tumors and have provided valuable information that has facilitated the eventual cloning of the suspected tumor suppressor genes involved. However, cytogenetic techniques clearly have limitations. Each human chromosome contains approximately 1 to 3×10^8 base pairs, with a single chromosome band representing about five to 10 percent of the total DNA of that chromosome, or about 10^7 base pairs (10 megabases). Therefore, deletions of as much as a megabase of DNA can go undetected by cytogenetic techniques; such deletions may encompass a dozen or more genes. Also, gross karyotypic deletions occur in a relatively small fraction of patients with heritable tumors. Despite these limitations, cytogenetic studies provided direct evidence that genetic loss frequently accompanies tumorigenesis; these findings yield further support for the existence of tumor suppressor genes.

Loss of Heterozygosity and RFLP Analysis

Loss of both alleles of a tumor suppressor gene is required for effects on cell phenotype to manifest. In familial tumors, the first of these losses occurs through inheritance of a mutant allele of a tumor suppressor gene that is passed through the germ line; in sporadic tumors, this loss may occur through somatic mutation. In both cases, the tumorigenic phenotype is usually realized only when a cell loses the surviving wild-type allele of the tumor suppressor gene.

Mutational inactivation of the second copy of the tumor suppressor gene may occur by several mechanisms. Independent mutational inactivation of the second copy of the gene is possible. However, somatic mutational events occur with a frequency of 10^{-6} to 10^{-7} per cell generation, and elimination of the second copy of a tumor suppressor gene by this mechanism is consequently a relatively rare event. However, several chromosomal mechanisms occurring at much higher frequencies (e.g., 10^{-3} to 10^{-4} per cell generation) are much more effective in eliminating the remaining wild-type allele. One of these changes is gene conversion, in which a break in a DNA strand of one chromosome leads to base pairing between that strand and the complementary strand on the homologous chromosome. After repair and replication, the two gene copies are rendered identical. In the case of certain tumor suppressor genes, a wild-type allele may be replaced by a duplicated copy of the mutant allele. A second chromosomal change is chromosomal nondisjunction with loss of the wild-type chromosome, resulting in *hemizygosity* at all loci on the affected chromosome. A third change is chromosomal nondisjunction with duplication of the chromosome containing the mutant tumor suppressor gene, resulting in *homozygosity* at all loci, as is seen after gene conversion. The last chromosomal change is mitotic recombination, occurring between the mutant tumor suppressor locus and the centromere. This phenomenon results in *heterozygosity* at loci in the proximal portions of the two chromosomes and homozygosity at loci distal to the point of crossover.

The important role of these genetic mechanisms in tumor suppressor gene inactivation is indicated by observations that in most tumors that lack functional copies of these genes, the tumor cells bear two identical mutant alleles of these genes. Thus, these loci have shown LOH and are therefore reduced to a homozygous mutant configuration.

The chromosomal mechanisms leading to LOH at the mutant tumor suppressor locus can also result in LOH or reduction to homozygosity of chromosomal regions that flank the suppressor gene. The technique of restriction fragment length polymorphism (RFLP) analysis has given researchers a way to identify LOH. RFLP analysis is based on the observation that variations in the DNA sequence of homologous chromosomes may exist at individual restriction endonuclease sites, thereby rendering these sites polymorphic with respect to each other. When a restriction site is present in the DNA of one chromosome but not the DNA of its companion chromosome, specific fragment length diversity exists when the DNA is cleaved with the relevant restriction enzyme. RFLPs can be inherited just as genes are and behave as mendelian codominant alleles in family studies. More than 3,000 such RFLP markers, spanning the entire human genome, are now known and form the basis for a linkage map of the human genome.

The mechanisms leading to LOH of a tumor suppressor gene can also lead to LOH of an RFLP marker, if the two genetic elements are closely linked. For example, in the case of retinoblastoma, LOH of specific RFLP markers mapping to chromosomal 13 at band q14 has been observed in approximately three quarters of such tumors, although no gross cytogenetic abnormalities at this locus could be detected in these cases. In addition, analysis of polymorphic markers in pedigree analysis revealed that the polymorphic alleles lost from the tumor genome originated in the chromosome derived from the unaffected parent. Thus, in these cases, the mutant allele inherited from an affected parent became duplicated in the tumor cell genome.[18]

Certain familial tumors, including retinoblastomas, also occur in a sporadic form. In these cases, inactivation of the first copy of the tumor suppressor gene occurs by a spontaneous somatic mutation that results in a single predisposed retinal cell. Elimination of the remaining wild-type allele by a second somatic mutation—often LOH—leads to the transformation of the phenotype.

In the inherited form of the disease, acquisition of a mutant copy of the tumor suppressor gene through the germ line renders all retinal cells susceptible to malignant transformation. Heterozygous retinal cells need only suffer a single somatic mutation in order for the tumor phenotype to manifest itself. Hence, retinal tumors are much more common in the hereditary form of the tumor syndrome than in the sporadic form. Southern blot analysis, in which probes for polymorphic RFLP markers linked to the wild-type tumor suppressor locus were used, allowed investigators to demonstrate that the aforementioned chromosomal mechanisms were indeed responsible for tumor suppressor gene inactivation in most tumors. The approach used is outlined in Figure 1.

Restriction fragment length polymorphism analysis has proved to be invaluable as a means of detecting somatic LOH in tumors. This technique has also been used to help investigators identify and localize novel genes that may be responsible for tumor formation. For example, investigators examining somatic mutations in colorectal cancer were able to demonstrate LOH on chromosome 18q in more than 70 percent of carcinomas and 50 percent of late adenomas.[19] This finding indicated that a putative tumor suppressor gene was located nearby and allowed these investigators to use the techniques of gene cloning to identify the responsible gene.[20] Likewise, RFLP analysis has proved to be a powerful technique for the study of familial cancers. Within a given kindred, comparison of the inheritance of a cancer trait with the inheritance of RFLP markers of known chromosomal location by linkage analysis has been used to yield information about the location of a putative tumor suppressor gene. This type of analysis has been extensively applied to the study of human tumors in the past decade. It has led to the identification and cloning of several tumor suppressor genes.[21] For example, the *NF*-1 gene responsible for certain forms of von Recklinghausen disease, which is characterized clinically by neurofibromas, skin abnormalities, and a predisposition to various malignancies, was cloned after it was mapped by linkage analysis to chromosome 17 at band q11.[22] A partial list of genomic regions that reproducibly display LOH in selected human tumors is provided in Table 2.

More recently, a new set of polymorphic markers has been used for performing linkage analysis more efficiently. This method takes advantage of the observation that the genomes of higher eukaryotes are uniformly interspersed with short segments of tandem repeat DNA sequences, which often include sequences denoted as $(G-T)_n$. These "microsatellite" repeats are highly polymorphic and can be analyzed by use of polymerase chain reaction techniques. Like RFLPs, microsatellite DNA units are inherited in mendelian dominant fashion. Second-generation maps of the human genome have now been constructed using these microsatellite DNA sequences and are widely used in linkage analysis in the study of human disease, including the chromosomal localization of tumor suppressor loci.[23]

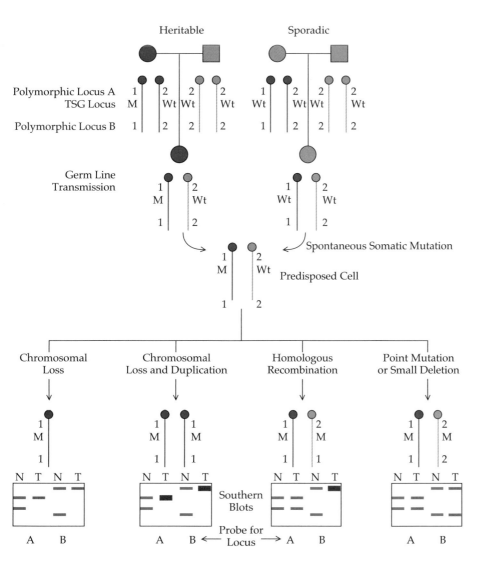

Figure 1 *Mechanisms resulting in loss of heterozygosity in human tumors. In heritable cancer syndromes, a mutant tumor suppressor allele (M)is passed through the germ line from parent to offspring (Knudson's "first hit"). The resulting predisposed cells have the genotype of M/Wt at the TSG locus. The tumor predisposition is unmasked by elimination of the remaining wild-type (Wt) allele by one of several mechanisms: chromosomal loss, chromosomal loss and duplication, homologous recombination, and point mutation or small deletion (Knudson's "second hit"). In the case of sporadic tumors, both parents pass on wild-type alleles of the TSG to their offspring. Spontaneous somatic mutation of one allele at the TSG locus of a single cell results in that cell's being predisposed to cancer. The predisposition is unmasked by mechanisms similar to those in heritable tumors. Southern blot analysis of normal (N) and tumor (T) DNA in which polymorphic probes are used for loci proximal (A) and distal (B) to the TSG locus allows for evaluation of the mechanism that led to the elimination of the remaining Wt allele. Normal DNA is informative for probes A and B in that the individual is heterozygous for the given restriction fragment length polymorphism (RFLP), one allele having been inherited from the father and the other allele from the mother(e.g., alleles 1 and 2 at locus A of the predisposed cell). In tumor DNA, loss of heterozygosity is observed when chromosomal loss with or without duplication or homologous recombination occurs. Quantitation of the probe signal allows for distinction of the mechanism involved.*

Table 2   Examples of Loss of Heterozygosity in Human Tumors

Tumor Type/Syndrome	Chromosomal Region	Tumor Suppressor Gene Involved
Breast cancer	13q14	*Rb*
	17p13	*p53*
	17q21	*BRCA1*
	13q12–13q13	*BRCA2*
	1p,1q,11p	Unknown
Colorectal cancer	2p	*hMSH2*
	3p21	*hMLH1*
	5q21	*APC*
	17p13	*p53*
	18q21	*DCC*
Retinoblastoma	13q14	*Rb*
Wilms' tumor	11p13	*WT*-1
Beckwith-Wiedemann syndrome	11p15	*WT*-2
Melanoma	9p21	*MTS1/p16*
	1p	Unknown
Multiple endocrine neoplasia		
MEN I	11q	Unknown
MEN II	10q11	*ret* proto-oncogene
Neurofibromatosis		
Type 1	17q11	Neurofibromin
Type 2	22q	Merlin/schwannomin
Renal cell carcinoma	3p25	*VHL*
	3p14	Unknown
Lung cancer	13q14	*Rb*
	17p13	*p53*
	3p14–3p21	Unknown
Prostate cancer	8p22,10q24	Unknown
Neuroblastoma	1p36,14q	Unknown
Brain tumors and gliomas	9p21	*MTS1/p16*
	17p13	*p53*
Meningiomas	1p,14q,17,22	Unknown

Retinoblastoma as a Paradigm for Familial Cancer

Retinoblastoma is the most common primary eye tumor of children; it has an annual incidence of one in 15,000 to 34,000 live births. Approximately 200 new cases are diagnosed in the United States each year, most of which occur before five years of age, with a mean age of presentation of 17 months. Before the advent of curative treatment, the disease was uniformly fatal, and death was linked to the development of distant metastases or direct intracranial extension via the optic nerve.

As curative therapy emerged, in the form of improved ophthalmologic evaluation for the detection of early tumors, surgical enucleation, and radiation therapy, two distinct clinical presentations of the disease became apparent. In the heritable form of retinoblastoma, afflicted children presented with multiple independent tumors involving both eyes. Approximately 40 percent of the cases are now known to fall into this category, which usually presents earlier in life than the sporadic form. In this disease entity, a positive family history is present in approximately one third of patients. In these retinoblastoma families, the disease is transmitted as a highly penetrant, autosomal dominant trait, and the offspring of an affected parent has a nearly 50 percent risk of developing retinoblastoma. In addition, these patients have an increased risk of developing second malignancies later in life. The incidence of second malignancies increases over time, and a second, nonocular tumor develops within 40 years of treatment of the retinoblastoma in 15 to 20 percent of patients. The most common second tumors include osteosarcoma, fibrosarcoma, Ewing's sarcoma, and Wilms' tumor.

The sporadic form of retinoblastoma accounts for 60 percent of cases. Children with the clinical presentation usually demonstrate unilateral eye involvement and a single tumor focus within the affected eye. In sporadic retinoblastoma, no family history is noted, and secondary malignancies do not occur later in life.

In 1970, DeMars proposed that cancer arises in predisposed individuals because they are heterozygous for a gene responsible for the predisposition and that tumors form when the normal allele of the gene is somatically mutated.[24] Knudson developed a mathematical model after a statistical analysis of the clinical presentation of sporadic and heritable retinoblastoma, which provided a genetic explanation for the two forms.[25] Knudson postulated that a common genetic mechanism is responsible for both forms and that disease production requires the advent of two critical mutations, most likely at a single locus. In sporadic retinoblastoma, two somatic mutations occur in a specific gene located in a single retinal cell that proliferates to form a tumor. As noted previously, two somatic mutations occurring in the same gene in the same cell is a rare event. So, affected patients tend to present with a single, unifocal tumor. In the heritable form of the disease, the first of these required mutations is inherited from one of the parents and present from conception.[25] Therefore, all of the cells in the newly formed retina would carry this mutation. The second necessary mutation occurs early in life. Because all retinal cells contain the first required mutation, tumorigenesis can occur at multiple sites in the retina; the second somatic mutagenic event leads to doubly mutated cells (i.e., potential tumor cells).

Knudson could only speculate that the two mutational events affected both alleles of a single gene rather than one allele of each of two independent target genes. As previously stated, clues to the location of the first of these genetic events came from cytogenetic analysis, which revealed deletions in the region of chromosome 13q14 in the leukocytes from patients with heritable retinoblastoma[16] and in the sporadic tumors of affected individuals.[17] These observations supported the prediction that sporadic cases were the result of mutations at the same genetic locus that contributed to the hereditary form of the disease.

Further support for the role of 13q14 in the etiology of retinoblastoma came from the observation of genetic linkage between retinoblastoma and the gene for the serum enzyme esterase D. In patients with retinoblastoma and visible deletions in chromosome 13, esterase D levels were reduced to 50 percent of normal in the patient's leukocytes, suggesting that the region of chromosome 13 that had been deleted contained both the esterase D and the retinoblastoma loci. The loci were found to be closely linked.[26] In no affected family was mitotic recombination noted between esterase D and the putative disease-producing gene. Direct evidence that hereditary retinoblastoma arises from the inactivation or elimination of the remaining wild-type allele of an inherited tumor suppressor gene came from a study of a retinoblastoma family in which a particular affected child revealed only one copy of chromosome 13.[27] No esterase D activity was found in the patient's tumor cells, indicating that the tumor contained only the mutant copy of chromosome 13, which lacked both the esterase D gene and the retinoblastoma gene. Hence, by following both the wild-type and the mutant chromosomes using polymorphic esterase D, it became clear that the wild-type chromosome had been lost. This result showed that loss of both functioning copies of the retinoblastoma gene, located on the long arm of chromosome 13, always occurs in retinoblastoma and suggested that the mutant alleles of the gene increase the potential for malignancy of retinal cells.

RFLP analysis provided additional evidence for the prediction that the two mutational events necessary for the retinoblastoma development occurs in a single gene (so-called Rb-1 [28,29]). Specifically, each of the known mechanisms of functional inactivation of the given gene was found to occur in retinoblastoma. LOH, achieved through chromosomal nondisjunction, proved to be the most frequent mechanism leading to elimination of the remaining wild-type allele.[29] Of particular importance was the fact that, in each case of heritable retinoblastoma, loss of Rb-1 gene function in the tumor cells was a product of inactivation/loss of the wild-type allele donated by the unaffected parent,[18] reinforcing Knudson's hypothesis.

Taken together, these results indicated that the retinoblastoma gene is a tumor suppressor gene and that loss of both copies of the gene predisposes to tumor formation. Conversely, a single wild-type copy of the Rb-1 gene is both necessary and sufficient to maintain normal cell growth, because the vast majority of retinal cells in patients with retinoblastoma exhibit a normal phenotype.

The cloning of the retinoblastoma (Rb-1) gene provided the proof that the genetic element that causes both the familial and the sporadic forms of this disease was indeed a tumor suppressor gene with many of the properties predicted from the indirect lines of evidence cited above. To isolate this gene, investigators constructed a chromosome 13 genomic library, from which a series of DNA markers were cloned. Markers that mapped to chromosome segment 13q14 were used to probe germ line and tumor DNA from retinoblastoma patients by Southern blot analysis. One such probe, designated H3-8, which was later shown to contain an exon of the Rb-1 gene, detected homozygous deletion of DNA sequences at 13q14 in three of

37 tumors.[30] This finding, in turn, led to the cloning of the gene by Friend and colleagues.[31]

Evidence for the authenticity of *Rb*-1 as the retinoblastoma susceptibility gene was subsequently provided by the demonstration of the presence of structural defects in both copies of the *Rb*-1 locus in the tumors of numerous retinoblastoma patients.[32] Moreover, studies of *Rb*-1 structure in the tumors and lymphocytes of patients with both familial and sporadic disease verified the Knudson hypothesis at the molecular level.[33] Further support came from the demonstration that tumor cell lines or short-term tumor cultures lacked an intact form of the protein product of this gene.[34] The inactivation of the *Rb*-1 gene occurs by various genetic alterations, the most common of which are point mutations or small deletions that result in truncated, unstable protein products[35] or splicing defects. Large deletions were detected in only 30 percent of tumors.

Corroboration of the role of *Rb*-1 in retinoblastoma was provided by the results of experiments in which a cloned wild-type *Rb*-1 allele was reintroduced into various retinoblastoma and *Rb*–/– osteosarcoma cell lines.[36-38] When plasmids expressing high levels of wild-type pRb were transfected into *Rb*–/– osteosarcoma cell lines (e.g., Saos-2) these cells arrested in the G_1 phase of the cell cycle, although they appeared to remain viable. In contrast, introduction of certain mutant *Rb* alleles into such cells had no such effect.

Function of Tumor Suppressor Genes

The discussion of the genetic mechanisms by which tumor suppressor genes are lost sheds little light on the biochemical mechanisms by which their protein products suppress cell proliferation. Approximately a dozen tumor suppressor genes have been identified and cloned [*see Table 3*]. The cellular functions of their respective protein products remains largely uncharacterized. However, as our knowledge has expanded, it has become increasingly clear that these proteins exhibit a wide variety of functions and act at many sites within the cell.

Proto-oncogenes encode proteins that deliver positive growth signals by various mechanisms at all known levels of cell growth–related signaling. The close regulation of proto-oncogene product function is essential to normal cell growth and differentiation. Therefore, it would not be surprising to find that tumor suppressor gene products, which antagonize cell growth, participate in these regulatory events as well. In keeping with this hypothesis, in several instances, a tumor suppressor gene product either directly or indirectly interacts with the product of an oncogene. In at least some instances, functional regulation of the oncogene product ensues.

In the following section, tumor suppressor proteins are examined from a functional point of view, and the ways in which they interact with specific signaling circuits in the cell are reviewed. The cellular localization and mechanisms of action of the known tumor suppressor proteins are listed in Table 3.

Tumor Suppressor Genes Active in Cell Cycle Control

The eukaryotic cell cycle can be divided into four distinct stages: the G_1 phase, or gap 1, the period between the previous period of nuclear division and the beginning of DNA synthesis; the S phase, the period of DNA synthesis during which chromosomal DNA replicates; the G_2 phase, or gap 2, the period between DNA replication and nuclear division; and the M phase, for mitosis, or the period of nuclear division [*see Chapter 2*]. In the M phase, chromosomes condense, line up, and pair along the metaphase plate; sister chromatids separate; and cytokinesis occurs, producing two daughter cells in the G_1 phase of the next cell cycle.

When G_1 cells have grown to a sufficient size and met other basic requirements, they become committed to progression through the cell cycle and division. This point of no return is called START in yeast and the restriction point in mammalian cells. The relatively constant amount of time required for different mammalian cells to progress through the restriction point and the S, G_2, and M phases suggests that events in these intervals are tightly regulated, as if run by a clock. Indeed, the phrase "cell cycle clock" is used to refer to the machinery that controls the pace at which a cell moves through the various intervals of the cycle.

At the molecular level, the progression through the cell cycle is governed by the formation and action of a series of regulatory protein kinase complexes composed of a catalytic subunit, termed a cyclin-dependent kinase (Cdk), and a regulatory protein subunit, called a cyclin. Certain cyclin-Cdk complexes form at specific points in the cell cycle, are activated, phosphorylate their various molecular targets, and then are inactivated. These cyclin-Cdk complexes constitute the core components of the cell cycle clock machinery.[39]

THE RETINOBLASTOMA PROTEIN

pRb, the product of the retinoblastoma susceptibility gene, is intimately involved in the operations of the cell cycle clock apparatus. Insights into the function of pRb come partly from the observation that certain oncoproteins encoded by three DNA tumor viruses, the adenovirus E1A protein, the SV40 virus large T antigen, and the E7 protein from human papilloma virus, interact with and functionally inactivate pRb.[40-42] These three viral proteins each contain a short sequence that is largely responsible for their ability to bind pRb. The integrity of this shared sequence is necessary for the transforming function of each of the viral oncoproteins.[41,43,44] This observation suggests that the transforming function of these oncoproteins is dependent on their ability to bind and inactivate the growth-suppressive function of pRb.

Further insights arose from the observation that pRb is phosphorylated in a cell cycle–dependent manner.[45-47] In G_1, pRb is underphosphorylated. In late G_1, pRb becomes extensively phosphorylated and remains hyperphosphorylated until mitotic anaphase, when it is rapidly dephosphorylated. The importance of phosphorylation in the control of pRb function was underscored by the observation that SV40 large T antigen binds only the underphosphorylated form of pRb and that this binding occurs in a cell cycle–dependent manner.[48,49] These observations suggested that the under-

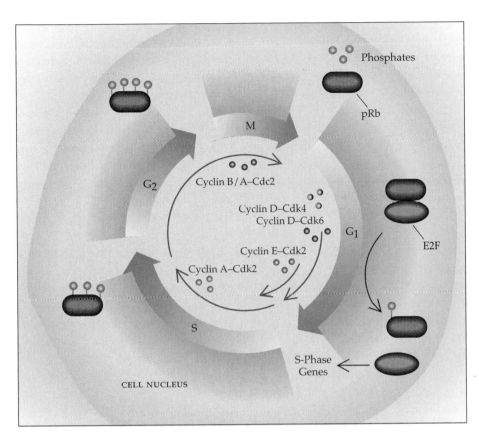

Figure 2   *The retinoblastoma protein (pRb) and the cell cycle. pRb is phosphorylated in a cell cycle–dependent manner. In G_1, pRb is underphosphorylated. In late G_1, pRb becomes extensively phosphorylated and remains hyperphosphorylated until the mitotic anaphase occurs, when it becomes rapidly dephosphorylated. The transcription factor E2F binds preferentially to underphosphorylated pRb in the G_1 phase of the cell cycle. Binding by pRb inhibits the ability of E2F to activate the promoters of several genes required for DNA synthesis. The pRb-E2F complex also appears to down-regulate numerous G_1 exit-promoting genes, including c-myc and c-myb. Phosphorylation of pRb, as well as E2F, by cyclin D–Cdk4 and cyclin E–Cdk2 complexes in late G_1 releases free E2F, which is then able to interact with the promoters of genes required for the S phase.*

phosphorylated form of pRb, which exists primarily in G_1, is the active growth-suppressing form of the protein.

The timing of pRb phosphorylation in G_1 suggests that pRb may be modified by components of the cell cycle clock [*see Figure 2*]. This has proved to be the case. When pRb-deficient cells were transfected with expression plasmids that encoded pRb and various combinations of G_1 cyclins, pRb phosphorylation occurred when the *Rb*-1 gene was cotransfected with cyclins D2 and D3. It also occurred when the *Rb*-1 was cotransfected with cyclins A or E.[38,50] In addition, pRb phosphorylation was accompanied by an override of the pRb-mediated G_1 block.

Additional evidence for the regulation of pRb phosphorylation by the cell cycle clock comes from analysis of the mechanism by which transforming growth factor–β (TGF-β) induces cell cycle arrest. TGF-β blocks cells in G_1, leading to the accumulation of underphosphorylated pRb.[51] TGF-β treatment of mink lung cells blocked synthesis of the Cdk4 kinase subunit in G_1, thus preventing the formation of cyclin D-Cdk4 complexes and, therefore, pRb phosphorylation in G_1.[52] Mink lung cells that overproduce Cdk4 overcome this block, a finding that suggests that down-regulation of Cdk4 expression plays a pivotal role in TGF-β growth suppression.

These experiments indicate how pRb function is modulated by components of the cell cycle clock, but they reveal nothing about the mechanisms by which pRb, in turn, controls cell cycle progression. Most current evidence suggests that this control is accomplished by pRb's binding to and regulating the activity of certain transcription factors. Much of this evidence has come from studies of the interaction between pRb and E2F, a transcription factor that was initially identified by its seemingly specific ability to activate the adenovirus E2 promoter.[53] E2F binds preferentially to underphosphorylated pRb in the G_1 phase of the cell cycle. Binding to pRb in G_1 inhibits the ability of E2F to activate the promoters of several genes required for DNA synthesis, thereby blocking activation of these genes. In addition, pRb-E2F complexes likely down-regulate the expression of many G_1 exit-promoting genes, including c-*myc* and c-*myb*. When pRb is phosphorylated in late G_1, it dissociates from E2F, allowing the latter to stimulate expression of various genes required for progression into the S phase. Viral oncoproteins also act by displacing E2F from pRb. Thus, phosphorylation or oncoprotein-mediated release of E2F from its negative regulator, pRb, contributes to cell cycle progression.

THE TUMOR SUPPRESSOR PROTEIN p53

Another tumor suppressor protein whose function appears to be linked to the cell cycle clock is p53. Like pRb, p53 is a nuclear phosphoprotein. It was originally identified through its interaction with the SV40 large T antigen. Indeed, all three of the DNA tumor viruses whose oncoproteins functionally inactivate p*Rb* also encode oncoproteins that functionally inactivate p53. However, the mechanisms by which this inactivation occurs are quite different than those described for pRb. Both the SV40 large T antigen and the adenovirus E1B oncoproteins appear to inactivate p53 by binding and sequestering it. The human papilloma virus E6 oncoprotein, in contrast, inactivates p53 by binding to it and targeting the protein for rapid destruction through the ubiquitin-dependent proteolytic pathway.[54]

The *p53* gene is the most frequently mutated gene in human cancer.[4,55,56] The nature of these mutations provided an exception to the paradigm for tumor suppressor genes established through the study of retinoblastoma. The *p53* gene encodes a protein of the same name that functions as a transcription factor. Most *p53* mutations in human tumors are missense mutations that occur at several sites that encode the sequence-specific DNA binding domain of the p53 protein; these missense mutations cause loss of DNA binding-ability by this protein. The biochemical importance of this region of the protein was recently revealed when the crystal structure of the p53-DNA complex showed these sites to be directly involved in supporting p53-DNA contacts.[57]

When introduced into cells bearing wild-type *p53* alleles, mutant alleles of *p53* can affect cell proliferation, apparently by interfering with wild-type p53 function. Their ability to affect cell proliferation indicates that these mutant alleles, rather than being recessive, null alleles, are functioning in a "dominant negative" function, compromising the activity of wild-type alleles that are coexpressed in the cell. This dominant negative mode of function could be explained by the observation that the p53 protein assembles into a tetramer. Therefore, mutant p53 subunits are able to form oligomeric complexes with coexpressed wild-type p53 subunits and compromise the growth-regulating functions of the latter, thereby contributing to the development of a neoplastic phenotype.[58-60]

Further support for the notion that the *p53* gene is a tumor suppressor comes from the study of families with a rare inherited disease, the Li-Fraumeni syndrome. Affected members manifest a wide variety of tumors that occur at an unusually early age. The components of Li-Fraumeni syndrome include breast carcinoma, soft tissue sarcoma, brain tumors, osteosarcoma, leukemia, and adrenocortical carcinoma. Germ line *p53* mutations were detected in five such families.[61] Interestingly, unlike most somatic mutations in *p53* described previously, these germ line mutations did not appear to produce amounts of mutant *p53* that were likely to exert a dominant negative effect on the remaining wild-type allele. From the wide variety of tumors seen in this syndrome, it appears that mutations in *p53* can predispose multiple tissue types to tumor formation.

p53 functions as a transcriptional activator. This property is responsible, at least in part, for its tumor-suppressing activity. Support for this concept comes from the observations that mutant viral oncoproteins (e.g., E1B) that are defective in transforming activity are all defective in blocking *p53*-induced transcription[62] and that naturally occurring mutations of the *p53* gene found in human tumors also inactivate this function. If transcriptional activity is responsible for the protein's growth suppressive effects, what are the biologically important genes that are regulated by p53, and do these genes mediate the p53 role in growth suppression?

Several investigators have shown that p53 induces transcription of a gene encoding a 21-kilodalton (kd) protein that interacts with and inhibits various cyclin-Cdk complexes.[63,64] Among the complexes that are inhibited are those containing Cdk2- and Cdk4, the kinase complexes that are responsible for phosphorylating, and thereby inactivating, pRb. Therefore, it would seem that at least one mechanism by which p53 induces a G_1 phase cell cycle arrest depends on its ability to keep pRb in its underphosphorylated, growth-inhibitory configuration.

The upstream signals that regulate p53 function are of interest because of their substantial clinical relevance. Cellular levels of p53 increase dramatically in response to DNA damage. For example, p53 is induced by ionizing or ultraviolet irradiation and certain cytotoxic anticancer agents. This increase in cellular levels of p53 causes the normal p53 protein to impose a G_1 arrest on the cell, a phenomenon that allows the cell to repair its DNA before proceeding on to S phase and DNA replication.[65] Cells that are deficient in p53 function do not arrest at G_1 and proceed to replicate damaged DNA. This situation may result in an increased number of mutations and genomic instability, thereby increasing the possibility of neoplastic transformation. In addition, p53 helps to trigger apoptosis—programmed cell death—after exposure to chemotherapeutic agents or irradiation.[66] Hence, p53-deficient cells exhibit a dramatically increased resistance to these agents, and malignant cells may acquire resistance to chemotherapy and radiation therapy through the development of *p53* gene mutations that interfere with the triggering of apoptosis.[67]

The p53 protein interacts with another protein of 90 kd; this protein appears to regulate the transcriptional activity of p53.[68] This protein is the product of the *mdm2* oncogene, originally identified as an amplified gene that is present on a double-minute chromosome from a transformed mouse cell line.[69] Although it is a nuclear phosphoprotein of unknown function, mdm2 possesses the structural properties of a transcription factor. It is a potent oncogene in cellular transformation assays, and it can confer a tumorigenic phenotype on properly conditioned cells. Importantly, mdm2 down-modulates p53 transcriptional activation and growth control function. The *mdm2* gene is amplified in certain human sarcomas and brain tumors bearing wild-type p53 function.[70] Therefore, at least part of the loss of growth control in these tumors may be a product of mdm2-dependent inhibition of p53 growth-controlling function.

THE CYCLIN-DEPENDENT KINASE INHIBITOR P16

p53 uses p21, an inhibitor of cyclin-Cdk complexes, to effect cell cycle arrest. p21 is only one of a set of Cdk inhibitors that regulate the cell cycle clock apparatus. Genes encoding such cyclin-Cdk inhibitors are attractive candidate tumor suppressor genes because their loss might be expected to result in overactive cyclin-Cdk complexes, which could lead to unrestrained cell proliferation. Indeed, this appears to be the case for at least one such Cdk inhibitor, p16.[39] p16 has been identified as a potent inhibitor of cyclin D–Cdk4 complexes.[71] It appears to antagonize the function of Cdk4 and the closely related Cdk6 by competing with cyclin D for binding to these Cdks. In vitro, these kinases can phosphorylate the product of the retinoblastoma tumor suppressor gene. p16 may therefore function as a tumor suppressor through the inhibition of phosphorylation and functional inactivation of pRB.

The possibility that the *p16* gene might be a tumor suppressor emerged when it was mapped to 9p21, a region known to contain deletions in some human tumors. Linkage studies of familial and sporadic melanoma had suggested the existence of a predisposing gene at 9p21, and LOH or homozygous deletion of the region was demonstrated in a wide variety of human tumors, including tumors of the brain, head and neck, bladder, and lung. Because of the many tumor types involved, the putative tumor suppressor at 9p21 was designated *MTS1*, for multiple tumor suppressor 1.

Although the *p16* gene was initially found to be inactivated in many human tumor cell lines,[72,73] recent results have shown that *p16* is mutated in a smaller number of primary tumors of the same tissue types, suggesting that *p16*-inactivating mutations in cell lines may be frequent secondary events that are selected for during the establishment of tumor cells in vitro. In addition, the level of this protein is greatly depleted in certain other human tumors including non–small cell lung carcinomas.[74] Further support for the role of *p16* as a tumor suppressor comes from the recent observation that it can suppress H-*ras* plus *myc* cotransformation of certain cultured primary cells.[75] It has been shown that overexpression of p16 in certain cell types leads to a G_1 cell cycle arrest.[76,77] This growth arrest is dependent on the cell containing functional pRb.[78] Several tumor-derived *p16* alleles that encode mutant forms of p16 are unable to growth-arrest cells or inhibit cyclin D–Cdk4 kinase activity in vitro. These data not only show that the presence of pRb is necessary for growth suppression by p16 but also suggest the pRb is the critical target of cyclin D–dependent kinases in the G_1 phase of the cell cycle. Thus, overexpression of D cyclins, loss or functional inactivation of pRb, and loss of p16 have similar effects on cell cycle progression at G_1 and may represent a common pathway toward tumorigenesis. Further support of this hypothesis come from the observation that mice carrying a targeted deletion of p16 are viable but develop spontaneous tumors at an early age.[79] These mice are also highly sensitive to carcinogenic agents.

Interestingly, a second gene, designated *MTS2*, with sequence homology to *p16*, is located close to *MTS1* on 9p21. The *MTS2* product closely resembles *p16* and is now designated $p15^{ink4b}(p15)$. Like p16, p15 inhibits Cdk4 and Cdk6.[80] However, unlike *p16*, TGF-β treatment of keratinocytes induces *p15* mRNA, resulting in a 30-fold increase in protein levels, which indicates that p15 may contribute to TGF-β–induced G_1 cell cycle arrest. Deletions of *MTS2* were also detected in some tumors. However, no point mutations in the *MTS2* gene were detected in melanoma cell lines that did not contain obvious homozygous deletions at 9p21, and deletions involving *MTS2* alone were not detected. Most homozygous deletions found at 9p21 in these tumors involved both *MTS1* and *MTS2* genes. Thus, the role of *MTS2* in tumorigenesis remains unclear. Recently, additional proteins that are structurally related to p15 and p16 have been identified,[81] implying that these proteins function as Cdk inhibitors that may also operate as tumor suppressor proteins.

Tumor Suppressor Genes as Transcriptional Regulators During Development: Wilms' Tumor

Wilms' tumor is a nephroblastoma of children that occurs in approximately one in 10,000 live births and accounts for five percent of all childhood cancers. Both familial and sporadic forms of the disease have been observed, with familial cases accounting for one percent of patients. In the former type of the disease, the trait is inherited in an autosomal dominant fashion with variable penetrance. Patients who present with unilateral tumors have a median age of 39 months at diagnosis; the corresponding time for those presenting with bilateral tumors is 26 months. Based on the differences in age of onset of unilateral versus bilateral tumors, Knudson and Strong proposed a two-hit genetic model similar to that of *Rb* to explain Wilms' tumor formation.[82]

The association between Wilms' tumor and several congenital anomalies has proved fruitful in identifying a responsible tumor suppressor gene. Wilms' tumor is often seen in the settings of WAGR syndrome (Wilms' tumor, aniridia, genitourinary abnormalities, and mental retardation), Beckwith-Wiedemann syndrome (in which gigantism and several other embryonal cancers occur), and Denys-Drash syndrome (in which severe genitourinary abnormalities occur). The observation that patients with WAGR syndrome have constitutional deletions of chromosome 11p13 provided the first clue to the location of the Wilms' tumor suppressor locus. Additional evidence was provided by the demonstration of LOH at 11p13 in sporadic tumors and the loss of tumorigenicity after the introduction of a normal chromosome 11 into a Wilms' tumor cell line by microcell fusion.[83] A candidate gene (WT-1) was cloned and found to encode a protein with sequence motifs that were characteristic of a transcription factor.[84] Evidence that WT-1 is involved in the cause of at least some Wilms' tumors was provided by the finding that the gene is deleted in 10 percent of sporadic tumors and in 100 percent of tumors occurring in Denys-Drash syndrome.[85]

Expression patterns of the WT-1 mRNA transcript suggest that WT-1 protein plays a prominent role in regulating genes that are involved in the development and function of the urogenital system.[86] What are the nature of these genes, and how does the absence of functional WT-1 protein contribute to tumor formation? An answer is suggested by the finding that the WT-1 transcription factor interacts with DNA in a sequence-specific manner and that the sequence it recognizes is similar to the binding site for EGR-1, a zinc finger transcription factor induced by mitogenic stimuli and responsible for the transactivation of several genes involved in cell proliferation. WT-1 has been shown to be a potent antagonist of EGR-1–activated transcription.[87] The target genes that are repressed by WT-1 and conversely activated by EGR-1 include the genes for several growth factors and their receptors. One of these growth factors, insulinlike growth factor–2 (IGF-2), is overproduced in 95 percent of Wilms' tumors, as is the IGF-1 receptor, suggesting an autocrine loop effect because IGF-2 is a known ligand of the IGF-1 receptor. Thus, one possibility is that deregulated expression of selected growth factor genes, such as IGF-2, at inappropriate times during development or in early life may contribute to renal tumorigenesis.

Another mechanism by which the WT-1 protein may play a role in tumorigenesis is suggested by the observation that WT-1 protein interacts with and stabilizes the p53 tumor suppressor protein.[88] This interaction results in increased steady-state levels of p53 by decreasing its degradation and prolonging its half-life. In addition, the WT protein enhances the DNA-binding activity of p53 and p53-mediated transcriptional activation while inhibiting p53-mediated transcriptional repression. Overexpression of WT-1 protein appears to inhibit p53-mediated apoptosis but does not appear to affect p53-mediated cell cycle arrest. The intriguing observation that Wilms' tumor specimens contain elevated levels of wild-type p53 suggests functional consequences to the WT-1 protein–p53 interaction.

Only 20 percent of Wilms' tumors can be attributed to a mutation in WT-1. Current evidence suggests that three distinct loci are involved in the development of Wilms' tumor. Patients with Beckwith-Wiedemann syndrome show chromosomal deletions in 11p15 instead of in 11p13, where WT-1 is located, and their tumors demonstrate LOH at 11p15 as well. The putative tumor suppressor at 11p15 has been designated WT-2. In addition, three large pedigrees with familial Wilms' tumor do not map to either 11p13 or 11p15, suggesting the existence of a third tumor suppressor locus in this disease.

Tumor Suppressor Proteins in Signal Transduction Pathways

Mutations that activate the *ras* proto-oncogenes exist in nearly 30 percent of all human tumors. The normal p21^{ras} proteins serve as molecular switches that regulate several signal transduction pathways in the cell [*see Chapters 4 and 5*]. When bound to guanosine triphosphate (GTP) in the form of GTP•p21^{ras}, p21^{ras} activates signaling. A p21^{ras}-associated GTPase activity leads to hydrolysis of GTP to guanosine diphosphate (GDP) and to the appearance of GDP•p21^{ras}, which cannot signal. GTPase-activating protein (rasGAP) stimulates the GTPase activity of p21^{ras}, thereby accelerating the conversion of GTP•p21^{ras} to the inactive form. In many tumors, mutations in the *ras* gene result in the loss of p21^{ras} -associated GTPase activity, thereby locking the protein into its active state and resulting in unregulated p21^{ras} signaling. This unregulated signaling, in turn, contributes to a transformed phenotype. Deregulated p21^{ras} signaling can also result from loss of GTPase-activating activity in a cell; this appears to explain the biochemical basis of type 1 neurofibromatosis.

von Recklinghausen disease, or neurofibromatosis type 1 (NF 1), is a commonly inherited genetic disorder that affects one in 3,500 individuals worldwide. The disease is transmitted as an autosomal dominant trait and is clinically characterized by neurofibromas involving the peripheral nervous system, café-au-lait spots, and Lisch nodules. In approximately three percent of cases, these neurofibromas undergo malignant transformation. Patients with neurofibromatosis type 1 also display a propensity to developing other tumors, including pheochromocytoma, rhabdomyosarcoma, Wilms' tumor, meningioma, and myelogenous leukemia. In half of all patients, a familial predisposition can be demonstrated; new germ line mutations account for the other half of cases.

The gene responsible for type 1 neurofibromatosis (*NF*-1) was mapped to chromosome 17q11.2 by linkage analysis and by the observation that two patients with neurofibromatosis type 1 had translocations involving this region. Cloning of the gene revealed it to encode a ubiquitous, 2,818-amino-acid protein with sequence homology to the catalytic domain of rasGAP [*see Chapter 5*]. [89] The functional implications of this homology were tested and verified, and it was shown that the catalytic domain of neurofibromin, the protein product of the *NF*-1 tumor suppressor gene, could stimulate intrinsic p21^{ras}•GTPase activity. This finding suggests that at least one important function of neurofibromin is regulation of the conversion of active GTP•p21^{ras} to inactive GDP•p21^{ras} and that mutations in *NF*-1 may alter the regulation of the p21^{ras} signaling pathways. Support for this mechanism of action is provided by the observation that schwannoma cell lines derived from patients with neurofibromatosis type 1 have increased levels of GTP•p21^{ras} and decreased levels of neurofibromin.[90]

Neurofibromin is likely to provide other regulatory functions as well. If its only role were to regulate the GTPase activity of p21^{ras}, one would predict that the clinical spectrum of tumors seen in neurofibromatosis might overlap considerably with that bearing acquired activating p21^{ras} mutations. This is not the case. In addition, recent studies in which neurofibromin was introduced into neurofibromin-deficient melanoma cell lines and into NIH 3T3 mouse fibroblasts have shown a growth-inhibitory and differentiation-promoting effect that is independent of p21^{ras}•GTPase-accelerating activity.[91] Overproduction of neurofibromin also inhibited transformation by v-*ras*, which is resistant to the GTPase activating function of rasGAP (e.g., neurofibromin), but not by v-*raf*, a kinase located downstream of ras in the signaling pathway, in NIH 3T3 cells. These results imply that neurofibromin inhibits growth signaling via the p21^{ras} pathway upstream of raf by at least two distinct mechanisms, one of which is independent of its GTPase-accelerating activity.

Many independent mutations in the coding region of *NF*-1 have been found in patients with neurofibromatosis, supporting the notion that *NF*-1 is the tumor suppressor gene in von Recklinghausen disease. However, *NF*-1 does not adhere precisely to the retinoblastoma paradigm. For example, some evidence suggests that only one of the *NF*-1 gene copies needs to be inactivated for the development of a neoplastic phenotype. Investigators have failed to detect LOH and inactivation of the second *NF*-1 allele in benign neurofibromas.[92] On the other hand, LOH at 17q has been demonstrated in malignant tumors of patients with neurofibromatosis type 1. Taken together, these results imply that loss of the second allele of *NF*-1 is not a necessary condition for the formation of benign neurofibromas and that a reduction in neurofibromin level to that encoded by a single allele predisposes to a neoplastic effect. It also suggests that a fully malignant phenotype of neurofibromatosis type 1 tumors depends on the inactivation of both *NF*-1 alleles.

Tumor Suppressor Proteins Located in the Plasma Membrane and Cytoplasm

As shown by the discussion regarding neurofibromatosis type 1, not all tumor suppressor proteins are transcription factors or are localized to the nucleus. The explosion in tumor suppressor gene research during the past decade has provided us with the insight that tumor suppressor proteins are localized throughout the cell and that their functions are varied. More recent work has identified several tumor suppressor genes whose protein products interact with, or are integral members of, the cell membrane or are located in the cytoplasm. Because the functions of these tumor suppressor proteins remain largely uncharacterized, they are only briefly discussed here.

Adenomatous Polyposis Coli (APC) Tumor Suppressor

Familial adenomatous polyposis is an autosomal dominant trait that has greater than 90 percent penetrance. It affects approximately one in 10,000 people in industrialized nations and is characterized by the appearance of hundreds, if not thousands, of clonal benign polyps of the colon. These polyps usually appear in the second decade of life. Invariably, colorectal cancer develops in all affected individuals who do not receive surgical intervention. A closely related disorder, Gardner syndrome, which is also inherited as an autosomal dominant trait, presents with adenomas involving the entire large and small bowel.

The gene responsible for familial adenomatous polyposis and Gardner syndrome was localized to chromosomal region 5q21 by cytogenetic and linkage analysis. A candidate gene, called *APC*, has been cloned and shown to be altered in the germ line of those with familial adenomatous polyposis and families with Gardner syndrome as well as in sporadic tumors, findings that strongly suggest that it is the gene responsible for these diseases. The *APC* gene encodes a 2,843-amino-acid protein whose amino terminus shows multiple sequence similarities to myosin, intermediate filaments, and plakoglobin, a cytoplasmic component of gap junctions. In addition, α-helical structures and heptad repeats (apolar-X-X-apolar-X-X-X) suggestive of regions that contribute to protein-protein interactions are present in the first 1,000 amino acids.[93] In fact, the first of these heptad repeats has recently been shown to be important for APC protein homodimer formation. Thus, it seems likely that the function of APC requires it to form homodimers or heterodimers in a coiled-coil arrangement, such as that seen with other structural proteins, including myosins, keratin, vimentin, and the nuclear lamins. Interestingly, a second gene on 5q, the mutated in colon carcinoma (*MCC*) gene, which is mutated in up to 55 percent of colorectal cancer patients, also contains these structures, and some investigators have suggested that the proteins may form heterodimers. However, much additional information is needed before the function of *APC* and its role in colorectal tumorigenesis is known.

DCC, *the Deleted in Colon Cancer Gene*

Allelic loss at chromosome 18q21 has been demonstrated by RFLP analysis in more than 70 percent of colorectal tumors and in 50 percent of late adenomas. Through the use of positional cloning techniques, a candidate gene (*DCC*) was isolated.[20] The gene encodes a 190-kd protein with the characteristics of a membrane-bound cell surface receptor that shows considerable homology to the neural cell adhesion molecule N-CAM. The protein contains a C-terminal cytoplasmic domain, a transmembrane hydrophobic domain, and an N-terminal extracellular domain that contains immunoglobulin and fibronectin homology regions. These characteristics suggest that *DCC* encodes a protein that may play a role in cell-cell or cell–extracellular matrix interactions. To date, no hereditary disease has been linked to a loss of *DCC* function. However, it likely has tumor suppressor function, given that introduction of a normal chromosome 18 into colorectal cell lines leads to loss of tumorigenic potential. Recent evidence suggests that the DCC protein may be involved in the process of differentiation. Colorectal tumors that have lost their capacity to differentiate into mucin-producing cells invariably lack expression of *DCC*.[94]

The Neurofibromatosis Type 2 Gene (NF-2)

Patients with neurofibromatosis type 1 present with neurofibromas involving the peripheral nervous system. A second type of heritable neurofibromatosis, neurofibromatosis type 2, has been characterized as a rare trait that is inherited in an autosomal dominant manner with incomplete penetrance. The hallmark of this disorder is the presence of central nervous system neurofibromas. Loss of the responsible gene predisposes affected individuals to acoustic nerve schwannomas, meningiomas, and gliomas. Neurofibromatosis type 2 was shown to be genetically distinct from neurofibromatosis type 1 when the gene responsible was mapped to chromosome 22q by cytogenetic and linkage analysis. The *NF-2* gene was cloned recently and shown to encode a 590-amino-acid phosphoprotein (called merlin or schwannomin). Merlin bears striking homology to members of the band 4.1 family of proteins that was originally detected in the erythrocyte membrane.[95] Evidence that the merlin gene is the responsible element in NF-2 disorder comes from the finding of *NF-2* germ line mutations in patients with neurofibromatosis type 2 and the observation of somatic mutations in sporadic schwannomas and meningiomas. Members of this family of proteins have been shown to stabilize spectrin-actin interactions in the cytoskeleton and to link the cytoskeleton to the plasma membrane. In addition, several members of the band 4.1 family have been shown to be phosphorylated on tyrosine residues, suggesting they may be involved in growth factor signaling pathways.[96] It will be interesting to see if the protein encoded by *NF-2* has a similar function.

von Hippel-Lindau Disease and Renal Cell Carcinoma

von Hippel-Lindau syndrome is a familial cancer syndrome that predisposes affected individuals to a variety of tumors, including hemangioblastomas of the retina and cerebellum, renal cell carcinoma, and pheochromocytoma. von Hippel-Lindau syndrome is an autosomal dominant disorder with almost complete penetrance that is seen in approximately one in 35,000 live births. Renal cell carcinoma is a prominent feature of this syndrome in 28 to 45 percent of affected individuals, and the kidney tumors tend to be multifocal and bilateral and to occur at a younger age than those of sporadic renal cell carcinoma. The *VHL* gene was localized to chromosome 3 at band p25 by linkage analysis and has been cloned.[97,98] Authentication of the cloned gene as the tumor suppressor responsible for the syndrome came from the demonstration of the inheritance of inactivating mutations in affected families and the detection of intragenic mutations in cell lines derived from sporadic renal cell carcinoma. The *VHL* gene appears to be expressed in all human tissues and is conserved throughout evolution from sea urchins to mammals.

The *VHL* gene encodes a 213-amino-acid protein that shows no significant homology to known proteins. Introduction of wild-type but not mutant *VHL* into renal carcinoma cells known to contain a *VHL* mutation inhibits their ability to form tumors in athymic mice.[99] Evidence suggests that a transcription elongation complex called elongin (SIII) is negatively regulated by the product of the *VHL* gene (pVHL). The elongin complex composed of a catalytic subunit, A, and two smaller subunits, B and C, which positively regulate the catalytic subunit, increases the rate of RNA polymerase II movement along the DNA template. In cells, elongin C in association with elongin B binds to elongin A.[100] pVHL competitively binds to the elongin B/C complex through a small linear domain it shares in common with elongin A.[101,102] Interestingly, this region of pVHL is frequently mutated in human tumors. The binding of pVHL to the elongin B/C complex disrupts elongin (SIII) function in vitro and suggests that regulation of elongin's transcriptional elongation activity by pVHL may be the basis of its tumor suppression function.

Tumor Suppressor Proteins and Maintenance of Genomic Integrity

The ability of a cell to repair DNA damage is paramount for the faithful transmission of the cell's genome from one generation to the next. We have seen that p53 is involved in the maintenance of genomic stability by inducing G_1 arrest when DNA is damaged and by allowing time for the cell to repair its DNA before progressing into the next replication cycle. This mechanism is aimed at limiting the propagation of heritable genetic errors. A common feature of cancer cells is their genomic instability, which is manifested by a myriad of abnormalities, including increased mutation rate, rearrangements, gene amplification, gross chromosomal defects, and even chromosomal loss. Therefore, it would not be surprising for loss of function of a DNA repair enzyme to present as a heritable trait that predisposes to a tumor syndrome, assuming that the enzyme defect were compatible with organismic viability.

Hereditary nonpolyposis colorectal cancer (HNPCC), or Lynch syndrome II, is characterized by the onset of tumors of the colon, ovary, breast, pancreas, endometrium, and stomach at an early age.[103] It is one of the commonest genetic syndromes that predisposes to cancer, affecting nearly one in 200 individuals in industrialized nations. HNPCC-linked colon cancers occur at multiple sites, typically in the proximal colon. This trait is inherited in an autosomal dominant manner and has been mapped to chromosome 2p by linkage analysis of large kindreds. An interesting feature of HNPCC tumors is the demonstration that they exhibit somatic alterations in repetitive "microsatellite" sequences that consist of dinucleotide or trinucleotide repeats found throughout the genome.[103] Similar phenomena were seen in a subset of sporadic, right-sided colon tumors, a finding that suggests that both heritable and sporadic tumors may have resulted from a molecular defect in DNA repair that manifests itself by replication errors (RER) in these microsatellites.

The first gene responsible for HNPCC was recently cloned and shown to be the human homolog of *mutS*, an *Escherichia coli* gene, and *MSH2*, a budding yeast gene. These genes encode proteins involved in the nucleotide mismatch repair pathway.[103,104] Authentication of the role of this gene (called *hMSH2*) in HNPCC was provided by the demonstration of *hMSH2* mutations, in the germ line of HNPCC kindreds, that segregate with the disease and by the finding of *hMSH2* mutations in both heritable and sporadic RER+ tumors. These effects of *hMSH2* mutations suggest that defects in the repair of mismatched nucleotides are linked to a future tumorigenic phenotype, perhaps by increasing the likelihood that certain tumor suppressor genes will be inactivated and oncogenes will be activated. Consistent with such a mechanism is the observation that colon tumors from patients with HNPCC contain mutations in the same genes (e.g., *APC*, *p53*, *ras*) as those found in sporadic colon tumors.[103] Given that tumors in patients with HNPCC also develop earlier in life than tumors in individuals without HNPCC, one can argue that somatic mutation rates are accelerated in these patients, thereby leading to an increase in the rate at which mutations in critical genes on the path toward tumor formation become clinically apparent.

Recently, it has been found that HNPCC may be caused by defects in other DNA repair genes. Linkage analysis of several HNPCC kindreds has revealed the disease to be linked to a gene on chromosome 3p21. Tumors from these families also exhibit dinucleotide repeat instability seen in other HNPCC kindreds with known *hMSH*2 mutations, a finding that suggests that a mutation in a second mismatch repair gene was a contributing factor in the pathogenesis of these particular tumors. The human homologue of the bacteria mismatch repair gene *mutL*, designated *hMLH*1, is located on chromosome 3p21, and it is specifically mutated in these HNPCC families.[105,106] In addition, two other homologues of the bacterial *mutL* gene, designated *hPMS*1 and *hPMS*2, have been cloned and have been found to be mutated in the germ line of certain patients with HNPCC.[107] In total, these results suggest HNPCC can result from mutations in one of several DNA mismatch repair genes.

Tumor Suppressor Genes and Breast Cancer Susceptibility

In industrialized nations, breast cancer develops in one in nine women by the ninth decade of life. Most of these cases are likely sporadic. However, it has long been observed that clustering of breast cancer occurs in certain families. Results of epidemiological studies suggest that hereditary factors that predispose a woman to an increased risk of the disease account for only a small number of all breast cancer cases, approximately five percent. However, hereditary factors may be responsible for as many as 25 percent of cases diagnosed before the age of 30.[108] Other primary tumors, most notably ovarian cancer, have also been found to arise in some of these breast cancer families.

The search for the gene or genes responsible for familial breast cancer advanced with the localization of a gene responsible for one form of breast cancer susceptibility on chromosome 17q21. This localization was accomplished by genetic linkage analysis of families with early-onset breast cancer.[109] Mutations in this gene, designated *BRCA*1, account for tumors in approximately 50 percent of families with overt susceptibility to breast cancer and in nearly 90 percent of families with susceptibility to both early-onset breast and ovarian cancer.[110] Recently, the *BRCA*1 gene has been isolated by analysis of mRNA sequences encoded by chromosome17q21 in individuals from kindreds marked by 17q-linked breast and ovarian cancer susceptibility.[111] The gene encodes a 1,863-amino-acid, ring-finger protein of unknown function. Interestingly, *BRCA*1 is not expressed solely in breast and ovarian tissue and is relatively abundant in testis, thymus, breast, ovary, and other organs. In this regard, it would not be unreasonable to suspect a linkage between the loss of *BRCA*1 function and the appearance of tumors in organs other than breast and ovary.

The evidence that a mutation of *BRCA*1 is, indeed, responsible for heightened susceptibility to breast and ovarian cancer is compelling. Initial evidence came from the observation of predisposing mutations in five of eight kindreds shown to demonstrate *BRCA*1 linkage.[111] Further support came from the observation of germ line mutations in four of 44 patients with putative sporadic breast or ovarian cancer.[112] A recent screen of 100 families with a history of multiple cases of breast and ovarian cancer revealed 31 cases of *BRCA*1 mutation, 22 of which were distinct.[113]

The Knudson hypothesis predicts that the remaining allele of a causative tumor suppressor gene for a given tumor contains an intragenic mutation, indicating inactivation of both alleles. The observation of allelic loss at 17q21 in many sporadic breast and ovarian cancers suggested that *BRCA*1 mutation would be involved in the cause of these tumors. Surprisingly, current data do not support this prediction. In a recent examination of 72 sporadic breast cancers and 21 ovarian cancers, nearly half of which demonstrated allelic loss of the *BRCA*1 region, only four of 44 tumors were found to contain mutations in the remaining *BRCA*1 allele, and all four of these proved to be germ line in nature.[112] These results suggest that *BRCA*1 may not play a major role in the development of most sporadic breast cancers and that yet another gene located at 17q21 might be involved through somatic mutation. *BRCA*1 mutation has been demonstrated in nearly one percent of women of Ashkenazi Jewish descent, a rate that is several times higher than the expected frequency in the general population.[114] It remains to be determined whether *BRCA*1 mutations in these individuals confer the same risk of breast and ovarian cancers as in individuals from high-risk families.

Linkage studies of breast cancer families have shown that *BRCA*1 is not linked to the disease in more than half of the cases. Recently, a new breast cancer susceptibility gene, *BRCA*2, has been localized to chromosome 13q12-13.[115] Mutation of *BRCA*2 is linked to an increased risk of early-onset

Table 3 Cloned Tumor Suppressor Genes and Their Functions

Cancer Syndrome	Gene	Primary Tumors	Cellular Location	Mode of Action
Li-Fraumeni	*p53*	Sarcomas, breast and brain tumors	Nucleus	Transcription factor/ regulator
Retinoblastoma	*Rb*	Retinoblastoma, osteosarcoma	Nucleus	Transcriptional regulator
Familial adenomatous polyposis	*APC*	Colon cancer	Cytoplasm	Unknown
Neurofibromatosis type 1	*NF-1*	Neurofibromas	Cytoplasm	$p21^{ras} \cdot$ GTPase activator
Neurofibromatosis type 2	*NF-2*	Schwannomas, meningiomas	Inner membrane	Cytoskeleton-membrane link
Wilms' Tumor	*WT-1*	Nephroblastoma	Nucleus	Transcription factor
von Hippel-Lindau	*VHL*	Renal cell carcinoma	Cytoplasm?	Inhibits transcription elongation
Familial breast cancer	*BRCA1*	Breast, ovary	Nucleus?	Transcription factor?
	BRCA2	Breast cancer	Unknown	Unknown
Colorectal cancer	*DCC*	Colon cancer	Membrane	Cell adhesion molecule
Familial melanoma	*p16*	Melanoma, many others	Nucleus	Cyclin-dependent kinase inhibitor
Hereditary nonpolyposis colon cancer	*hMSH2*	Colon cancer	Nucleus	Nucleotide mismatch repair
	hMLH1	Colon cancer	Nucleus	Nucleotide mismatch repair
	hPMS1	Colon cancer	Nucleus	Nucleotide mismatch repair
	hPMS2	Colon cancer	Nucleus	Nucleotide mismatch repair

breast cancer in women and to an increased risk of breast cancer in men. A candidate gene for *BRCA2* has been cloned and shown to contain germ line mutations that disrupt the open reading frame in six different breast cancer families.[116] The *BRCA2* gene encodes a 2,329-amino-acid protein that contains no sequence homology to known proteins. Thus, its function remains to be elucidated.

Future Directions

Tumor suppressor gene research has not only provided us with a better understanding of the genetic basis of cancer, it has also led to new insights into the events that control normal cell growth and proliferation. Despite the burst of knowledge during the past decade, the field of tumor suppressor gene research is still in its infancy. To date, relatively few tumor suppressor genes have been cloned [*see Table 3*], and our knowledge of the function of their protein products is highly limited. The techniques used to identify the retinoblastoma gene (e.g., LOH detection, RFLP analysis) have been applied to other familial cancers and have mapped another half dozen tumor suppressor loci whose genes have yet to be cloned. However, as Knudson pointed out, "the most common conditions are those that are mapped first, and it already appears that the remaining hereditary cancers will be so rare as to render linkage analysis difficult."[5] New approaches will be needed if most newly suspected tumor suppressor genes are to be discovered and cloned in the future.

The paradigm of tumor suppressor genes and the proteins they encode provides a new opportunity for cancer therapy research. For example, the development of drugs that either mimic tumor suppressor function or block downstream events elicited by the absence of function of a given tumor suppressor is, as might be expected, an active area of pharmaceutical research.

One does not, however, have to wait for the future to begin reaping the rewards of ongoing tumor suppressor gene research. Diagnostic tests with prognostic significance are already beginning to be used at the clinical level; for example, the presence of a mutant *p53* allele appears to correlate with increased relapse rate and decreased survival in node-negative breast cancer.[56] Presymptomatic diagnosis of predisposition of individuals in cancer families has, in several instances, identified those who require close surveillance and has relieved others of the psychological burden of fearing that they will develop cancer at an early age. In principle, the observation that the same genes are mutated in some familial and sporadic tumors of the same cell type may lead to the early detection of a healthy fraction of common tumors and to successful follow-up after primary tumor detection and removal.

References

1. Hofstra RMW, Landsvater RM, Ceccherini I, et al: A mutation in the RET proto-onco-gene associated with multiple endocrine neoplasia type 2B and sporadic medullary thyroid carcinoma. *Nature* 367:375, 1994

2. Eng C, Ponder BAJ: The role of gene mutations in the genesis of familial cancers. *FASEB J* 7:910, 1993

3. Klein G: Genes that can antagonize tumor development. *FASEB J* 7:821, 1993

4. Levine AJ: The tumor suppressor genes. *Annu Rev Biochem* 62:623, 1993

5. Knudson AG: Antioncogenes and human cancer. *Proc Natl Acad Sci USA* 90:10914, 1993

6. Weinberg RA: Tumor suppressor genes. *Science* 254:1138, 1991

7. Weinberg R: Tumor suppressor genes. *Neuron* 11:191, 1993

8. Harris H, Miller OJ, Klein G, et al: Suppression of malignancy by cell fusion. *Nature* 223:363, 1969

9. Klein G, Bregula U, Wiener F, et al: The analysis of malignancy by cell fusion. *J Cell Sci* 8:659, 1971

10. Anderson MJ, Stanbridge EJ: Tumor suppressor genes studied by cell hybridization and chromosome transfer. *FASEB J* 7:826, 1993

11. Stanbridge EJ, Flandermeyer RR, Daniels DW, et al: Specific chromosome loss associated with the expression of tumorigenicity in human cell hybrids. *Somatic Cell Mol Genet* 7:699, 1981

12. Benedict WF, Weissman BE, Mark C, et al: Tumorigenicity of human HT1080 fibrosarcoma X normal fibroblast hybrids: chromosome dosage dependency. *Cancer Res* 44:3471, 1984

13. Fournier REK, Ruddle FH: Microcell-mediated transfer of murine chromosomes into mouse, Chinese hamster, and human somatic cells. *Proc Natl Acad Sci USA* 74:319, 1977

14. Saxon PJ, Srivatsan ES, Leipzig GV, et al: Selective transfer of individual human chromosomes to recipient cells. *Mol Cell Biol* 5:140, 1985

15. Knudson AG Jr: Hereditary cancer, oncogenes, and antioncogenes. *Cancer Res* 45:1437, 1985

16. Yunis J, Ramsay N: Retinoblastoma and subband deletion of chromosome 13. *Am J Dis Child* 32:161, 1978

17. Balaban G, Gilbert F, Nichols W, et al: Abnormalities of chromosome 13 in retinoblastoma from individduals with normal constitutional karyotypes. *Cancer Genet Cytogenet* 6: 213, 1982

18. Hansen MF, Koufos A, Gallie BL, et al: Osteosarcoma and retinoblastoma: a shared chromosomal mechanism revealing recessive predisposition. *Proc Natl Acad Sci USA* 82:6216, 1985

19. Vogelstein B, Fearon ER, Hamilton SR, et al: Genetic alterations during colorectal-tumor development. *N Engl J Med* 319:525, 1988

20. Fearon ER, Cho KR, Nigro JM, et al: Identification of a chromosome 18q gene that is altered in colorectal cancers. *Science* 247:49, 1990

21. Lasko D, Cavenee W, Nordenskjold M: Loss of constitutional heterozygosity in human cancer. *Annu Rev Genet* 25:281, 1991

22. Xu G, O'Connell P, Viskochill D, et al: The neurofibromatosis type 1 gene encodes a protein related to GAP. *Cell* 62:599, 1990

23. Weissenbach J, Gyapay G, Dib C, et al: A second-generation linkage map of the human genome. *Nature* 359:794, 1992

24. DeMars R: *Fundamental Cancer Research: 23rd Annual Symposium.* Williams & Wilkins, Baltimore, 1970

25. Knudson AG Jr: Mutation and cancer: statistical study of retinoblastoma. *Proc Natl Acad Sci USA* 68:820, 1971

26. Sparkes RS, Murphree AL, Lingua RW, et al: Gene for hereditaryy retinoblastoma assigned to human chromosome 13 by linkage to esterase D. *Science* 219:971, 1983

27. Benedict WF, Murphree AL, Manerjee A, et al: Patient with chromosome 13 deletion: evidence that retinoblastoma gene is a recessisve cancer gene. *Science* 219:973, 1983

28. Dryja TP, Cavenee W, White R, et al: Homozygosity of chromosome 13 in retinoblastoma. *N Engl J. Med* 310:550, 1984

29. Cavenee WK, Dryja TP, Phillips RA, et al: Expression of recessive alleles by chromosomal mechanisms in retinoblastoma. *Nature* 305:779, 1983

30. Dryja TP, Rapaport JM, Joyce JM, et al: Molecular detection of deletions involving band q14 of chromosome 13 in retinoblastomas. *Proc Natl Acad Sci USA* 83:7391, 1986

31. Friend SH, Bernards R, Rogelj S, et al: A human DNA segment with properties of the gene that predisposes to retinoblastoma and osteosarcoma. *Nature* 323:643, 1986

32. Fung Y-KT, Murphree AL, T'Ang A, et al: Structural evidence for the authenticity of the

human retinoblastoma gene. *Science* 236:1657, 1987

33. Dunn JM, Phillips RA, Becker AJ, et al: Identification of germ line and somatic mutations affecting the retinoblastoma gene. *Science* 241:1797, 1988

34. Horowitz JM, Park S, Bogenmann E, et al: Frequent inactivation of the retinoblastoma anti-oncogene is restricted to a subset of human tumor cells. *Proc Natl Acad Sci USA* 87:2775, 1990

35. Kaye FJ, Kratzke RA, Gerster JL, et al: A single amino acid substitution results in a retinoblastoma protein defective in phosphorylation and oncoprotein binding. *Proc Natl Acad Sci USA* 87:6922, 1990

36. Huang H-JS, Yee J-K, Shew J-Y, et al: Suppression of the neoplastic phenotype by replacement of the RB gene in human cancer cells. *Science* 242:1563, 1988

37. Qin X-Q, Chittenden T, Livingston DM, et al: Identification of a growth suppression domain within the retinoblastoma gene product. *Genes Dev* 6:953, 1992

38. Hinds PW, Mittnacht S, Dulic V, et al: Regulation of retinoblastoma protein functions by ectopic expression of human cyclins. *Cell* 70:993, 1992

39. Hunter T, Pines J: Cyclins and cancer II: cyclin d and cdk inhibitors come of age. *Cell* 79:573, 1994

40. Whyte P, Buchkovich KJ, Horowitz JM, et al: Association between an oncogene and an antioncogene: the adenovirus E1A proteins bind to the retinoblastoma gene product. *Nature* 334:124, 1988

41. DeCaprio JA, Ludlow JW, Figge J, et al: SV40 large T antigen forms a specific complex with the product of the retinoblastoma susceptibility gene. *Cell* 54:275, 1988

42. Dyson N, Howley PM, Munger K, et al: The human papilloma virus-16 E7 oncoprotein is able to bind to the retinoblastoma gene product. *Science* 243:934, 1989

43. Chen S, Paucha E: Identification of a region of simian virus 40 large T antigen required for cell transformation. *J Virol* 64:3350, 1990

44. Whyte P, Ruley HE, Harlow E: Two regions of the adenovirus early region 1A proteins are required for transformation. *J Virol* 62:257, 1988

45. DeCaprio JA, Ludlow JW, Lynch D, et al: The product of the retinoblastoma susceptibility gene has properties of a cell cycle regulatory element. *Cell* 58:1085, 1989

46. Buchkovich K, Duffy LA, Harlow E: The retinoblastoma protein is phosphorylated during specific phases of the cell cycle. *Cell* 58:1097, 1989

47. Chen P, Scully P, Shew J, et al: Phosphorylation of the retinoblastoma gene product is modulated during the cell cycle and cellular differentiation. *Cell* 58:1193, 1989

48. Ludlow JW, DeCaprio JA, Huang C, et al: SV40 large T antigen binds preferentially to an underphosphorylated member of the retinoblastoma susceptibility gene product family. *Cell* 56:57, 1989

49. Ludlow JW, Shon J, Pipas JM, et al: The retinoblastoma susceptibility gene product undergoes cell cycle-dependent dephosphorylation and binding to and release from SV40 large T. *Cell* 60:387, 1990

50. Ewen ME, Sluss HK, Sherr CJ, et al: Functional interactions of the retinoblastoma protein with mammalian D-type cyclins. *Cell* 73:487, 1993

51. Laiho M, DeCaprio JA, Ludlow JW, et al: Growth inhibition by TGF-β linked to suppression of retinoblastoma protein phosphorylation. *Cell* 62:175, 1990

52. Ewen ME, Sluss HK, Whitehouse LL, et al: TGFβ1 inhibition of cdk4 synthesis is linked to cell cycle arrest. *Cell* 74:1009-1020, 1993

53. Nevins JR: E2F: A link between the Rb tumor suppressor protein and viral oncoproteins. *Science* 258:424, 1992

54. Werness BA, Levine AJ, Howley PM: Association of human papillomavirus types 16 and 18 E6 proteins with p53. *Science* 248:76, 1990

55. Barak Y, Oren M: Enhanced binding of a 95 KDa protein to p53 in cells undergoing p53-mediated growth arrest. *EMBO J* 11:2115, 1992

56. Harris CC, Hollstein M: Clinical implications of the p53 tumor-suppressor gene. *N Engl J Med* 329:1318, 1993

57. Cho Y, Gorina S, Jeffrey PD, et al: Crystal structure of a p53 tumor suppressor-DNA complex: understanding tumorigenic mutations. *Science* 265:346, 1994

58. Michalovitz D, Halevy O, Oren M: Conditional inhibition of transformation and of cell proliferation by a temperature-sensitive mutant of p53. *Cell* 62:671, 1990

59. Martinez J, Georgeoff I, Martinez J, et al: Cellular localization and cell cycle regulation by a temperature-sensitive p53 protein. *Genes Dev* 5:151, 1991

60. Levine AJ, Momand J, Finlay CA: The p53 tumor suppressor gene. *Nature* 351:453, 1991

61. Malkin D, Li FP, Strong LC, et al: Germ line p53 mutations in a familial syndrome of breast cancer, sarcomas, and other neoplasms. *Science* 250:1233, 1990

62. Yew PR, Berk AJ: Inhibition of p53 transactivation required for transformation by adenovirus early E1B protein. *Nature* 357:82, 1992

63. el-Deiry WS, Tokino T, Velculescu VE, et al: WAF1, a potential mediator of p53 tumor suppression. *Cell* 75:817, 1993

64. Harper JW, Adami GR, Wei N, et al: The p21 cdk-interacting protein CIP1 is a potent inhibitor of G1 cyclin-dependent kinases. *Cell* 75:805, 1993

65. Kastan MB, Zhan Q, el-Deiry WS, et al: A mammalian cell cycle checkpoint pathway utilizing p53 and GADD45 is defective in ataxia-telangiectasia. *Cell* 71:587, 1992

66. Lowe SW, Ruley HE, Jacks T, et al: p53-dependent apoptosis modulates the cytotoxicity of anticancer agents. *Cell* 74:957, 1993

67. Lane D: p53, guardian of the genome. *Nature* 358:15, 1992

68. Momand J, Zambetti GP, Olson DC, et al: The mdm-2 oncogene product forms a complex with the p53 protein and inhibits p53-mediated transactivation. *Cell* 69:1237, 1992

69. Cahilly-Snyder L, Yang-Feng T, Francke U, et al: Molecular analysis and chromosomal mapping of amplified genes isolated from a transformed mouse 3T3 cell line. *Somat Cell Mol Genet* 13:235, 1987

70. Oliner JD, Kinzler KW, Meltzer PS, et al: Amplification of a gene encoding a p53-associated protein in human sarcomas. *Nature* 358:80, 1992

71. Serrano M, Hannon G, Beach D: A new regulatory motif in cell-cycle control causing specific inhibition of cyclin D/CDK4. *Nature* 366:704, 1993

72. Kamb A, Gruis N, Weaver-Feldhaus J, et al: A cell cycle regulator potentially involved in genesis of many tumor types. *Science* 264:436, 1994

73. Nobori T, Miura K, Wu D, et al: Deletions of the cyclin-dependent kinase-4 inhibitor gene in multiple human cancers. *Nature* 368:753, 1994

74. Mori T, Miura K, Aoki T, et al: Frequent somatic mutation of the MTS1/CDK4I (multiple tumor suppressor/cyclin-dependent kinase 4 inhibitor) gene in esophageal squamous cell carcinoma. *Cancer Res* 54:3396, 1994

75. Serrano M, Gomez-Lahoz E, DePinho RA, et al: Inhibition of ras-induced proliferation and cellular transformation by p16INK4. *Science* 267:249, 1995

76. Lukas J, Parry D, Aagaard L, et al: Retinoblastoma-protein-dependent cell-cycle inhibition by the tumor suppressor p16. *Nature* 375:503, 1995

77. Koh J, Enders G, Dynlacht BD, et al: Tumor-derived p16 alleles encoding proteins defective in cell-cycle inhibition. *Nature* 375:505, 1995

78. Medema R, Herrera R, Lam F, et al: Growth suppression by p16ink4 requires functional retinoblastoma protein. *Proc Natl Acad Sci USA* 92:6289, 1995

79. Serrano M, Lee H-W, Chin L, et al: Role of the INK4a locus in tumor suppression and cell mortality. *Cell* 85:27, 1996

80. Hannon GJ, Beach D: p15INK4B is a potential effector of TGF-β-induced cell cycle arrest. *Nature* 371:257-261, 1994

81. Guan K-L, Jenkins CW, Li Y, et al: Growth suppression by p18, a p16 INK4/MTS1 and p14 INK4B/MTS1-related CDK6 inhibitor, correlates with wild-type pRB function. *Genes Dev* 8:2939, 1994

82. Knudson AG, Strong LC: Mutation and cancer: a model for Wilms' tumor of the kidney. *J Natl Cancer Inst* 48:313, 1972

83. Weissman BE, Saxon PJ, Pasquale SR, et al: Introduction of a normal chromosome 11 into a Wilms' tumor cell line controls its tumorigenic expression. *Science* 236:175, 1987

84. Lichter P, Tang CJ, Call K, et al: High-resolution mapping of human chromosome 11 by in situ hybridization with cosmid clones. *Science* 247:64, 1990

85. Coppes MJ, Cambell CE, Williams BRG: The role of WT1 in Wilms tumorigenesis. *FASEB J* 7:886, 1993

86. Rauscher FJ III: The WT1 Wilms tumor gene product: a developmentally regulated transcription factor in the kidney that functions as a tumor suppressor. *FASEB J* 7:896, 1993

87. Madden SL, Cook DM, Morris JF, et al: Transcriptional repression mediated by the WT1 tumor gene product. *Science* 253:1550, 1991

88. Maheswaran S, Englert C, Bennett P, et al: The WT1 gene product stabilizes p53 and inhibits p53-mediated apoptosis. *Genes Dev* 9:2143, 1995.

89. Viskochil D, White R, Cawthon R: The neurofibromatosis type 1 gene. *Annu Rev Neurosci* 16:183, 1993

90. DeClue JE, Papageorge AG, Fletcher JA, et al: Abnormal regulation of mammalian p21^{ras} contributes to malignant tumor growth in von Recklinghausen (type 1) neurofibromatosis. *Cell* 69:265, 1992

91. Johnson MR, DeClue JE, Felzmann S, et al: Neurofibromin can inhibit ras-dependent growth by a mechanism independent of its GTPase-accelerating function. *Mol Cell Biol* 14:641, 1994

92. Skuse G, Kosciolek B, Rowley P: The neurofibroma in von Recklinghausen neurofibromatosis has a unicellular origin. *Am J Hum Genet* 49:600, 1991

93. Groden J, Thliveris A, Samowitz W, et al: Identification and characterization of the familial adenomatous polyposis coli gene. *Cell* 66:589, 1991

94. Hedrick L, Cho KR, Fearon ER, et al: The DCC gene product in cellular differentiation and colorectal tumorigenesis. *Genes Dev* 8:1174, 1994

95. Trofatter JA, MacCollin MM, Rutter JL, et al: A novel moesin-, ezrin- radixin-like gene is a candidate for the neurofibromatosis 2 tumor suppressor. *Cell* 72:791, 1993

96. Fazioli F, Wong WT, Ullrich SJ, et al: The ezrin-like family of tyrosine kinase substrates: receptor-specific pattern of tyrosine phosphorylation and relationship to malignant transformation. *Oncogene* 8:1335, 1993

97. Latif F, Tory K, Gnarra J, et al: Identification of the von Hippel-Lindau disease tumor suppressor gene. *Science* 260:1317, 1993

98. Linehan WM, Lerman MI, Zbar B: Identification of the von Hippel-Lindau (VHL) Gene. *JAMA* 273:564, 1995

99. Iliopoulos O, Kibel a, Gray s, et al: Tumour suppression by the human von Hippel-Lindau gene product. *Nature Med* 1:822, 1995

100. Aso T, Lane WS, Conaway JW, et al: Elongin (SIII): a multisubunit regulator of elongation by RNA polymerase II. *Science* 269:1439, 1995

101. Duan DR, Pause A, Burgess WH, et al: Inhibition of transcription elongation by the VHL tumor suppressor protein. *Science* 269:1402, 1995

102. Kibel A, Iliopoulos O, DeCaprio JA, et al: Binding of the von Hippel-Lindau tumor supressssor protein to elongin B and C. Science 269, 1444, 1995

103. Leach FS, Nicolaides NC, Papadopoulos N, et al: Mutations of a mutS homolog in hereditary nonpolyposis colorectal cancer. *Cell* 75:1215, 1993

104. Fishel R, Lescoe MK, Rao MRS, et al: The human mutator gene homolog MSH2 and its association with hereditary nonpolyposis colon cancer. *Cell* 75:1027, 1993

105. Bronner CE, Baker SM, Morrison PT, et al: Mutation in the DNA mismatch repair gene homologue hMLH1 is associated with hereditary non-polyposis colon cancer. *Nature* 368:258, 1994

106. Papadopoulos N, Nicolaides NC, Wei Y, et al: Mutation of a mutL homolog in hereditary colon cancer. *Science* 263:1625, 1994

107. Nicolaides NC, Papadopoulos N, Liu B, et al: Mutations of two PMS homologues in hereditary nonpolyposis colon cancer. *Nature* 371:75, 1994

108. Claus EB, Risch N, Thompson WD: Genetic analysis of breast cancer in the cancer and steroid hormone study. *Am J Hum Genet* 48:232, 1991

109. Hall JM, Lee MK, Newman B, et al: Linkage of early-onset familial breast cancer to chromosome 17q21. *Science* 250:1684, 1990

110. Easton DF, Bishop DT, Ford D, et al: Genetic linkage analysis in familial breast and ovarian cancer: results from 214 families. The Breast Cancer Linkage Consortium. *Am J Hum Genet* 52:678, 1993

111. Miki Y, Swensen J, Shattuck ED, et al: A strong candidate for the breast and ovarian cancer susceptibility gene BRCA1. *Science* 266:66, 1994

112. Futreal PA, Liu Q, Shattuck-Eidens D, et al: BRCA1 mutations in primary breast and ovarian carcinomas. *Science* 266:120, 1994

113. Friedman LS, Ostermeyer EA, Szabo CI, et al: Confirmation of BRCA1 by analysis of germ line mutations linked to breast and ovarian cancer in ten families. *Nature Genet* 8:399, 1994

114. Struewing JP, Abeliovich D, Peretz T, et al: The carrier frequency of the BRCA1 185delAG mutation is approximately 1 percent in Ashkenazi Jewish individuals. *Nature Genet* 11:198, 1995

115. Wooster R, Neuhausen SL, Mangion J, et al: Localization of a breast cancer susceptibility gene, BRCA2, to chromosome 13q12-13. *Science* 265:2088, 1994

116. Wooster R, Bignell G, Lancaster J, et al: Identification of the breast cancer gene *BRCA2*. *Nature* 378:789, 1995

Acknowledgments

Figure 1   Talar Agasyan.
Figure 2   Dimitry Schidlovsky.

CHAPTER 7

Genetic Lesions in Human Cancer

Eric R. Fearon, M.D., Ph.D.

Human cancer has long been hypothesized to have a genetic basis. However, only over the past two decades has direct evidence been obtained to support this proposal. A widely held consensus is that cancers arise through a multistep evolutionary process that is driven by mutation of cellular genes and clonal selection of variant progeny that have increasingly aggressive growth properties. The targets for these mutations are proto-oncogenes, tumor suppressor genes, and DNA repair genes. A relatively small subset of the mutations may be present in the germ line of individuals and may predispose to various cancer types. Most of the mutations that contribute to the cancer cell phenotype, however, are of somatic origin and hence are present only in the neoplastic cells of patients.

The relationship between proto-oncogenes and oncogenes, as well as their functions, was reviewed in Chapters 4 and 5, and the identification and function of various tumor suppressor genes were reviewed in Chapter 6. Recent studies have highlighted the critical role of mutations that involve a third class of genes in the cancer process—the DNA repair genes. Like the tumor suppressor genes, these genes are targeted by loss-of-function mutations. However, the DNA repair genes differ in their normal functions from the tumor suppressor genes in critical ways. The protein products of some tumor suppressor gene products may transduce growth-inhibitory signals or may induce differentiation responses. Other tumor suppressor gene products may mediate programmed cell death (apoptosis) after DNA damage or cell cycle perturbations. Inactivation of DNA repair genes probably does not directly affect the normal processes that control growth. Rather, their inactivation appears to result in an increased rate of mutations in other cellular genes, including proto-oncogenes and tumor suppressor genes. Because the accumulation of mutations in these two classes of growth-regulating genes appears to be the rate-limiting step in tumorigenesis, DNA repair gene inactivation greatly accelerates the process of tumor progression.

It is not possible to elaborate all of the mutations that have been identified in human tumor cell genomes. Rather, the primary goals of this chapter are twofold: to summarize past and present strategies for the identification of genetic lesions in human cancers and to review the proto-oncogenes, tumor suppressor, and DNA repair genes that are frequently mutated in human tumors. The focus of this chapter is on how the emerging knowledge of genetic lesions in human tumors has led to new and powerful insights into the pathogenesis and biologic behavior of cancer.

Strategies for the Identification of Genetic Lesions in Human Cancer

Oncogene Identification

Gene transfer techniques have been a particularly powerful means for discovering a small number of tumor-associated oncogenes, particularly activated alleles of the *ras* gene family [*see Chapter 4*].[1,2] Nevertheless, despite the successes of these techniques in identifying novel oncogenic alleles in human cancer, problems existed with the approach, including its labor-intensive nature. Moreover, many of the alleles identified were generated by point mutations or DNA rearrangements occurring during the in vitro manipulation of the tumor-derived DNA and did not actually exist in the cancers from which the DNA was prepared.

The nonrandom chromosomal translocations frequently observed in leukemias, lymphomas, and other tumors have proved to be a rich source for the identification of oncogenes.[1,3] Many of the translocations are characteristic of particular tumor types and even of specific histopathologic subtypes. In many hematopoietic and lymphoid neoplasms, the chromosomal abnormalities involve juxtaposition of an immunoglobulin (*Ig*) or T cell receptor (*TCR*) locus with novel gene sequences.[3] The proximity of the novel gene to well-characterized *Ig* or *TCR* sequences has also often allowed rapid cloning and identification of the activated proto-oncogene.

Other translocations do not involve *Ig* and *TCR* locus sequences but may nonetheless deregulate proto-oncogene expression.[3] These translocations also generate chimeric oncogenes by fusing sequences from one side of the translocation breakpoint to sequences on the other side of the breakpoint. In many cases, the chimeric oncogenes have been identified because they contain sequences from cellular homologues of v-*onc* genes or from proto-oncogenes targeted by other activation mechanisms in cancer. In other cases, in which known proto-oncogenes are not found to be affected by the chromosomal translocation, chromosome microdissection techniques and positional cloning approaches have been needed for the identification of the novel chimeric oncogene. Fluorescence in situ hybridization–based techniques and polymerase chain reaction (PCR)–based methodology are expected to increasingly supplant conventional cytogenetic and positional cloning approaches in the search for proto-oncogenes activated by chromosomal translocations.

Amplification of DNA can also activate proto-oncogenes.[1,2] Several hundred thousand base pairs of flanking DNA sequences are often coamplified with the proto-oncogene; the entire amplified unit is referred to as an amplicon. The amplicons, often manifested in karyotypic analyses as extrachromosomal elements termed double-minute chromosomes or as novel banding regions termed homogeneously staining regions on chromosomes, may be present in as many several hundred copies per cell. In some tumors, more than one proto-oncogene may be contained in the amplified sequences. In many cases, the amplified proto-oncogenes represent cellular homologues of v-*onc* genes or proto-oncogenes targeted by other activation mechanisms in cancer, although powerful recombinant DNA techniques are now available for the identification of novel proto-oncogenes amplified in human cancers.

Identification of Tumor Suppressor Genes

The identification of oncogenic alleles in human tumors has been greatly facilitated by several of their features, including the prior identification of the v-*onc* genes, the ability of some oncogenes to generate tumorigenic properties when transferred to nontumorigenic recipient cells, and the molecular cloning and characterization of novel oncogene sequences at translocation breakpoints. By contrast, the direct identification of tumor suppressor genes has proved to be far more difficult.[1] Functional strategies for their identification have many practical problems. For example, although the successful transfer of a functional copy of tumor suppressor gene to a tumor cell might be expected to revert aspects of its phenotype, such as its anchorage-independent growth, contact inhibition, or altered morphology, the identification of such reverted cells in the midst of a background of fully transformed cells has proved to be a particularly arduous experimental task. Hence, the strategies for the identification of tumor suppressor genes and the specific mutations present in these genes in human cancers have been somewhat more circuitous.

Among the strategies that have been successfully applied to tumor suppressor gene localization are cytogenetic studies for the identification of deletions in the normal or tumor cells of patients with cancer, loss of heterozygosity (LOH) or allelic loss studies of human tumors, and DNA linkage approaches for the localization of genes involved in the inherited predisposition to cancer. All of these approaches ultimately require positional cloning strategies for the identification and isolation of tumor suppressor genes from the chromosomal region. Although aspects of tumor suppressor gene localization strategies were discussed in Chapter 6, because of the general importance of these strategies to tumor suppressor gene discovery in human cancer, several aspects of the approaches are also emphasized here.

Cytogenetic studies have often been critical to the initial localization of tumor suppressor genes. The rationale for such an approach is that chromosomal deletions, as well as some translocations, might be predicted to inactivate one of the two copies of a tumor suppressor gene. Although chromosomal abnormalities in tumors are common, the sheer number and complexity of the chromosomal aberrations in many cancers has been an obstacle to deciphering the identity of the chromosomes involved and to determining the significance of any one observation. In contrast, although only a very small subset of cancer patients have been found to harbor gross chromosomal abnormalities in their normal cells, when noted, the anomalies have proved to be extremely valuable for highlighting particular regions that are likely to contain tumor suppressor genes. In a small number of patients with retinoblastoma, cytogenetic studies of peripheral blood lymphocytes or skin fibroblasts have revealed interstitial deletions involving band q14 of chromosome 13.[4] Patients with the constellation of findings termed WAGR (Wilms' tumor, aniridia, genitourinary abnormalities, and mental retardation) have often been found to have interstitial deletions of chromosome 11p13.[5] In addition, cytogenetic studies of a mentally retarded man with hundreds of adenomatous intestinal polyps revealed that the patient had an interstitial deletion involving chromosome 5q and suggested that mutant alleles of a gene that predisposed to these polyps might map to chromosome 5q.[6] Furthermore, in some cancer patients, balanced translocations have been noted, such as those involving chromosome 17q in a subset of patients with neurofibromatosis type 1, suggesting the presence of the NF-1 gene on this chromosome.[7,8]

Nevertheless, although recurrent constitutional deletions of specific chromosomal regions in patients with a particular type of cancer provide compelling evidence that a tumor predisposition gene may reside there, isolation of the tumor predisposition gene ultimately requires much additional work. Moreover, the identification of a single cancer patient with a constitutional deletion of a particular chromosomal region, such as the patient with the chromosome 5q deletion and polyposis, does not alone constitute definitive proof that a tumor predisposition gene maps to the region. In such cases, linkage analysis must be used to document the fact that genetic markers from the implicated chromosomal region cosegregate with the inheritance of the disease phenotype in numerous large, multigenerational kindreds with a specific inherited cancer syndrome. Although linkage analysis can pinpoint the region that contains the tumor suppressor gene to a domain much smaller than a chromosomal band, identification of the tumor suppressor gene ultimately requires positional cloning approaches and detailed mutational analyses. In several cancer syndromes, including familial polyposis and von Hippel-Lindau syndrome, localization and eventual identification of each of the tumor suppressor genes was greatly aided by the fact that some patients had interstitial chromosomal deletions that although not detectable in conventional cytogenetic analysis, were readily detectable by such techniques as pulsed-field electrophoresis.[9-11]

Genetic analysis of somatically mutated alleles of a candidate suppressor gene can supplement and reinforce the information derived from analysis of germ line mutations. One of the most fruitful approaches has been the determination of whether the chromosomal region carrying a putative cancer-predisposing gene is affected somatically by LOH.[12,13] The relevance of LOH to the cancer process is that inactivation of the remaining normal copy of a predisposition/tumor suppressor gene often results from a discarding (i.e., LOH) of a sizable portion of the chromosomal arm carrying the gene [see Chapter 6]. Hence, LOH affects not only the suppressor gene but also many linked marker genes. Identification of LOH events affecting the chromosomal region that carries a tumor predisposition gene in many independent tumor samples implies that the predisposition gene is likely to function as a tumor suppressor gene. Moreover, both copies of the tumor suppressor gene may also be inactivated by somatic mutations in sporadic cancers with LOH of the chromosomal region.

Although some tumor suppressor genes are inactivated by both germ line and somatic mutations, others may contribute to tumor development only as a result of somatic mutations. LOH analysis might be used for the identification and localization of these suppressor genes as well. Unfortunately, in most cases, LOH may affect many or all of the markers on a particular chromosomal arm. For this reason, precise localization of a tumor suppressor gene is difficult to achieve by LOH analysis alone. Candidate tumor suppressor genes from several chromosomal regions frequently targeted by LOH, but for which no inherited tumor predisposition syndrome has been localized, remain to be identified.[13] Among these is a gene or genes on 10q in prostate cancers and gliomas; on 8p in colorectal, breast, prostate, and other cancers; and 1p in neuroblastomas, colorectal cancer, and numerous other tumors.

Oncogene Lesions in Human Cancer

More than 50 proto-oncogenes have been identified through many experimental approaches [*see Chapter 4*]. Nevertheless, most of these 50 genes were discovered in experimental models of cancer, often involving animal retroviruses, and only a subset of such proto-oncogenes are actually activated by somatic mutations in human cancer. Only the most common and instructive oncogenic alleles seen in human cancers are reviewed in this chapter. Examples of oncogene activation by point mutation (H-*ras*, K-*ras*, and N-*ras*), chromosomal translocation (*myc*, *bcl*-2, *CYCD*1, *E2A-pbx*1, and *bcr-abl*), and gene amplification (*myc*, N-*myc*, L-*myc*, *neu*, *EGFR*, and *CYCD*1) are discussed. Somatic mutations in oncogenes that are commonly seen in various human cancers are summarized in Table 1. The germ line mutations that confer cancer susceptibility are typically tumor suppressor and DNA repair gene defects [*see Chapter 6*]. Only one proto-oncogene, *ret*, has been found to be mutated in the germ line of those with inherited predisposition to cancer.[14]

Point Mutations: ras

Three human *ras* genes exist: H-*ras* on chromosome 11p, K-*ras* on 12q, and N-*ras* on 1p [*see Chapters 4 and 5*]. Only a very limited subset of the possible mutations that could arise in the *ras* genes are seen in human cancers. To date, only codons 12, 13, and 61 have been found to be mutated in human tumors.[15,16] These sites appear to be the most effective in activating the transforming activity of the Ras protein. This observation implies that in the screening for mutant *ras* alleles in human tumor samples, only a few *ras* gene codons need be screened for mutations. PCR-based methods are now routinely used to determine whether tumor specimens harbor mutant *ras* alleles, and one such strategy is outlined in Figure 1. Mutations in K-*ras* are much more commonly seen in human cancers than are mutations in H-*ras*

Table 1   Representative Oncogenic Alleles in Human Cancers

Gene	Activation Mechanism	Protein Properties	Tumor Type
K-*ras*	Point mutation	p21 GTPase	Pancreatic, colorectal, lung, and other cancers, leukemia
N-*ras*	Point mutation	p21 GTPase	Myeloid leukemia
H-*ras*	Point mutation	p21 GTPase	Bladder and other cancers
EGFR (*erb-b*)	Amplification, rearrangement	Growth factor receptor	Gliomas, carcinomas
neu (*erb-b*2)	Amplification	Growth factor receptor	Breast, ovarian, and other carcinomas
myc	Chromosome translocation, amplification	Transcription factor	Burkitt's lymphoma, small cell lung cancer (SCCL) and other cancers
N-*myc*	Amplification	Transcription factor	Neuroblastoma, SCCL
L-*myc*	Amplification	Transcription factor	SCCL
bcl-2	Chromosome translocation	Antiapoptosis protein	B cell lymphoma (follicular type)
CYCD1	Amplification, chromosome translocation	Cyclin D (G_1 phase?)	Breast and other cancers, B cell lymphoma, parathyroid adenomas
bcr-abl	Chromosome translocation	Chimeric nonreceptor tyrosine kinase	CML, ALL (T cell)
ret	Rearrangement	Chimeric receptor tyrosine kinase	Thyroid cancer (papillary)
trk	Rearrangement	Chimeric receptor tyrosine kinase	Colorectal cancer
hst	Amplification	Growth factor (FGF-like)	Gastric cancer
APL-RARa	Chromosome translocation	Chimeric transcription factor	Acute promyelocytic leukemia
*E2A-pbx*1	Chromosome translocation	Chimeric transcription factor	Pre–B cell ALL
MDM2	Amplification	p53 binding protein (nuclear)	Sarcomas
gli	Amplification	Transcription factor	Sarcomas, gliomas
ttg	Chromosome translocation	Transcription factor	T cell ALL
Cdk4	Amplification	Cyclin-dependent kinase	Sarcomas

GTPase—guanosine triphosphatase; FGF—fibroblast growth factor; CML—chronic myelogenous leukemia; ALL—acute lymphocytic leukemia.

or N-*ras*. K-*ras* mutations are present in about 50 percent of colorectal cancers, 75 to 90 percent of pancreatic cancers, 30 percent of lung adenocarcinomas, and 20 to 25 percent of endometrial cancers.[16] Codon 12 is the target of most mutations, but codons 13 and 61 are mutated in some tumors. The N-*ras* gene is mutated in about 25 to 30 percent of acute nonlymphocytic leukemias and very infrequently in epithelial cancers, such as colorectal cancer. H-*ras* is mutated in about 10 to 15 percent of bladder cancers and infrequently in some other epithelial cancers, including breast and prostate cancer.[16]

The relationship of *ras* gene mutations to various steps of tumor development has been most extensively studied in colorectal tumors.[17] A sizable body of clinical and histopathologic evidence indicates that most colorectal carcinomas arise from adenomatous polyps. Furthermore, adenomatous polyps greater than 1 cm in diameter or with more marked abnormalities in cellular architecture (i.e., high-grade dysplasia) are more likely to progress to cancer than are adenomas lacking these features. About 50 percent of colorectal carcinomas and a similar percentage of adenomas that are greater than 1 cm in diameter or that have high-grade dysplasia have been found to have K-*ras* mutations. Fewer than 10 percent of adenomas that are less than 1 cm in diameter or that have low-grade dysplasia have been found to have K-*ras* mutations. Hence, K-*ras* gene mutations may be responsible for the progression of small adenomas to larger and more aggressive adenomas. Finally, *ras* mutations appear to have clinical significance when they are present in some tumors. About 30 percent of lung adenocarcinomas have mutant K-*ras* alleles, and patients whose tumors have a mutant K-*ras* allele have a poorer prognosis than those patients whose tumors do not have a mutant K-ras allele.[18] Unfortunately, no definitive evidence indicates that *ras* mutation status is related to prognosis in other cancers.

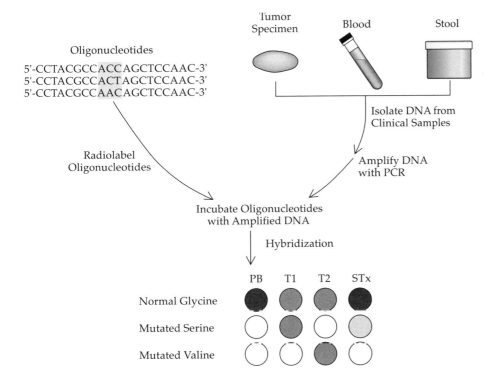

Figure 1 K-ras *mutation detection by allele-specific oligonucleotide hybridization. DNA is isolated from a tumor specimen (T1 or T2), a blood sample (PB), or a stool specimen (ST). To greatly increase the sensitivity of the detection of mutations, the K-ras gene sequence of interest is amplified with respect to its copy number in total DNA by use of the polymerase chain reaction (PCR). The amplified DNA preparations are then spotted onto nylon filters and hybridized with a series of radiolabeled oligonucleotides that specifically recognize either the normal glycine codon (ACC) at K-ras codon 12 or single base pair substitutions that would result in a mutated serine codon (ACT) or mutated valine codon (AAC). The oligonucleotide detecting the normal glycine codon hybridizes to DNA from all four samples tested. The oligonucleotide detecting the serine mutation at codon 12 hybridizes to DNA from T1 and ST, and the oligonucleotide detecting the valine mutation hybridizes to DNA from T2. Although only two examples are shown, oligonucleotides specific for all possible amino acid substitutions at the* ras *codon under study can be prepared.*

Chromosomal Translocations: myc, bcl-*2,* CYCD*1, and* bcr-abl

Although chromosomal translocations that activate oncogenes have been studied extensively in leukemias, lymphomas, and some solid tumors, including Ewing's sarcoma and rhabdomyosarcoma, little is known about the role of translocations in most epithelial cancers.[1,3] This lack of information may reflect the fact that translocations arise more frequently in the cells that give rise to the former group of tumors, perhaps because of defective somatic recombination events mediated by the immunoglobulin–T cell receptor (Ig-TCR) recombinase enzymes in B and T cells. However, the apparent increased frequency of translocation detection in leukemias, lymphomas, and some pediatric solid tumors may also reflect the fact that these malignancies can be induced to divide in culture more readily than can many adult solid tumors, thereby yielding the metaphase chromosomes that are essential for most types of karyotypic analysis.

Among the genes activated by juxtaposition with the *Ig* and *TCR* loci are *myc*, *bcl*-1 (also known as *PRAD*1, cyclin D1, or *CYCD*1), and *bcl*-2.[3] Other genes activated in particular subsets of lymphoid tumors include genes that encode transcription factors, such as *ttg*-1, *ttg*-2, *lyl*-1, *hox*-11, *bcl*-6, and *tal*-1 [*see Table 2*].[3] Perhaps the common theme in these genes is that many are normally expressed in a tissue-specific fashion, such as in neural tissues or the developing embryo. Instead of being expressed in a tissue-specific fashion or in response to particular physiologic stimuli, their expression in affected cells is now constant and often excessive. Such deregulation of their expression presumably leads to inappropriate expression of other cellular genes and, ultimately, defects in the proliferation and/or differentiation of the affected lymphoid cells. Finally, some of the genes, such as *tal*-1, can apparently be activated by Ig-TCR recombinase–mediated chromosomal translocations that, although they do not affect *Ig* or *TCR* locus sequences, involve genomic sequences bearing similarity to the Ig-like consensus[3,19]

The analysis of translocations involving *myc* provided the first molecular evidence for activation of a proto-oncogene by chromosomal translocation [see *Chapter 4*]. In brief, translocations involving the *myc* gene on chromosome 8 and one of the *Ig* loci are of three types.[3] Roughly 80 percent of cases involve translocation between *myc* sequences and *Ig* heavy-chain locus sequences on chromosome 14q. The remainder involve translocations between *myc* and *Ig* light-chain sequences on chromosomes 2p or 22q. The translocations between the *myc* and *Ig* loci are associated with a fairly heterogeneous group of B cell neoplasms, including B cell non-Hodgkin's lymphoma of both Burkitt's and non-Burkitt's types; acquired immunodeficiency syndrome associated non-Hodgkin's lymphoma; and B cell acute lymphocytic leukemia (ALL). A small number of T cell ALL cases have translocations involving *myc* and sequences from the *TCR* α or δ loci.[3] The common theme in all cases is that *myc* expression is deregulated because its transcription is now controlled by immunoglobulin or *TCR* regulatory elements. Unfortunately, the mechanisms by which increased *myc* expression deregulates cell proliferation remain poorly understood.

Although the genes encoding transcription factors are often the targets of the translocations involving *Ig* or *TCR* locus sequences, *bcl*-2 and cyclin D1

Table 2   Chromosomal Translocation Breakpoints and Genes: Nonfusions and Hematopoietic Tumors

Type	Affected Gene	Disease	Rearranging Gene
Basic helix-loop-helix			
t(8; 14)(q24; q32)	c-*myc* (8q24)	BL, BL-ALL	*IgH, IgL*
t(2; 8)(q12; q24)			
t(8; 22)(q24; q11)			
t(8; 14)(q24; q11)	c-*myc* (8q24)	T cell ALL	*TCR-α*
t(8; 12)(q24; q22)	c-*myc* (8q24)	B cell CLL/ALL	—
	BTG (12q22)		
t(7; 19)(q35; p13)	*lyl*-1 (19p13)	T cell ALL	*TCR-β*
t(1; 14)(p32; q11)	*tal*-1/*scl* (1p32)	T cell ALL	*TCR-α*
t(7; 9)(q35; q34)	*tal*-2 (9q34)	T cell ALL	*TCR-β*
LIM proteins			
t(11; 14)(p15; q11)	*RBTN1/ttg*-1 (11p15)	T cell ALL	*TCR-δ*
t(11; 14)(p13; q11)	*RBTN2/ttg*-2 (11p13)	T cell ALL	*TCR-δ/α/β*
t(7; 11)(q35; p13)			
Homeobox protein			
t(10; 14)(q24; q11)	*hox*-11 (10q24)	T cell ALL	*TCR-α/β*
t(7; 10)(q35; q24)			
Zinc finger protein			
t(3; 14)(q27; q32)	*laz*-3/*bcl*-6 (3q27)	NHL/DLCL	*IgH*
t(3; 4)(q27; p11)	*laz*-3/*bcl*-6 (3q27)	NHL	—
Others			
t(11; 14)(q13; q32)	*bcl*-1/(*PRAD*1) (11q13)	B cell CLL and others	*IgH*
t(14; 18)(q32; 21)	*bcl*-2 (18q21)	FL	*IgH, IgL*
inv14 and t(14; 14)(q11q32)	*tcl*-1 (14q32.1)	T cell CLL	*TCR-Cα*
t(10; 14)(q24; q32)	*lyt*-10 (10q24)	B cell lymphoma	*IgH*
t(14; 19)(q32; q13.1)	*bcl*-3 (19q13.1)	B cell CLL	*IgH*
t(5; 14)(q31; q32)	*IL*-3 (5q31)	pre–B cell ALL	*IgH*
t(7; 9)(q34; q34.3)	*tan*-1 (9q34.3)	T cell ALL	*TCR-β*
t(1; 7)(p34; q34)	*lck* (1p34)	T cell ALL	*TCR-β*
t(X; 14)(q28; q11)	*C6.1b* (Xq28)	T cell PLL	*TCR-α*

ALL—acute lymphocytic leukemia; BL—Burkitt's lymphoma; CLL—chronic lymphocytic leukemia; DLCL—diffuse large cell lymphoma; FL—follicular lymphoma; NHL—non-Hodgkin's lymphoma; PLL—prolymphocytic leukemia.

(*CYCD*1) are clear-cut exceptions to this generalization. The *bcl*-2 gene was identified by molecular cloning of the chromosome 18q sequences involved in translocation between 18q and the *Ig* heavy-chain locus in the t(14;18)(q32;q21) translocation.[3,20] This translocation is the most common chromosomal abnormality in B cell non-Hodgkin's lymphoma. Virtually all cases of follicular lymphoma, as well as a small subset of diffuse lymphomas, display this translocation.[20] The translocation places the *Ig* transcriptional regulatory elements downstream of *bcl*-2 gene sequences, resulting in deregulation of *bcl*-2 expression. Approximately 70 percent of the breakpoints at the *bcl*-2 locus are clustered within a minimal breakpoint cluster region, and PCR-based strategies can thus often be used to detect the t(14;18) translocation. *bcl*-2 function appears to promote cell survival and to oppose apoptosis [*see Chapter 5*].[20] The pattern of *bcl*-2 expression in normal lymphoid cells suggests that it may function in the generation of mem-

Table 3   Chromosomal Breakpoints and Genes: Fusions and Hematopoietic Tumors

Type	Affected Gene	Protein Domain	Fusion Protein	Disease
inv14 (q11; q32)	TCR-α (14q11)	TCR-Cα	VH-TCR-Cα	T/B cell lymphoma
	VH (14q32)	Ig VH		
t(9; 22)(q34; q11)	C-abL (9q34)	Tyrosine kinase	Serine + tyrosine kinase	CML/ALL
	bcr (22q11)	Serine kinase		
t(1; 19)(q23; p13.3)	pbx1 (1q23)	HD	AD + HD	pre–B cell ALL
	E2A (19p13.3)	AD-b-HLH		
t(17; 19)(q22; p13)	HLF (17q22)	bZIP	AD + bZIP	pre–B cell ALL
	E2A (19p13)	AD-b-HLH		
t(15; 17)(q21-q11-22)	PML (15q21)	Zinc finger	Zinc finger + RAR DNA and ligand binding	APL
	RARa (17q21)	Retinoic acid receptor-α		
t(11; 17)(q23; q21.1)	PLZF (11q23)	Zinc finger	Zinc finger + RAR DNA and ligand binding	APL
	RARa (17q21)	Retinoic acid receptor-α		
t(4; 11)(q21; q23)	MLL (11q23)	A-T hook/zinc finger	A-T hook + Ser-Pro	ALL/pre–B cell ALL/ANLL
	AF4 (4q21)	Ser-pro rich		
t(9; 11)(q21; q23)	MLL (11q23)	A-T hook/zinc finger	A-T hook + Ser-Pro	ALL/pre–B cell ALL/ANLL
	AF9/MLLT3 (9p22)	Ser-Pro rich		
t(11; 19)(q23; p13)	MLL (11q23)	A-T hook/zinc finger	A-T hook + Ser-Pro	pre–B cell ALL/T cell ALL/ANLL
	ENL (19p13)	Ser-Pro rich		
t(X; 11)(q13; q23)	MLL (11q23)	A-T hook/zinc finger	A-T hook + Ser-Pro	T cell ALL
	AFX1 (Xq13)	(Ser-Pro rich)		
t(1; 11)(p32; q23)	MLL (11q23)	A-T hook/zinc finger	A-T hook + ?	ALL
	AF1P (1p32)	Eps-15 homologue		

ALL—acute lymphocytic leukemia; AML—acute myelogenous leukemia; ANLL—acute nonlymphocytic leukemia; APL—acute promyelocytic leukemia; AUL—acute undifferentiated leukemia; CML—chronic myelogenous leukemia; CMML—chronic myelomonocytic leukemia; NHL—non-Hodgkin's lymphoma.
AD—transcriptional activation domain; bHLH—basic helix-loop-helix; bZIP—basic region leucine zipper; HD—homeodomain; IL—interleukin; PB—paired box; Ph—Philadelphia chromosome; RARa—retinoic acid receptor-α; TM—TM sequence; ZIP—leucine zipper motif.

ory B cells. Results of many in vitro experiments as well as studies of transgenic mice that overexpress bcl-2 indicate that bcl-2 activation alone is not sufficient to generate lymphomas. Consistent with this proposal, bcl-2 has been found to be translocated in rare populations of cells in nearly 50 percent of lymph nodes and tonsils with follicular hyperplasia.[21] In both of these benign settings, although bcl-2 is activated by translocation, the risk of subsequent lymphoma development is very low.

The bcl-1 locus was originally defined as a breakpoint site on chromosome 11q in B cell neoplasms with translocations between 11q and Ig heavy-chain locus sequences from chromosome 14q.[3,22] Characteristically, translocations involving bcl-1 are seen in 50 percent of centrocytic lymphomas (also known as mantle zone or intermediate lymphocytic lymphomas).[3,23] Despite the identification of the translocation breakpoint on 11q many years ago, only in the recent past was the proto-oncogene CYCD1 at the bcl-1 locus identified.[3,24]

CYCD1 is an important element in regulating cell cycle progression [see Chapter 5]. In addition to its activation by translocation with Ig locus sequences in a subset of lymphomas, CYCD1 is activated by juxtaposition

Table 3 continued

Type	Affected Gene	Protein Domain	Fusion Protein	Disease
t(6; 11)(q27; q23)	MLL (11q23)	A-T hook/zinc finger	A-T hook + ?	ALL
	AF6 (6q27)	myosin homologue		
t(11; 17)(q23; q21)	MLL (11q23)	A-T hook/zinc finger	A-T hook + leucine zipper	AML
	AF17 (17q21)	Cys rich/leucine zipper		
t(8; 21)(q22; q22)	AML1/CBF-α (21q22)	DNA binding/runt homology	DNA binding + zinc fingers	AML
	ETO/MTG8 (8q22)	Zinc finger		
t(3; 21)(q26; q22)	AML1 (21q22)	DNA binding	DNA binding + zinc fingers	CML
	cvi-1 (3q26)	Zinc finger		
t(3; 21)(q26; q22)	AML1 (21q22)	DNA binding	DNA binding + out-of-frame EAP	Myelodysplasia
	EAP (3q26)	Sn protein		
t(16; 21)(p11; q22)	fus (16p11)	Gln-Ser-Tyr/Gly rich/RNA binding	Gln-Ser-Tyr + DNA binding	Myeloid
	erg (21q22)	Ets-like DNA binding		
t(6; 9)(p23; q34)	dek (6p23)	?	? + ZIP	AML
	can (9q34)	ZIP		
9; 9?	set (9q34)	?	? + ZIP	AUL
	can (9p34)	ZIP		
t(4; 16)(q26; p13)	IL-2 (4q26)	IL-2	IL-2/TM	T cell lymphoma
	8cm (16p13.1)	?/TM domain		
inv(2; 2)(p13; p11.2-14)	rel (2p13)	DNA binding-activator	DNA binding + ?	NHL
	nrg (2p11.2-14)	Not known		
inv(16)(p13q22)	Myosin-myh-11 (16p13)		DNA binding?	AML
	C8F-β (16q22)			
t(5; 12)(q33; p13)	PDGF-β (5q33)	Receptor kinase	Kinase + DNA binding	CMML
	tel (12p13)	Ets-like DNA binding		
t(2; 5)(2p23; q35)	npm (5q35)	Nucleolar phosphoprotein	N-terminal NPM + kinase	NHL
	alk (2p23)	Tyrosine kinase		

with parathyroid hormone gene sequences in some parathyroid adenomas.[25]

Although the predominant effect of the aforementioned translocations (e.g., *myc* and *bcl-2*) is deregulation of gene expression, many of the chromosomal translocations in hematopoietic malignancies result in the synthesis of novel fusion proteins that contain sequences from two different proteins [*see Tables 2 and 3*]. The first and most well-known example of a chimeric oncogene that encodes a novel fusion protein product was provided by the elucidation of the Philadelphia (Ph) chromosome. The Ph chromosome was first described by Nowell and Hungerford in 1960 as a minute chromosome seen in their karyotypic analysis of bone marrow cells from a patient with chronic myelogenous leukemia.[26] It was subsequently found that the Ph chromosome resulted from translocation between chromosome 9q and 22q.[27] About 95 percent of patients with chronic myelogenous leukemia, 10 percent of patients with ALL, and five percent of patients with acute myelogenous leukemia have a Ph chromosome in their neoplastic cells.[28] The translocation juxtaposes *abl* sequences from 9q with sequences from a 22q locus termed *bcr*. The first four exons of the *bcr* gene are joined in the same transcriptional orientation to the second exon of the *abl* gene [*see Figure 2*]. The chimeric gene encodes a hybrid Bcr-Abl protein termed p210, which has N-terminal sequences from the *bcr* gene and retains the tyrosine kinase catalytic domain of *abl*.[28] In a subset of patients with ALL, translocation between the *bcr* and *abl* genes can be detected, but the breakpoints occur in a different region of *bcr*, leading to the synthesis of a p190 Bcr-Abl protein.[28] Nevertheless, although the p210 and p190 proteins differ subtly in their function, both proteins retain tyrosine kinase activity and have altered functional activity because of the replacement of N-terminal *abl* regulatory sequences with sequences from the Bcr protein. In vitro and animal studies with chimeric *bcr-abl* gene constructs have provided strong support for the causal role of *bcr-abl* in leukemogenesis.[28]

Other translocations that create chimeric proteins encode transcription factors [*see Tables 2 through 4*].[3] For example, about 25 percent of pre–B cell ALL neoplasms harbor a t(1;19)(q23;p13) translocation, making this the most common translocation seen in childhood ALL.[29] The *E2A* gene, which encodes two alternatively spliced transcription factors of the basic helix-loop-helix family, is consistently found at the breakpoint site on chromosome 19p.[30] As a result of the translocation, *E2A* sequences are juxtaposed with those from a chromosome 1q homeobox gene termed *pbx*1. The resulting *E2A-pbx*1 chimeric gene generated encodes a fusion protein in which the E2A transcriptional regulatory domain and the Pbx1 sequences necessary for specific DNA binding are now present in the same novel protein molecule.[30] Thus, the novel chimeric transcription factor generated has

Table 4 Chromosomal Breakpoints and Genes: Fusions and Solid Tumors

Type	Affected Gene	Protein Domain	Fusion Protein	Disease
inv10(q11.2; q21)	*ret* (10q11.2)	Tyrosine kinase	Unknown + tyrosine kinase	Papillary thyroid carcinoma
	D10S170 (q21)	Uncharacterized		
t(11; 22)(q24; q12)	*fli-1* (11q24)	Ets-like DNA binding	Gln-Ser-Tyr + DNA binding	Ewing's sarcoma
	EWS (22q12)	Gln-Ser-Tyr/Gly rich/ RNA binding		
t(21; 22)(?; q12)	*erg* (21q22)	Ets-like DNA binding	Gln-Ser-Tyr + DNA binding	Ewing's sarcoma
	EWS (22q12)	Gln-Ser-Tyr/Gly rich/ RNA binding		
t(12; 22)(q13; q12)	*ATF1* (12q13)	bZIP	Gln-Ser-Tyr + bZIP	Melanoma of soft parts
	EWS (22q12)	Gln-Ser-Tyr/Gly rich/ RNA binding		
t(12; 16)(q13; p11)	*CHOP* (12q13)	(DNA binding?)/ZIP	Gln-Ser-Tyr + (DNA binding?)/ZIP	Liposarcoma
	fus (16p11)	Gln-Ser-Tyr/Gly rich/ RNA binding		
t(2; 13)(q35; q14)	*pax3* (2q35)	Paired box/homeodomain	PB/HD + DNA binding	Rhabdomyosarcoma
	FKHR (13q14)	Forkhead domain		
t(X; 18)(p11.2; q11.2)	*syt* (18q11.2)	None identified		Synovial sarcoma
	ssx (Xp11.2)	None identified		

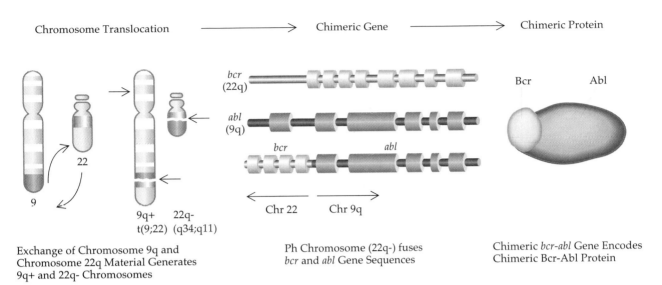

Chromosome Translocation ⟶ Chimeric Gene ⟶ Chimeric Protein

bcr (22q)

abl (9q)

bcr   *abl*

Bcr   Abl

⟵ Chr 22 ⟶ Chr 9q ⟶

9q+   22q-
t(9;22) (q34;q11)

Exchange of Chromosome 9q and Chromosome 22q Material Generates 9q+ and 22q- Chromosomes

Ph Chromosome (22q-) fuses *bcr* and *abl* Gene Sequences

Chimeric *bcr-abl* Gene Encodes Chimeric Bcr-Abl Protein

Figure 2 *Philadelphia chromosome translocation [t(9;22)(q34;q11)] fuses* bcr *and* abl *gene sequences and results in the synthesis of a chimeric bcr/abl protein.*

an altered structure and is likely to have altered functional activity. Furthermore, although *E2A* is ubiquitously expressed, *pbx*1 is not normally expressed in lymphoid cells. The E2A-Pbx1 chimeric protein presumably alters growth, therefore, by inappropriately activating the expression of Pbx1-regulated genes in lymphoid cells. Further support for the critical role of the *E2A-pbx*1 chimeric gene in leukemia has been provided by studies demonstrating that *E2A-pbx*1 gene transfer causes transformation in experimental model systems.[31]

Gene Amplification: **myc, N-myc, L-myc, neu, EGFR, and CYCD1**

Although point mutations and translocations are the most common mechanisms for the generation of oncogenic alleles in many human cancers, in other tumor types, such as neuroblastomas, breast cancers, and glioblastomas, the most common known mechanism of proto-oncogene activation is DNA amplification.[1]

The *myc* gene is frequently amplified in small-cell lung cancer and much less frequently in glioblastomas and epithelial cancers, including breast and colorectal cancer.[1,32] Two *myc*-related genes, known as N-*myc* and L-*myc*, encode proteins that are closely related to the Myc protein. These two genes were initially identified partly because they are amplified in such tumors as neuroblastoma and small-cell lung cancer. In fact, about 30 to 40 percent of small-cell lung cancer tumors have amplification of *myc*, N-*myc*, or L-*myc*.[32] Although L-*myc* has not been found to be amplified in tumors other than small-cell lung cancer, N-*myc* is amplified in a sizable fraction of neuroblastomas and in a subset of glioblastomas.[1] In addition to differences in the spectrum of tumors in which each gene is amplified, *myc*, N-*myc*, and L-*myc* have unique patterns of expression in development and exhibit subtle differences in assays of their oncogenic functions in vitro. The net effect of the various amplifications is that the levels of the respective gene products are increased and are no longer responsive to normal physiologic regulation. As a consequence, many *myc*-regulated cellular genes are apparently deregulated, and cell growth regulation is altered. The relationship of N-*myc* gene amplification to the biologic and clinical behavior of neuroblastoma is addressed in Chapter 9.

The *neu* (also known as the *HER*-2 or *erb*-B2) gene, which encodes a protein related to the epidermal growth factor receptor (EGFR), was initially found to be activated by point mutation in rodent tumors.[1,33] Although *neu* point mutations have not yet been identified in studies of human tumors, *neu* is amplified and overexpressed in 10 to 30 percent of breast, gastric, and ovarian cancers.[34] A small subset of other epithelial cancers, such as colorectal, pancreatic, and endometrial cancer, also have amplification and overexpression of *neu*. Studies have attempted to ascertain whether *neu* expression levels can be used as a prognostic marker or indicator in breast cancer and other cancers [*see Chapter 9*].

Amplification and overexpression of the *EGFR* gene has been seen in nearly 40 percent of glioblastomas, the highest grade of glioma.[1,35] *EGFR* amplification is much less common in lower-stage gliomas. Thus, the data suggest that overexpression of *EGFR* may be associated with tumor progression in brain tumors. Amplification of *EGFR* is also seen in a subset of epithelial cancers. In addition, apparent overexpression of *EGFR* in the absence of *EGFR* gene amplification is seen in some epithelial cancers. For example, although the *EGFR* gene is amplified in a very small subset of breast cancers, there are many more breast cancers with EGFR overexpression than with amplification of the gene.[36]

The *CYCD*1 and *CYCE* genes have each been found to be amplified in a small percentage of epithelial cancers, such as breast and colorectal cancers.[37,38] In addition, recent studies suggest that the *Cdk*-4 gene on chromosome 12q, which encodes one of the catalytic cyclin-dependent kinases that associates with CYCD1 is amplified in 10 to 20 percent of gliomas and in a small percentage of several other tumors, including childhood sarcomas.[39,40] Presumably, alterations in the expression of the cyclin and the cyclin-dependent kinase (Cdk) proteins, caused by gene amplification and overexpression, drive inappropriate transit of tumor cells through the G_1-S checkpoint.

Oncogene Mutations in Inherited Cancer Predisposition: ret

Germ line mutations generating dominant, oncogenic alleles might be predicted to interfere with normal embryonic and fetal development. For many years, this prediction was supported by the absence of any evidence that germ line mutations in proto-oncogenes contributed to inherited predisposition to cancer or that such mutations were even present in any patients with cancer. However, recent studies have demonstrated that germ line mutations in the *ret* proto-oncogene are associated with inherited predisposition to endocrine neoplasia.

An activated allele of the *ret* gene was first identified through DNA transformation studies of papillary thyroid cancer DNA samples.[41] These studies revealed that in about 30 percent of such specimens, the extracellular domain *ret* sequences had been removed as a result of a chromosomal translocation, and the remaining tyrosine kinase domain sequences of *ret* underwent fusion to protein fragments from various other genes. Although the thyrocytes from which papillary thyroid cancers arise do not normally express the *ret* gene, subsequent studies demonstrated that *ret* was expressed at high levels in some cancers, including medullary thyroid cancers and pheochromocytomas. In addition, the chromosome 10 region containing the *ret* gene was found to be genetically linked to cancer predisposition in several inherited endocrine neoplastic syndromes associated with these tumors, including familial medullary thyroid cancer and multiple endocrine neoplasia (MEN) types IIA and IIB.

Germ line mutations in the *ret* gene have now been identified in patients with familial medullary thyroid cancer, MEN IIA, and MEN IIB.[14,42,43] All patients with mutations are heterozygous and carry one wild-type and one mutant *ret* allele. The *ret* mutations seen thus far in those with MEN IIA and familial medullary thyroid cancer alter any one of four conserved cysteines in the *ret* extracellular domain, whereas those with the more severe, MEN IIB syndrome alter amino acids other than the conserved cysteines. Recent studies have demonstrated that the mutant *ret* alleles seen in patients with familial medullary thyroid cancer, MEN IIA, and MEN IIB transform rodent fibroblasts, a finding that provides further support that the mutant *ret* alleles function as dominant oncogenes. Presumably, the *ret* gene mutations in those with the MEN syndromes may mimic the effect of ligand binding to the Ret receptor. The resultant constitutive activation of Ret in the cell types that normally express the *ret* gene, including parathyroid C cells and other neural crest–derived cells, presumably causes a hyperproliferative phenotype. Malignant tumors presumably arise from the hyperproliferative cells after additional somatic mutations. Interestingly, loss-of-function mutations in the *ret* gene appear to predispose to Hirschsprung's disease,[14] or congenital megacolon, in which there is a congenital absence of ganglion cells in the colon and a consequent loss of peristalsis.

Tumor Suppressor Gene Lesions in Cancer

Less than a dozen well-established and candidate tumor suppressor genes have been identified [*see Chapter 6*]. For some genes, such as the retinoblastoma (*Rb*-1), *p53*, Wilms' tumor (*WT*-1), and adenomatous polyposis coli (*APC*) genes, much is known about the inherited and somatic mutations in the genes and the spectrum of human cancers in which mutations are most frequently found. For others, like the neurofibromatosis type 1 (*NF*-1), neurofibromatosis type 2 (*NF*-2), *VHL*, and *p16/MTS*1 genes, much less is known about the nature and prevalence of mutations in various tumor types. It is not possible to review in detail all of the mutations that have been identified in these tumor suppressor genes and other candidate suppressor genes, such as the *DCC* gene on chromosome 18q, the *MCC* gene on 5q, and the E-cadherin gene on 16q. Rather, this discussion focuses primarily on the genetic alterations that are most instructive with regard to the pathogenetic mechanisms underlying various forms of cancer. Finally, the functions of several of the tumor suppressor genes are addressed briefly in this chapter; the reader is referred to Chapter 6 for more detailed descriptions of tumor suppressor gene function.

Rb-1 Mutations

The *Rb*-1 gene was localized and isolated by molecular cloning in 1986 [*see Chapter 6*].[44] *Rb*-1 is a large gene with 27 exons, spanning greater than 200 kilobases (kb) of genomic DNA. Although gross deletions, of either inherited or somatic origin, affect the *Rb*-1 gene in some retinoblastomas and osteosarcomas (<10 percent), gross rearrangements of the gene do not occur in most tumors. Most mutations that inactivate *Rb*-1 are point mutations or small insertions and deletions that result in premature truncation of the protein product, although splicing mutations impairing the formation of the *Rb*-1 messenger RNA (mRNA) and missense mutations affecting the amino acid sequences of its protein product have also been identified.[44-49] These more subtle changes in DNA sequence have been found at many sites in this very large gene. This wide dispersion of mutations greatly complicates attempts at discovering the specific mutation responsible for inactivating the *Rb*-1 gene. As predicted by the Knudson hypothesis, both *Rb*-1 alleles are inactivated by inherited mutations, somatic mutations, or both, in retinoblastomas and osteosarcomas.

Although germ line inactivation of *Rb*-1 in humans predisposes almost exclusively to the development of retinoblastomas in childhood and osteosarcomas during adolescence, somatic mutations in *Rb*-1 have been identified in a fairly broad spectrum of adult tumors.[49] The *Rb*-1 mutations in adult tumors are similar to the germ line and somatic mutations observed in retinoblastomas and osteosarcomas and include frameshift, nonsense, and splicing mutations, as well as deletions. Because most *Rb*-1 mutations lead to the loss of stable production of p105-Rb protein, it is now possible to use immunoblotting approaches or even immunohistochemistry with anti–p105-Rb antibodies to screen primary tumors for loss of p105-Rb expression. This is an important advance for the analysis of clinical specimens because identification of specific mutations in *Rb*-1 is not always practical. The prevalence of *Rb*-1 mutations varies markedly from one tumor type to another.[49] Although roughly 90 percent of small-cell lung cancers have *Rb*-1 mutations, only about 25 to 35 percent of non–small cell lung cancers have *Rb*-1 mutations. Roughly 10 to 30 percent of breast, bladder, prostate, head and neck, and pancreatic cancers have *Rb*-1 mutations, and a small subset of human leukemias, predominantly those of myeloid type, may harbor *Rb*-1 mutations. In some cancers, such as colorectal cancer, *Rb*-1 mutations are present in fewer than five percent of tumors. It remains unclear why *Rb*-1 germ line mutations predispose to a different set of tumors than are provoked later in life by somatic mutation of the gene.

A subset of the human papilloma viruses (HPVs) appear to have a causal role in cervical cancer. These are the so-called high-risk HPVs and include types 16 and 18.[50] The E7 proteins from HPV types 16 and 18 complex more tightly with p105-Rb than do the E7 proteins from "low-risk" viruses (e.g., HPV types 6 and 11) [*see Chapter 6*]. More than two thirds of cervical cancers harbor HPV types 16 and 18, and thus p105-Rb inactivation has been implicated in the development of these cancers. Interestingly, those few cervical cancers that do not harbor high-risk HPV genomes appear to have *Rb*-1 mutations.[51] Thus, the data suggest that *Rb*-1 inactivation, either through mutation of the cellular gene or sequestration of its product by a viral oncoprotein, may be common to all cervical cancers.

p53 *Mutations*

Evidence that *p53* might frequently be inactivated in human cancers was initially provided by studies demonstrating that LOH for the chromosome 17p region containing *p53* was common in many tumors, including colorectal, breast, bladder, and lung cancer.[13,52,53] Sequence analysis of the *p53* alleles retained in cancers with 17p LOH demonstrated that the remaining *p53* allele was mutated in most cases.[53,54] Based on the types of tumors in which mutations have been found and the prevalence of mutations in those tumor types, *p53* is believed to be among the most frequently mutated genes in human cancer.[54] Although gross rearrangements of the *p53* gene are seen in some pediatric tumors, like osteosarcoma and rhabdomyosarcoma, and splicing mutations are seen in some small-cell lung cancers, most of the somatic mutations in *p53* in human cancers are missense mutations [*see Figure 3*].[54] These missense mutations are scattered throughout the central core domain of the *p53* coding region (exons 5 to 9). The missense mutations all appear to have marked effects on the ability of the p53 transcription factor to bind to its cognate DNA recognition sites through either of two mechanisms.[55] Some mutations (e.g., mutations at codons 248 and 273) alter p53 sequences that are directly responsible for sequence-specific DNA binding. Others (e.g., codon 175) appear to affect the folding of p53 and thus indirectly affect its ability to bind to DNA.

Additional compelling evidence that *p53* mutations are critical to human cancer has been provided by the identification of germ line *p53* mutations in patients with the Li-Fraumeni syndrome, as well as in some children with soft tissue sarcomas or osteosarcomas who do not meet rigorous clinical criteria for the diagnosis of Li-Fraumeni syndrome.[56,57] Those affected by Li-Fraumeni syndrome show greatly elevated risk for the development of various tumors, including soft tissue sarcomas, osteosarcomas, brain tumors, breast cancers, and leukemias. Nearly two thirds of those with the Li-Fraumeni syndrome have germ line mutations in the central core domain of the *p53* coding sequences (exons 5 to 9); these mutations resemble the somatic mutations frequently seen in *p53*. However, about one third of patients with Li-Fraumeni syndrome have mutations outside of the *p53* coding region, and many of these mutations appear to result in loss of transcripts from the affected allele.

Detailed characterization of the mutations present in the *p53* gene in particular types of cancer has provided some particularly striking results with regard to the mutational mechanisms that underlie cancer development.[54] For example, many of the *p53* mutations in colorectal cancers appear to have arisen as a result of deamination of methylated cytosine bases. In lung cancer and in head and neck cancer, many of the *p53* mutations appear to have arisen as a result of direct interactions between *p53* sequences and car-

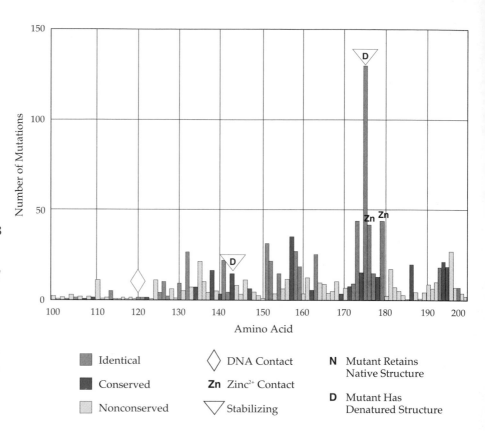

Figure 3 *Structure-function comparison for the central regions of p53. Codons 100 to 300 encode the site-specific DNA-binding core domain of the protein. The number of missense mutations identified at each codon in studies of human tumors is indicated. Some mutations inactivate p53 function while either retaining the overall structure of the protein (N) or disrupting global stability (D). Other mutations affect specific p53 protein sequences involved in DNA binding, Zn²⁺ atom contacts, or stabilizing protein structure. Amino acids that are identical, conserved, or not conserved among p53 proteins of diverse species are indicated.*

cinogens present in tobacco smoke. The study of *p53* mutations from squamous cell skin cancers arising in ultraviolet light–exposed body regions has demonstrated that ultraviolet light–induced pyrimidine dimer lesions may be responsible for the generation of mutant alleles. Finally, the *p53* mutations present in hepatocellular cancers in individuals from geographic areas with very high exposure to aflatoxin have been shown to occur at sites known to be altered by aflatoxin in studies in vitro.

Although *p53* is most commonly inactivated by somatic mutations, in some tumor types, *p53* function is inactivated by other mechanisms.[58] Most cervical cancers contain high-risk or cancer-associated HPV genomes. The p53 protein in these tumors has been found to be complexed with, and degraded by, a second distinct protein, termed E6, made by the high-risk viruses.[50] Low-risk HPVs also encode E6 proteins, but the E6 proteins of low-risk viruses fail to cause p53 depletion. Most cervical cancers that do not harbor high-risk HPV genomes have instead somatic mutations in the *p53* gene. In the rare instances in which a cancer-associated HPV E6 protein and a somatic *p53* mutation are both present in a cervical cancer specimen, data suggest that such cancers may behave more aggressively.[50]

In a subset of soft tissue sarcomas, a cellular *p53*-binding protein, known as Mdm2, is overexpressed as a result of DNA amplification.[58,59] Mdm2 has been shown to function as an oncogene in vitro when it is overexpressed. Presumably, one of the mechanisms by which *mdm2* overexpression may alter cell growth and promote tumorigenesis is by complexing and inactivating *p53* function. Consistent with this proposal, sarcomas with *mdm2*

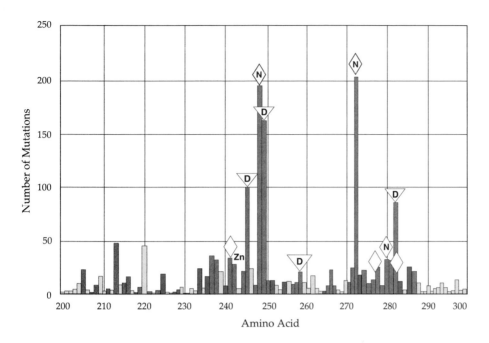

amplification have not been found to harbor somatic mutations in *p53*.

APC *Mutations*

Hereditary colorectal cancer is usually divided into polyposis and nonpoly-posis subtypes. The genetics of the nonpolyposis types are addressed later in this chapter. Familial adenomatous polyposis, or adenomatous polyposis coli, is the most common of the polyposis types. This syndrome is an auto-somal dominant disorder in which hundreds to thousands of adenomatous (benign) polyps arise in the colon and rectum by the third to fourth decades of life. *APC* is a large gene with at least 15 exons. It encodes a protein of 2,843 amino acids that is expressed in many adult tissues.[60] The predicted APC protein product is a cytoplasmic protein of unknown function. How-ever, recent studies have shown that APC complexes through its C-terminal sequences with microtubules, and its more N-terminal sequences are in-volved in binding to α- and β-catenin, two adherens junction proteins that may be involved in mediating cell-cell interactions in epithelial cells.[60]

In greater than two thirds of patients with polyposis, germ line mutation of one of the *APC* alleles has been identified by use of various combinations of recombinant DNA–based techniques.[60-63] The germ line *APC* mutations observed include gross deletions of the gene, mutations that affect its tran-scription or splicing, and missense mutations. However, more than 90 per-cent of the germ line *APC* mutations identified thus far cause premature truncation of the protein product, as a result of either a frameshift or a non-sense mutation [*see Figure 4*]. Thus, a rapid screening strategy for mutations that cause premature truncation of the APC protein product, termed the in vitro protein synthesis or the in vitro transcription translation assay, has been introduced [*see Figure 5*].[63] Characterization of the germ line *APC* mu-tations in families with variant polyposis syndromes, such as Gardner syn-

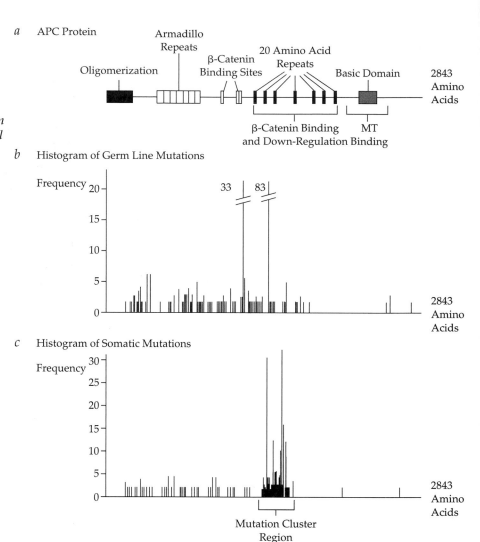

a APC Protein

Oligomerization

Armadillo
Repeats

β-Catenin
Binding Sites

20 Amino Acid
Repeats

Basic Domain

2843
Amino
Acids

β-Catenin Binding
and Down-Regulation Binding

MT

b Histogram of Germ Line Mutations

Frequency

33 | 83 |

2843
Amino
Acids

c Histogram of Somatic Mutations

Frequency

2843
Amino
Acids

Mutation Cluster
Region

Figure 4 *Linear representation of APC protein with mutational histograms. (a) A putative domain involved in homo-oligomerization of the APC protein is located at the N-terminal. Also noted are a series of repeats of unknown function with similarity to the* Drosophila *armadillo protein, several sites known to mediate binding to β-catenin, and a region near the C-terminal of the protein that appears to facilitate complexing with microtubules (MT). (b) Germ line mutations in the APC gene (predominantly chain-terminating mutations) are dispersed throughout the 5' half of the sequence, with two apparent "hot spots" at codons 1061 and 1309. (c) Somatic mutations in the APC gene in colorectal cancer appear to cluster in a region termed the "mutation cluster region," and mutations at codons 1309 and 1450 are the most common.*

drome, attenuated adenomatous polyposis coli, and Turcot's syndrome has yielded only a few clues to the genetic basis of the variability in disease phenotype.[60,64,65] One clue concerns the site of the mutation within the *APC* allele: hundreds to thousands of polyps usually develop in patients who harbor germ line mutations that cause truncation of the APC protein to one third to one half of its usual length. In contrast, attenuated adenomatous polyposis coli usually develops in those who have mutations that lead to the synthesis of severely truncated APC polypeptides of less than 200 amino acids. Unfortunately, the molecular genetic studies carried out thus far have not provided definitive insights into the bases for the predisposition to jaw osteomas and desmoid tumors in patients from kindreds with Gardner syndrome or for the predisposition to brain tumors in some individuals from kindreds with Turcot's syndrome.

Germ line mutations in *APC* may account for only about 0.5 percent of the total colorectal cases that occur annually. Far more common are the somatic mutations in *APC* that arise in 70 to 75 percent of all colorectal adenomatous polyps and cancers. Similar to the germ line mutations, the overwhelming majority of somatic *APC* mutations in colorectal tumors cause premature truncation of the protein product [*see Figure 4*].[60,66] The mutations appear to be present in nearly the same percentage of early-stage adenomas as in advanced cancers, suggesting that *APC* mutations may be an initiating event in the generation of most preneoplastic and neoplastic colorectal lesions. In the few detailed studies that have been conducted, the data suggest that both *APC* alleles are inactivated, either as the result of one inherited and one somatic mutation in lesions arising in those with polyposis, or as the result of two somatic mutations in sporadic tumors. Somatic *APC* mutations have also been identified in tumors arising outside the colon and rectum.[60]

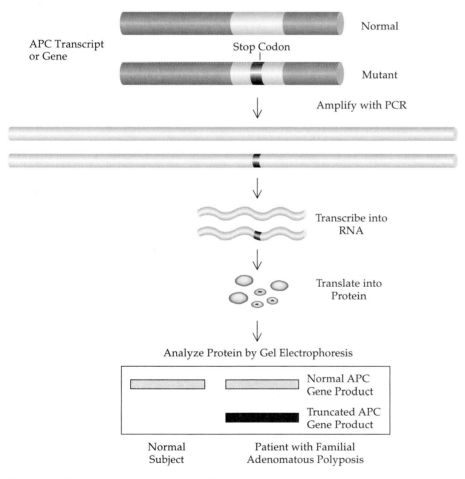

Figure 5 *APC mutation detection by the in vitro synthesized protein assay (also known as the protein truncation test). The* APC *gene is divided into overlapping segments that encompass the entire coding region of the gene. These regions are amplified with specifically designed polymerase chain reaction (PCR) primers that place the necessary transcriptional and translational regulatory sequences at the 5' end of the PCR product. Radiolabeled APC protein is synthesized in vitro from these surrogate genes in a simple one-step coupled transcription-translation reaction (illustrated as two steps). Truncating mutations can then be identified when smaller protein products are visualized after gel electrophoresis and autoradiography. The stop codon represents a typical* APC *mutation, resulting in premature truncation of the protein product (e.g., a small insertion or deletion resulting in a frameshift in protein translation).*

The data suggest that upwards of 40 percent of gastric cancers may have mutations that lead to premature truncation of the APC protein, and similar mutations may be present in some esophageal, breast, and brain tumors.

p16/MTS*1 Mutations*

Loss of heterozygosity affecting chromosome 9p has been found to be common in a wide spectrum of tumors, including melanomas, gliomas, and non–small cell lung, bladder, and head and neck cancers, as well as leukemias.[67] Moreover, some primary tumors of these types and a much higher percentage of tumor cell lines were found to have homozygous (complete) deletions of variable extents on chromosome 9p, often involving the interferon α gene cluster and flanking sequences.[67-70] In addition to common somatic alterations on 9p in cancers, linkage studies of some families with an inherited predisposition to melanoma established that a melanoma predisposition gene mapped to chromosome 9p.[71]

These data motivated the successful effort to identify and isolate the responsible gene, which was termed *MTS*1 (for multiple tumor suppressor gene).[72,73] Of great interest, *MTS*1 was found to be identical to the *p16* (*Cdk-N2*) gene, which was already known to encode a protein that functions as a specific inhibitor of cyclin-dependent kinases (i.e., Cdk4 and Cdk6). Further studies revealed that *p16* was commonly mutated in many tumor cell lines adapted for growth in culture.[72-74] However, *p16* mutations were found to be less common in primary human tumor samples.[74-76] For example, although about 55 to 60 percent of bladder cancer cell lines had *p16* mutations, only about 30 percent of primary tumors harbored mutations. Similarly, although up to 60 percent of breast cancer cell lines exhibited homozygous deletions of *p16*, very few mutations had been found in primary breast cancers. These findings suggested that in at least some instances, *p16* gene inactivation permits the adaptation of tumor cells for growth in vitro and is thus not present in the tumor cell genomes in vivo. The *p16* findings, therefore, are particularly useful for illustrating the potential difficulties in reaching conclusions about the nature and significance of mutations solely from studies of cancer cell lines, rather than of primary tumors. Nevertheless, *p16* mutations do appear to be present in a sizable number of primary tumors of some types, including esophageal, pancreatic, and bladder cancers and gliomas. In some gliomas, homozygous deletions affecting *p16* also affect the *p15/MTS2* gene, which encodes a presumptive Cdk protein inhibitor that is very closely related to p16 protein.[77] Recent studies have suggested that *p16* may be inactivated in some cancers by methylation of its regulatory (i.e., promoter/enhancer) sequences, a situation that often results in a loss of gene expression.[78,79] Although further studies of *p16* inactivation by DNA methylation are needed, the observations raise questions regarding the generality and the significance of DNA methylation as a mechanism for inactivation of tumor suppressor gene function. Moreover, should DNA methylation prove to be a common mechanism of tumor suppressor gene inactivation, new techniques may be needed for the identification of inactivated tumor suppressor genes.

Based on the findings obtained thus far, germ line mutations in the *p16/MTS*1 gene appear to account for only a subset of inherited melanoma cases, and other genes, perhaps even other genes on chromosome 9p, may play an important role.[71] Moreover, further studies are needed to address more definitively the prevalence, mechanisms, and functional consequences of *p16/MTS*1 inactivation in primary cancers.

WT-*1 Mutations*

Some Wilms' tumor patients have constitutional chromosomal deletions that affect one copy of chromosome 11, at band 11p13.[5] On the basis of this observation and the precedent established from studies of chromosome 13q deletions in retinoblastoma, it was inferred that inactivation of a gene—the *WT*-1 gene—at 11p13 predisposed to Wilms' tumor. The *WT*-1 gene was localized in 1990 by virtue of germ line deletions affecting chromosome 11p13 in the small subset of patients with Wilms' tumor and WAGR congenital abnormalities [see Identification of Tumor Suppressor Genes].[80,81] Subsequent studies established that somatic mutations in both *WT*-1 alleles were present in some Wilms' tumors in patients without obvious congenital abnormalities or a family history of Wilms' tumor. The *WT*-1 gene is encoded by 10 exons, its mRNA is subject to a relatively complex pattern of alternative splicing, and the mRNAs encode proteins with molecular masses of 45-49,000.[82] The WT-1 proteins have four zinc finger motifs at their C-terminal and appear to function as transcriptional repressors, perhaps suppressing the expression of growth-inducing genes like the early growth response (*EGR*1), insulinlike growth factor–2 (*IGF*-2), and platelet-derived growth factor A chain (*PDGF-A*) genes.[82]

The germ line mutations identified thus far in *WT*-1 include gross deletions of the gene in patients with the WAGR triad and more localized alterations, such as missense mutations in the zinc finger domains, in some patients.[82,83] Somatic mutations in *WT*-1, including deletions, splice mutations, and frameshift, nonsense, and missense mutations, have been identified in only about 10 percent of sporadic Wilms' tumors and in one non–asbsestos-related mesothelioma arising in the abdomen. The *WT*-1 gene has also been found to be involved in a translocation with the Ewing's sarcoma (*EWS*) gene on chromosome 11q in a rare pediatric tumor known as desmoplastic small round cell tumor.[84] Similar to the chimeric genes present in some leukemias, the *EWS–WT-1* translocation generates a novel fusion protein with the C-terminal *WT*-1 DNA binding domain and the N-terminal transcriptional activation sequences from *EWS*. The net result is that genes that may normally be repressed by *WT*-1 may be activated in cells expressing the EWS–WT-1 fusion protein.

Although *WT*-1 inactivation contributes to about 10 percent of all Wilms' tumors, much evidence suggests most Wilms' tumors arise through inherited and somatic mutations in other genes—some of which may also be located on chromosome 11.[83] For example, LOH on chromosome 11p in Wilms' tumors most often affects band 11p15.5 and not the *WT*-1 gene in band p13. In addition, the 11p15 region contains a gene responsible for Beckwith-Wiedemann syndrome (BWS), a congenital syndrome in which affected individuals are predisposed to embryonic tumors, such as Wilms' tumor and hepatoblastoma. Finally, linkage studies of three large kindreds with dominant inheritance of Wilms' tumor have established that the predisposition gene in these families does not map to any region of chromosome 11p. Results like these suggest that at least three different genes (*WT-1*, the *BWS* gene, and a non–chromosome 11p gene) exist that predispose to the development of Wilms' tumor when the genes are mutated in the germ line.[83] It will be interesting to determine if a combination of inherited and somatic mutations in more than one of these genes is required for Wilms' tumor development.

NF-*1*, NF-*2*, VHL, *and* BRCA1 *Mutations*

Many other tumor suppressor genes, including *NF-1*, *NF-2*, *VHL*, and *BRCA*1, have been identified [*see Chapter 6*]. Patients with germ line mutations in the neurofibromatosis type 1 (*NF-1*) gene are predisposed to benign neurofibromas of peripheral nerves and malignant tumors, including pheochromocytomas, schwannomas, neurofibrosarcomas, brain tumors, and leukemias. Although neurofibromatosis type 1 is thought to be a genetically homogenous disease, germ line mutations have been identified in the *NF-1* gene in only about 25 percent of patients with neurofibromatosis type 1.[85] This may be partly the result of the practical problems associated with the mutational analyses of a gene with the size and complexity of *NF-1*. Somatic mutations in *NF-1* have been identified in some tumors in patients without neurofibromatosis, including colorectal cancer, melanomas, and neuroblastomas, and bone marrow specimens from those with the myelodysplastic syndrome.[85] Nevertheless, questions about *NF-1* mutations remain, including the nature of germ line mutations in many patients with neurofibromatosis and the spectrum and prevalence of somatic mutations in various tumor types.

Patients with neurofibromatosis type 2 usually present with benign schwannomas affecting the eighth cranial nerve, although they are at greatly increased risk for the development of other tumors, including meningiomas, spinal schwannomas, and ependymomas. Germ line mutations in the *NF-2* gene, including deletions, nonsense, frameshift, and occasional missense mutations, have been identified in many patients with neurofibromatosis type 2.[86,87] Somatic mutations in the *NF-2* gene have also been identified in meningiomas, ependymomas, and mesotheliomas in patients without neurofibromatosis type 2.[86,87] The prevalence of *NF-2* somatic mutations in other, more common, cancer types remains to be determined. However, in this regard, although chromosome 22q is affected by LOH in a large number of other tumor types, such as colorectal and breast cancer,[13] no *NF-2* mutations have been described in these tumor types, suggesting that chromosome 22q may contain more than one tumor suppressor gene.

Those with the von Hippel-Lindau syndrome are predisposed to renal cell cancer, hemangioblastomas of the central nervous system and retina, and pheochromocytomas. Germ line mutations inactivating *VHL* gene function have been identified in many patients with von Hippel-Lindau syndrome and include deletions, frameshifts, nonsense, and missense mutations.[11] Somatic mutations in the *VHL* gene have also been detected in the overwhelming majority of sporadic clear-cell renal cancers.[88] Interestingly, about 20 percent of sporadic clear-cell renal cancers do not harbor a detectable mutation in the *VHL* gene. In many of these cases, *VHL* may be inactivated by methylation of its transcriptional regulatory sequences.[89] The prevalence of *VHL* inactivation by somatic mutations or by other mechanisms (e.g., methylation of the *VHL* promoter) in other tumor types appears to be low.

The identification of families with syndromes that predispose to rare cancers is often more straightforward than is the definitive identification of those with predisposition to a common cancer. For example, although family history was long known to be a major risk factor for breast cancer, studies in the 1980s were the first to provide definitive evidence that predisposition to premenopausal breast cancer could be attributed to a highly penetrant autosomal dominant allele. In 1990, a breast cancer predisposition gene (termed *BRCA1*) was localized to chromosome 17q21.[90] Subsequent studies established that the *BRCA1* gene, when mutated in the germ line, predisposes women not only to breast cancer but also to ovarian cancer.[91] After an intensive positional cloning effort focused on genes at 17q21, the *BRCA1* gene was recently isolated.[92,93] The gene has at least 24 exons and encodes a protein product of unknown function.

Germ line mutations in *BRCA1* have been identified in many patients with premenopausal breast cancer, ovarian cancer, or both, and the mutations appear to be scattered throughout the gene.[92-94] However, although nonsense, frameshift, and missense mutations in *BRCA1* have all been seen, precise details on the nature and frequency of germ line mutations in patients with breast and ovarian cancer are still emerging. The best estimates are that about half of the families with apparent autosomal dominant transmission of breast and ovarian cancer susceptibility and an average age of onset of younger than 45 years may harbor germ line mutations in *BRCA1*. Unexpectedly, preliminary studies suggest that somatic mutations in coding regions of *BRCA1* may be very uncommon in nonfamilial breast cancers and ovarian cancers.[93,95] In this sense, *BRCA1* does not behave like most other tumor suppressor genes that are known to be involved in the genesis of both hereditary and sporadic forms of specific tumors. Despite the absence of mutations in the *BRCA1* gene in most breast and ovarian cancers, results of a recent study suggest that the BRCA1 protein may be mislocalized in nearly all breast and ovarian cancers,[96] implying that the growth pathways regulated by BRCA1 protein may be altered in most breast and ovarian cancers. The prevalence and spectrum of *BRCA1* mutations in other tumor types have not yet been determined.

Another gene, termed *BRCA2*, that predisposes to premenopausal breast cancer has recently been identified from a region of chromosome 13q.[97] Current estimates are that *BRCA1* and *BRCA2* are each responsible for fewer than five percent of breast cancer cases occurring annually in the United States. Additional, novel tumor suppressor genes may be mutated in the germ lines of others with breast cancer.

Candidate Tumor Suppressor Genes: DCC, MCC, *E-cadherin*

Some tumor suppressor genes that have critical roles in human cancer may not give rise to an obvious cancer predisposition phenotype when they are present in mutant forms in the germ line. One approach to the identification of genes with such properties has been the mapping of chromosomal regions for which allelic losses can be commonly observed in sporadic cancers of a particular type [*see Table 3*]. For example, chromosome 18q is affected by LOH in greater than 70 percent of colorectal cancers, suggesting that it may contain one or more tumor suppressor genes.[98] Unfortunately, because in most colorectal cancers, the entire chromosomal arm is affected by LOH, it is difficult to localize the region or regions on 18q that are likely to contain the tumor suppressor gene or genes. A candidate tumor suppressor gene from 18q, termed *DCC* (for deleted in colorectal cancer), has been identified. *DCC* is an enormous gene with more than 29 exons spanning

Table 5   Tumor Suppressor Gene Alterations in Selected Human Tumor Types or Tumor Syndromes

Tumor Type/Tumor Syndrome	Chromosomal Region	Evidence
Retinoblastoma	13q14	LA, LOH, *Rb*-1 mutation
Osteosarcoma	13q14	LA, LOH, *Rb*-1 mutation
	17p13	LA, LOH, *p53* mutation
Wilms' tumor	11p13	LA, LOH, *WT*-1 mutation
	11p15	LA,LOH
	16q	LOH
	Other(s)	LA
Rhabdomyosarcoma	17p13	LA, LOH, *p53* mutation
	11p15	LOH
Hepatoblastoma	11p15	LOH
Colorectal	1p	LOH
	5q21	LA, LOH, *APC* mutation
	8p	LOH
	17p13	LOH, *p53* mutation
	18q21	LOH, *DCC* mutation
	Others	LOH
Breast	17p13	LA, LOH, *p53* mutation
	17q	LA, LOH, *BRCA*1 mutation
	16q	LOH, E-cadherin mutation
	11p15	LOH
	11q	LOH
	13q	LA (*BRCA2*)
	13q	LOH
	13q	*Rb*-1 mutation
	Others	LOH
Lung (small cell)	3p	LOH
	13p14	LOH, *Rb*-1 mutation
	17p	LOH, *p53* mutation
	Others	LOH

LA—linkage analysis; LOH—loss of heterozygosity.

more than 1,350 kb, and it encodes a transmembrane protein of largely unknown function.[98] Specific somatic mutations in *DCC* have been identified in only a very small number of cases, although this paucity may reflect the difficulties associated with screening for mutations in a gene the size of *DCC*. Nonetheless, in most colorectal cancers and cancer cell lines, *DCC* expression is markedly reduced or absent, a finding that is consistent with the proposal that loss of its function may contribute to tumorigenesis.[98]

In the search for the *APC* gene at chromosome 5q21, the *MCC* gene (for mutated in colorectal cancer) was identified.[99] *MCC* was found to be somatically mutated in about 10 percent of colorectal cancers, and the mutations

Table 5   continued

Tumor Type/Tumor Syndrome	Chromosomal Region	Evidence
Lung (non–small cell)	3p	LOH
	17p13	LOH, *p53* mutation
	Others	LOH
Bladder (transitional cell)	9p21	LOH, *p16* (*Cdk*-N2) mutation
	9q	LOH
	11p15	LOH
	17p13	LOH, *p53* mutation
	Others	LOH
Kidney (renal cell)	3p	LA, LOH, *VHL* mutation
	17p13	LOH, *p53* mutation
	Others	LOH
Glioblastoma	9p21	LOH, *p16* (*Cdk*-N2) mutation
	10q	LOH
	17p13	LOH, *p53* mutation
	Others	LOH
Melanoma	9p21	LA, LOH, *p16* (*Cdk*-N2) mutation
	17q	*NF*-1 mutation
	Others	LOH
Ovarian	16q	LOH, E-cadherin mutation
	17q	LOH, *BRCA*1 mutation
	Others	LOH
Gastric	5q	LOH, *APC* mutation
	16q	LOH, E-cadherin mutation
	17p	LOH, *p53* mutation
	18q	LOH
Neurofibromatosis type 1	17q	LA, LOH, *NF*-1 mutation
Neurofibromatosis type 2	22q	LA, LOH, *NF*-2 mutation
Meningioma	22q	LOH, *NF*-2 mutation

included missense mutations, splicing mutations, and gross rearrangement of the gene. *MCC* encodes a protein product of 829 amino acids that bears little similarity to previously identified proteins. Because *MCC* was not mutated in the germ line of those with familial polyposis, further studies on the gene have essentially ceased. Estimates of the prevalence and the nature of somatic mutations in *MCC* in other tumor types, as well as more definitive insights into the role of *MCC* in human cancer, await the results of renewed studies of this gene.

The gene encoding E-cadherin, a calcium-dependent transmembrane protein involved in epithelial cell-cell interactions, has also been suggested as a candidate tumor suppressor.[100] Decreased or undetectable levels of E-cadherin expression have been noted in many immunohistochemical studies of epithelial cancers, including one third or more of breast, bladder, prostate, stomach, and esophageal cancers.[100] The E-cadherin gene is located on chromosome 16q in a region that is frequent affected by LOH in breast and prostate cancers. Somatic mutations in the gene have been identified in more than one third of gastric cancers of diffuse subtype, in about five to 10 percent of endometrial and ovarian cancers, and in about 10 percent of breast cancer cell lines. The mutations identified include missense, nonsense, and splice mutations.[100] Nevertheless, in most tumors with altered E-cadherin expression, little is known about the mechanisms underlying its reduced or absent expression. E-cadherin function appears to depend on its ability to link to the submembrane cytoskeletal matrix through interactions with adherens junction proteins, such as α- and β-catenin. Some recent studies have shown α-catenin expression is commonly decreased or absent in epithelial cancers.[100] A prostate cancer cell line and two lung cancer lines have been found to have mutations affecting both of their α-catenin alleles. Further studies are necessary to address the prevalence and functional consequences of alterations in E-cadherin and the catenins in cancer.

A caveat needs to be expressed about premature designation of a gene as a tumor suppressor. An increasing number of genes with decreased or absent expression in cancer cells are being discovered. In response, these genes are sometimes termed tumor suppressor genes. Genes that antagonize the tumorigenic growth properties of tumor cell lines may also be termed tumor suppressors. Undoubtedly, some of these genes may ultimately prove to be critically involved in growth regulation and may also be targets for loss-of-function mutations in human cancer. However, the altered expression of many genes in cancers may not result from specific inactivation by mutational mechanisms, but may simply reflect the altered growth properties of the cells. Finally, as is the case for the gene that encodes the retinoblastoma cousin p107 and the *p21/WAF*1/*CIP*1 gene, some genes may have particularly potent growth suppressive properties in cancer cells but may be rarely if ever mutated in human cancer. In the end, the totality of the mutational and functional data must evaluated before a gene is designated a tumor suppressor.

DNA Repair Pathway Lesions in Cancer

Mutations in human cancer have been identified in three different classes of genes—proto-oncogenes, tumor suppressor genes, and DNA repair genes. Given that both tumor suppressor and DNA repair genes are affected by loss-of-function mutations, why then has a distinction been made here between them? The rationale is that the protein products of tumor suppressor genes are presumed to function directly in the regulation of cell growth. In contrast, DNA repair genes influence cell proliferation only indirectly through their effects on the structure of growth-controlling genes, notably proto-oncogenes and tumor suppressor genes. Although several rare, recessive cancer predisposition syndromes result from inactivation of genes involved in DNA repair, including xeroderma pigmentosum, Cockayne syndrome, and ataxia telangiectasia, this chapter focuses on the gene defects in a more common clinical syndrome—hereditary nonpolyposis colorectal cancer.

Hereditary Nonpolyposis Colorectal Cancer

Familial clustering of colorectal cancer has long been noted. The relative risk of colorectal cancer for any individual is elevated about threefold if a first-degree relative has had colorectal cancer. Indeed, familial adenomatous polyposis is a particularly striking example of familial clustering and inherited predisposition to colorectal cancer. However, germ line mutations in the *APC* gene are present in only about one in 10,000 individuals, and familial adenomatous polyposis accounts for fewer than one percent of all colorectal cancer cases. In contrast, about two to five percent of colorectal cancers are thought to arise in those with hereditary nonpolyposis colorectal cancer (HNPCC).[101] Diagnosis of the HNPCC syndromes on a clinical basis alone is problematic for at least two reasons. First, the likelihood of chance clustering for a common malignancy like colorectal cancer exists within families because colorectal cancer will develop in about four percent of the United States population. In addition, those affected by HNPCC lack characteristic overt premalignant clinical lesions, such as intestinal polyposis. However, the following diagnostic criteria for HNPCC have been agreed on: (1) exclusion of polyposis; (2) colorectal cancer in at least three relatives, and one of them should be a first-degree relative of the others; (3) two of more successive generations should be affected; and (4) at least one of the affected individuals should be younger than 50 years at diagnosis. In addition to colorectal cancer, other cancers are often seen in families affected by HNPCC, including endometrial, urinary tract, and hepatobiliary tract cancers. These other cancers, however, are not included in the diagnostic criteria for HNPCC.

After the involvement of many of the known tumor suppressor genes in HNPCC was excluded, linkage studies of numerous large, unrelated HNPCC families were carried out by use of polymorphic markers scattered throughout the genome. On the basis of these studies, one HNPCC gene was mapped to chromosome 2p and another to chromosome 3p, and several families with HNPCC showed no linkage to either 2p or 3p.[102,103] A critical set of observations on an entirely new type of mutation in human cancer considerably facilitated the identification of the responsible genes, thereby avoiding the laborious positional cloning strategies usually required.

Specifically, cancers from patients with HNPCC were found to have characteristic alterations in simple repeated DNA sequences, termed microsatellites.[104] Each microsatellite is composed of a mononucleotide, dinucleotide, trinucleotide, or tetranucleotide repeat tract of variable length [e.g., $(A)_N$, $(CA)_N$, $(CAG)_N$, or $(CAGT)_N$], and microsatellites are dispersed widely throughout the genome. In the tumors of patients with HNPCC, expansions or contractions of the microsatellite repeats were seen and led to the generation of alleles not found in the normal cells of the same patient. This "microsatellite instability" was found to occur at many different microsatellite tracts, suggesting that the tumor cells of patients with HNPCC might harbor thousands or even tens of thousands of mutations, some of which might affect proto-oncogenes or tumor suppressor genes. Interestingly, microsatellite instability had previously been noted in about 15 percent of tumors in patients without a family history of colorectal cancer.[105, 106] The instability in microsatellite sequences was hypothesized to result from replication errors caused by defects in DNA synthesis or repair. Moreover, of keen interest were the observations that bacterial and yeast mutants with defects in DNA proofreading ("mismatch repair") displayed a replication error phenotype that was very similar to that of the tumor cells.[107]

Provoked by these similarities, investigators cloned the human homologue of the yeast *mutS* mismatch repair gene, termed *MSH*2, and localized it to chromosome 2p.[108] Subsequent studies revealed constitutional mutations in one *MSH*2 allele in affected individuals from many families in which the disease-causing HNPCC mutation had been localized to chromosome 2p.[109] The second *MSH*2 allele was found to be inactivated by somatic mutations in the colorectal cancers that arose in these patients. Present data suggest that affected individuals from about 30 to 35 percent of the colorectal cancer families meeting the classic clinical criteria for HNPCC harbor germ line mutations in an *MSH*2 allele.[107] After the *MSH*2 studies were conducted, a human homologue of the yeast *mutL* DNA mismatch repair gene, termed *MLH*1, was identified and localized to chromosome 3p.[107] Constitutional mutations in *MLH*1 appear to account for cancer predisposition in about 35 to 40 percent of HNPCC cases. Cancer predisposition in the remaining 25 to 35 percent of HNPCC cases appears to result from germ line mutations in one allele of other DNA mismatch repair genes, such as the *PMS*1 gene on chromosome 2q, the *PMS*2 gene on chromosome 7p, or perhaps other yet-to-be-identified genes.[107]

In the normal cells of patients with HNPCC, DNA repair is not impaired, because the cells retain one normal allele of the affected DNA repair gene. However, inactivation of this wild-type allele can occur as the result of a somatic mutation in a cell population that is initiated for tumor formation. The exact stage of tumorigenesis at which this inactivation of the wild-type DNA repair allele occurs is not yet well understood. Regardless, such a cell has lost, as a consequence, a vital component of the machinery required for the maintenance of its genomic integrity. The cell and its descendants will then accumulate genomic mutations at a high rate. Although many of the mutations that arise may be detrimental to cell growth and survival, some of the mutations may activate proto-oncogenes or inactivate tumor suppressor genes, thereby accelerating the normally slow rate of tumor progression.

Several questions remain unanswered concerning the nature and the role of mutations in the DNA repair genes in cancer. First, given the apparently ubiquitous expression of the DNA mismatch repair genes in adult tissues, the basis for the specific predisposition to colorectal cancer and to cancers of only a few other organs in those with HNPCC is not well understood. Second, although the HNPCC syndromes are thought to account for only about two to five percent of all colorectal cancer cases, about 15 percent of colorectal cancers display the replication error phenotype.[105,106] In addition, a sizable percentage of several other cancer types, including endometrial and ovarian cancer, also display the replication error phenotype.[107] However, in most cancers in patients who do not have a family history that meets the clinical criteria for diagnosis of HNPCC, somatic mutations in the *MSH2*, *MLH1*, *PMS1*, and *PMS2* genes have not been identified.[107] Presumably, germ line mutations, somatic mutations, or both, in other genes involved in DNA damage repair may generate somewhat similar cellular phenotypes.

Summary and Future Directions

Enormous progress has been made in the past two decades in identifying the genetic alterations present in human cancer. We now know that germ line and somatic mutations in three classes of genes—proto-onocogenes, tumor suppressor genes, and DNA damage repair genes—are critical to the initiation, progression, and biologic behavior of cancers. Undoubtedly, many additional discoveries on the nature and significance of various genetic alterations in human cancers await. For example, additional proto-oncogenes, tumor suppressor genes, and DNA repair genes that are targeted by somatic mutations in particular human tumors remain to be identified. Further studies will identify additional genes that are responsible for the inherited predisposition to cancer. Genes that modify the risk of cancer development in genetically predisposed individuals, as well as perhaps the general population, remain to be discovered. In addition, further studies may help to decipher further the relationships between dietary and environmental factors and particular somatic mutations. An optimistic view is that future studies of the genetic alterations in human cancer will lead not only to further understanding of the pathogenesis of cancer but also to insights that fundamentally alter the care and treatment of patients with cancer.

References

1. Bishop JM: Molecular themes in oncogenesis. *Cell* 64:235, 1991
2. Weinberg RA: Oncogenes, anti-oncogenes, and the molecular bases of multistep carcinogenesis. *Cancer Res* 49:3713, 1989
3. Rabbitts TH: Chromosomal translocations in human cancer. *Nature* 372:143, 1994
4. Francke U: Retinoblastoma and chromosome 13. *Cytogenet Cell Genet* 16:131, 1976
5. Riccardi VM, Hitter HM, Francke U, et al: The aniridia-Wilm's association: the clinical role of chromosome band 11p13. *Cancer Cytogenet* 2:131, 1980
6. Herrera L, Kakati S, Gibas L, et al: Brief clinical report: Gardner syndrome in a man with an interstitial deletion of 5q. *Am J Med Genet* 25:473, 1986

7. Fountain JW, Wallace MF, Bruce MJ, et al: Physical mapping of a translocation breakpoint in neurofibromatosis. *Science* 244:1085, 1989

8. O'Connell P, Leach R, Cawthon R, et al: Two von Recklinghausen neurofibromatosis translocations map within a 600 kb segment of 17q. *Science* 244:1087, 1989

9. Joslyn G, Carlson M, Thlivers A, et al: Identification of deletion mutations and three new genes at the familial polyposis locus. *Cell* 66:601, 1991

10. Groden J, Thlivers A, Samowitz W, et al: Identification and characterization of the familial adenomatous polyposis coli gene. *Cell* 66: 589, 1991

11. Latif F, Tory K, Gnarra J, et al: Identification of the von Hippel-Lindau disease tumor suppressor gene. *Science* 260:1317, 1993

12. Cavenee WK, Dryja TP, Phillips RA, et al: Expression of recessive alleles by chromosomal mechanisms in retinoblastoma. *Nature* 305:779, 1983

13. Lasko D, Cavenee WK, Nordenskjold M: Loss of constitutional heterozygosity in human cancer. *Annu Rev Genet* 25:281, 1991

14. van Heyningen V: One gene: four syndromes. *Nature* 367:319, 1994

15. Barbacid M: *ras* genes. *Annu Rev Biochem* 56:779, 1987

16. Bos JL: *ras* oncogenes in human cancer: a review. *Cancer Res* 49:4682, 1989

17. Fearon ER: K-*ras* mutation as a pathogenetic and diagnostic marker in human cancer. *J Natl Cancer Inst* 85:1978, 1993

18. Slebos RJ, Kibdelaar RE, Dalesio O, et al: K-*ras* activation as a prognostic marker in adenocarcinoma of the lung. *N Engl J Med* 323:561, 1990

19. Aplan PD, Lombardi DP, Ginsberg AM, et al: Disruption of the human SCL locus by "illegitimate" V-(D)-J recombinase activity. *Science* 250:1426, 1990

20. Korsmeyer SJ: *Bcl-2* initiates a new category of oncogenes: regulators of cell death. *Blood* 80:879, 1992

21. Limpens J, de Jong D, van Krieken JH, et al: Bcl-2/J_H rearrangements in benign lymphoid tissues with follicular hyperplasia. *Oncogene* 6:2271, 1991

22. Tsujimoto Y, Jaffe ES, Cossman J, et al: Clustering of breakpoints on chromosome 11 in human B-cell neoplasms with the t(11;14) chromosome translocation. *Nature* 315:340, 1985

23. Raffeld M, Jaffe ES: *bcl-1*, t(11;14) and mantle zone lymphoma. *Blood* 78:259, 1991

24. Motokura T, Bloom T, Goo KH, et al: A novel cyclin encoded by a *bcl-1* linked candidate oncogene. *Nature* 350:512, 1991

25. Motokura T, Arnold A: Cyclin D and oncogenesis. *Curr Opin Genet Dev* 3:5, 1993

26. Nowell PC, Hungerford DA: A minute chromosome in human granulocytic leukemia. *Science* 132:1497, 1960

27. Rowley JD: A new consistent chromosomal abnormality in chronic myelogenous leukemia. *Nature* 243:290, 1973

28. Sawyers CL, Denny CT, Witte ON: Leukemia and the disruption of hematopoiesis. *Cell* 64:337, 1991

29. Raimondi SC, Behm FG, Robertson PK, et al: Cytogenetics of pre-B acute lymphocytic leukemia with emphasis on prognostic implications of the t(1;19). *J Clin Oncol* 8:1380, 1990

30. Kamps MP, Murre C, Sun X-H, et al: A new homeobox gene contributes the DNA binding domain of the t(1;19) translocation protein in pre-B ALL. *Cell* 60:547, 1990

31. Kamps MP, Look AT, Baltimore D: The human t(1;19) translocation in pre-B ALL produces multiple nuclear E2A/PBX1 fusion proteins with differing transforming potential. *Genes Dev* 5:528, 1991

32. Takahashi T, Obata Y, Sekido Y, et al: Expression and amplification of *myc* gene family in small cell lung cancer and its relation to biological characteristics. *Cancer Res* 49:2683, 1989

33. Bargmann CI, Hung M-C, Weinberg RA: Multiple independent activations of the *neu* oncogene by a point mutation altering the transmembrane domain of p185. *Cell* 45:649, 1986

34. Bougall WC, Qian X, Peterson NC, et al: The *neu*-oncogene: signal transduction pathways, transformation mechanisms and evolving therapies. *Oncogene* 9:2109, 1994

35. Leon SP, Zhu J, Black PM: Genetic aberrations in human brain tumors. *Neurosurgery* 34:708, 1994

36. Klign JGM, Berns PMJJ, Schmitz PIM, et al: The clinical significance of epidermal growth factor receptor (EGF-R) in human breast cancer: a review of 5232 patients. *Endocr Rev* 13:3, 1992

37. Gillett C, Fantl V, Smith R, et al: Amplification and overexpression of cyclin D1 in breast cancer detected by immunohistochemical staining. *Cancer Res* 54:1812, 1994

38. Leach FS, Elledge SJ, Cherr CJ, et al: Amplification of cyclin genes in colorectal carcinomas. *Cancer Res* 53:1986, 1993

39. Khatib ZA, Matsushime H, Valentine M, et al: Coamplification of the *CDK4* gene with *MDM2* and *GLI* in human sarcomas. *Cancer Res* 53:5535, 1993

40. Schmidt EE, Ichimura K, Reifenberger G, Collins VP: *CDKN2 (p16/MTS1)* gene deletion or *CDK4* amplication occurs in the majority of glioblastomas. *Cancer Res* 54:6321, 1994

41. Grieco M, Santoro M, Berlingieri MT, et al: *PTC* is a novel rearranged form of the *ret* proto-oncogene and is frequently detected in vivo in human thyroid papillary carcinomas. *Cell* 60:557, 1990

42. Mulligan LM, Kwok JBJ, Healey CS, et al: Germ-line mutation of the *RET* proto-oncogene in multiple endocrine neoplasia type 2A. *Nature* 363:458, 1993

43. Hofstra RMW, Landsvater RM, Ceccherini I, et al: A mutation in the *RET* proto-oncogene associated with multiple endocrine neoplasia type 2B and sporadic medullary thyroid cancers. *Nature* 367, 375, 1994

44. Friend SH, Bernards R, Rogel S, et al: A human DNA segment with the properties of a gene that predisposes to retinoblastoma and osteosarcoma. *Nature* 323:643, 1986

45. Lee WH, Bookstein R, Hong F, et al: Human retinoblastoma susceptibility gene: cloning, identification and sequence. *Science* 235:1394, 1987

46. Fung Y-KT, Murphree AL, T-Ang A, et al: Structural evidence for the authenticity of the human retinoblastoma gene. *Science* 236:1657, 1987

47. Yandell D, Campbell TA, Dayton SH, et al: Oncogenic point mutations in the human retinoblastoma gene: their application to genetic counseling. *N Engl J Med* 321:1689, 1989

48. Horowitz J, Yandell DW, Parks S-H, et al: Point mutational inactivation of the retinoblastoma antioncogene. *Science* 243:937, 1989

49. Horowitz JM, Park S, Bogenmann E, et al: Frequent inactivation of the retinoblastoma anti-oncogene is restricted to a subset of human tumor cells. *Proc Natl Acad Sci USA* 87:2775, 1990

50. Munger K, Scheffner M, Huibregtse JM, Howley PM: Interactions of HPV E6 and E7 oncoproteins with tumour suppressor gene products. *Cancer Surv* 12:197, 1992

51. Scheffner M, Munger K, Byrne JC, et al: The state of the *p53* and retinoblastoma genes in human cervical carcinoma cell lines. *Proc Natl Acad Sci USA* 88:5523, 1991

52. Baker SJ, Fearon ER, Nigro JM, et al: Chromosome 17 deletions and *p53* gene mutations in colorectal carcinomas. *Science* 244:217, 1989

53. Levine AJ, Momand J, Finlay CA: The *p53* tumor suppressor gene. *Nature* 351:453, 1991

54. Greenblatt MS, Bennett WP, Hollstein M, Harris CC: Mutations in the *p53* tumor suppressor gene: clues to cancer etiology and molecular pathogenesis. *Cancer Res* 54:4855, 1994

55. Cho Y, Gorina S, Jeffrey PD, Pavletich NP: Crystal structure of the p53 tumor suppressor-DNA complex: understanding tumorigenic mutations. *Science* 265:334, 1994

56. Malkin D, Li FP, Strong LC, et al: Germ line *p53* mutations in a familial syndrome of breast cancer, sarcomas, and other neoplasms. *Science* 250:1233, 1990

57. Birch JM, Hartley AL, Tricker KJ, et al: Prevalence and diversity of constitutional mutations in the *p53* gene among 21 Li-Fraumeni families. *Cancer Res* 54:1298, 1994

58. Vogelstein B, Kinzler KW: p53 function and dysfunction. *Cell* 70:523, 1992

59. Oliner JD, Kinzler KW, Meltzer PS, et al: Amplification of a gene encoding a p53-associated protein in human sarcomas. *Nature* 358:80, 1992

60. Polakis P: Mutations in the *APC* gene and their implication for protein structure and function. *Curr Opin Genet Dev* 5:66, 1995

61. Nagase H, Nakamura Y: Mutations of the *APC* (adenomatous polyposis coli) gene. *Hum Mutat* 2:425, 1993

62. Madl M, Paffenholz R, Freidl W, et al: Frequency of common and novel inactivating *APC* mutations in 202 families with familial adenomatous polyposis. *Hum Mol Genet* 3:181, 1994

63. Powell SM, Petersen GEM, Krush AJ, et al: Molecular diagnosis of familial adenomatous polyposis. *N Engl J Med* 329:1982, 1993

64. Spirio L, Olschwang S, Groden J, et al: Alleles of the *APC* gene: an attenuated form of familial polyposis. *Cell* 75:951, 1993

65. Hamilton SR, Liu B, Parsons RE, et al: The molecular basis of Turcot's Syndrome. *N Engl J Med* 332:839, 1995

66. Miyaki M, Konishi M, Kikuchi-Yanoshita R, et al: Characteristics of somatic mutations of the adenomatous polyposis coli gene in colorectal tumors. *Cancer Res* 54:3011, 1994

67. Olopade OI, Bohlander SK, Pomykala H, et al: Mapping of the shortest region of overlap of deletions of the short arm of chromosome 9 associated with human neoplasia. *Genomics* 14:437, 1992

68. Fountain JW, Karayiorgou M, Ernstoff MS, et al: Homozygous deletions within human chromosome band 9p21 in melanoma. *Proc Natl Acad Sci USA* 89:10557, 1992

69. James CD, Collins VP, Allaluni-Turner MJ, Days RS: Localization of chromosome 9p homozygous deletions in glioma cell lines with markers constituting a continuous linkage map. *Cancer Res* 53:3674, 1993

70. Weaver-Feldhaus J, Gruis NE, Neuhausen S, et al: Localization of a putative tumor suppressor gene by using homozygous deletions in melanomas. *Proc Natl Acad Sci USA* 91:7563, 1994

71. Wainwright B: Familial melanoma and *p16*: a hung jury. *Nature Genet* 8:3, 1994

72. Kamb A, Gruis NA, Weaver-Feldhaus J, et al: A cell cycle regulator potentially involved in genesis of many tumor types. *Science* 264:436, 1994

73. Noburi T, Miura K, Wu DJ, et al: Deletions of the cyclin-dependent kinase-4 inhibitor gene in multiple human cancers. *Nature* 368:753, 1994

74. Cairns P, Mao L, Merlo A, et al: Rates of *p16* (*MTS1*) mutations in primary tumors with 9p loss. *Science* 265:415, 1994

75. Spruck CHL, Gonzalez-Zuleta M, Shibata A, et al: *p16* gene in uncultured tumors. *Nature* 370:183, 1994

76. Bonnetta L: Tumour suppressor genes: open questions on *p16*. *Nature* 370:180, 1994

77. Jen J, Harper JW, Bigner SH, et al: Deletion of *p16* and *p15* genes in brain tumors. *Cancer Res* 54:6353, 1994

78. Merlo A, Herman JG, Mao L, et al: 5'CpG island methylation is associated with transcriptional silencing of the tumor suppressor *p16/CDKN2/MTS1* in human cancers. *Nat Med* 1:686, 1995

79. Gonzalez-Zulueta M, Bender CM, Yang AS, et al: Methylation of the 5'CpG island of the *p16/CDKN2* tumor suppressor gene in normal and transformed human tissues correlates with gene silencing. *Cancer Res* 55:4531, 1995

80. Call KM, Glaser T, Ito CY, et al: Isolation and characterization of a zinc finger polypeptide gene at the human chromosome 11 Wilms' tumor locus. *Cell* 60:509, 1990

81. Gessler M, Poutska A, Cavenee WK, et al: Homozygous deletion in Wilms' tumors of a zinc-finger gene identified by chromosome jumping. *Nature* 343:774, 1990

82. Rauscher FJ III: The WT1 Wilms' tumor gene product: a developmentally regulated transcription factor in the kidney that functions as a tumor suppressor. *FASEB J* 7:896, 1993

83. Coppes MJ, Haber DA, Grundy PE: Genetic events in the development of Wilms' tumor. *N Engl J Med* 331:586, 1994

84. Ladanyi M, Gerald W: Fusion of the *EWS* and *WT1* genes in desmoplastic small round cell tumor. *Cancer Res* 54:2837, 1994

85. Viskochil D, White R, Cawthon R: The neurofibromatosis type 1 gene. *Annu Rev Neurosci* 16:183, 1993

86. Trofatter J, MacCollin M, Rutter J, et al: A novel moesin-, ezrin-, radixin-like gene is a candidate for the neurofibromatosis 2 tumor suppressor. *Cell* 72:791, 1993

87. Rouleau GA, Merel P, Luchtman M, et al: Alteration in a new gene encoding a putative membrane-organizing protein causes neurofibromatosis type 2. *Nature* 363:515, 1993

88. Shuin T, Kondo K, Torigoe S, et al: Frequent somatic mutations and loss of heterozygosity of the von Hippel-Lindau tumor suppressor gene in primary human renal cell carcinomas. *Cancer Res* 54:2852, 1994

89. Herman JG, Latif F, Weng Y, et al: Silencing of the *VHL* tumor-suppressor gene by DNA methylation in renal carcinoma. *Proc Natl Acad Sci USA* 91:9700, 1994

90. Hall JM, Lee MK, Newman B, et al: Linkage of early onset breast cancer to chromosome 17q21. *Science* 250:1684, 1990

91. Easton DF, Bishop DT, Ford D, Crockford GP: Genetic linkage analysis in familial breast and ovarian cancer: result from 214 families. *Am J Hum Genet* 52:678, 1993

92. Miki Y, Swensen J, Shattuck-Eidens D, et al: A strong candidate for the breast and ovarian cancer susceptibility gene *BRCA1*. Science 266:66, 1994

93. Futreal PA, Lui Q, Shattuck-Eidens D, et al: *BRCA1* mutations in primary breast and ovarian carcinomas. *Science* 266:120, 1994

94. Gayther SA, Warren W, Mazoyer S, et al: Germ line mutations of the *BRCA1* gene in breast and ovarian cancer families provide evidence for a genotype-phenotype correlation. *Nature Genet* 11:428, 1995

95. Vogelstein B, Kinzler KW: Has the breast cancer gene been found? *Cell* 79:1, 1994

96. Chen Y, Chen C-F, Riley DJ, et al: Aberrant subcellular localization of BRCA1 in breast cancer. *Science* 270:789, 1995

97. Wooster R, Bigness G, Lancaster J, et al: Identification of the breast cancer susceptibility gene BRCA2. Nature 378:789, 1995

98. Cho KR, Fearon ER: *DCC*: linking tumor suppressor genes and altered cell surface interactions in cancer? *Curr Opin Genet Dev* 5:72, 1995

99. Kinzler KW, Nilbert MC, Vogelstein B, et al: Identification of a gene located at chromosome 5q21 that is mutated in colorectal cancers. *Science* 251:1366, 1991

100. Birchmeier W, Hulsken J, Behrens J: Adherens junction proteins in tumour progression. *Cancer Surv* 24:129, 1995

101. Lynch HT, Smyrk RC, Watson P, et al: Genetics, natural history, tumor spectrum, and pathology of hereditary nonpolyposis colorectal cancer: an updated review. *Gastroenterology* 104:1535, 1993

102. Peltomaki P, Aaltonen LA, Sistonen P, et al: Genetic mapping of a locus predisposing to human colorectal cancer. *Science* 260:810, 1993

103. Lindblom A, Tannergard P, Werelius B, Nordenskjold M: Genetic mapping of a second locus predisposing to hereditary nonpolyposis colorectal cancer. *Nature Genet* 5:279, 1993

104. Aalton LA, Peltomaki P, Leach FS, et al: Clues to the pathogenesis of familial colorectal cancer. *Science* 260:812, 1993

105. Thibodeau SN, Bren G, Schaid D: Microsatellite instability in cancer of the proximal colon. *Science* 260:816, 1993

106. Ionov YM, Peinado A, Malkhosyan S, et al: Ubiquitous somatic mutations in simple repeated sequences reveal a new mechanism for colonic carcinogenesis. *Nature* 363:558, 1993

107. Modrich P: Mismatch repair, genetic stability, and cancer. *Science* 266:1959, 1994

108. Fishel R, Lescoe MK, Rao MRS, et al. The human mutator gene homolog *MSH2* and its association with hereditary nonpolyposis colon cancer. *Cell* 75:1027, 1993

109. Leach FS, Nicolaides NC, Papadopoulos N, et al: Mutations of a *MutS* homolog in hereditary non-polyposis colorectal cancer. *Cell* 75:1215, 1993

Acknowledgments

Figure 1   Kathy Konkle. Adapted from "The Genetics of Colorectal Tumor Development: The Emerging Picture and Clinical Implications," by E. R. Fearon, in *Seminars in Colon and Rectal Surgery* 2:253, 1991. Used by permission.

Figure 2   Kathy Konkle. Adapted from "Oncogenes and Tumor Suppressor Genes," by E. R. Fearon, in *Clinical Oncology*, edited by M. D. Abeloff, J. O. Armitage, A. S. Lichter, and J. E. Niederhuber. Churchill Livingstone, New York, 1995, p 11. Used by permission.

Figure 3   Marcia Kammerer. Adapted from "p53: A Glimpse at the Puppet Behind the Shadow Play," by S. H. Friend, in *Science* 265:334, 1994. Used by permission.

Figure 4   Talar Agasyan. Adapted from "Mutations in the APC Gene and their Implications for Protein Structure and Function," by P. Polakis, in *Current Opinion in Genetics and Development* 5:66, 1995. Used by permission.

Figure 5   Kathy Konkle.

Table 1   Adapted from "Oncogenes and Tumor Suppressor Genes," by E. R. Fearon, in *Clinical Oncology*, edited by M. D. Abeloff, J. O. Armitage, A. S. Lichter, and J. E. Niederhuber. Churchill Livingstone, New York, 1995, p 11. Used by permission.

Tables 2 through 4   Adapted from "Chromosomal Translocations in Human Cancer," by T. H. Rabbitts, in *Nature* 372:143, 1994. Used by permission.

CHAPTER 8

The Molecular Pathogenesis of Cancer

Robert A. Weinberg, Ph.D., Douglas Hanahan, Ph.D.

T he extensive descriptions of oncogenes and tumor suppressor genes that have preceded this chapter represent a revolution in our understanding of the genetic and molecular mechanisms that underlie cancer pathogenesis. The findings described in the preceding chapters have been obtained by use of a variety of experimental models, many of which were designed to reveal the actions of single cancer-causing genes operating amid the complex genetic background that is present in all cells. Although these experimental strategies have proved to be enormously fruitful, they leave the impression that tumorigenesis is a simple process in which one or another mutant gene succeeds in redirecting the growth program of a hitherto normal cell, thereby transforming it into a malignant derivative.

Such simplicity is an illusion; tumorigenesis in humans is a complex process of multiple steps that incrementally convert a fully normal cell into one that is highly neoplastic in its growth properties. This chapter discusses the evidence of the multistep nature of tumorigenesis and the roles played by the individual steps in the creation of a fully malignant tumor.

This tension between experimental models of tumor pathogenesis and the experience gained from the study of actual human tumors is most apparent after review of the results of gene transfer experiments in which activated, mutant oncogenes were used. Introduction of mutant *ras* oncogenes into nontransformed NIH3T3 mouse fibroblasts results in the malignant transformation of these cells, seemingly in a single step. Similarly, numerous tumor viruses transform infected cells from a normal to a malignant growth phenotype in a single step.

These gene transfer (transfection) experiments illustrate the powers of cell and viral oncogenes, but they are difficult to reconcile with the complex histopathology of premalignant and malignant tissues in humans. This far greater complexity becomes most apparent in the study of tissues that are anatomically accessible and therefore provide ample opportunity for biopsy at various stages during the process of tumor development. Most striking in this regard are observations deriving from the colon. Colonoscopy reveals the presence of many distinct histopathologic tissue entities that deviate to differing extents from the normal intestinal epithelium.

Among these growths are hyperplastic epithelium, dysplastic epithelium, several classes of adenomatous polyps, localized carcinomas, and finally carcinomas that have invaded underlying basement membrane and have begun to metastasize via lymphatics or blood vessels to distant sites. Similar catalogues, usually less extensive, have been compiled for growths that are present in other organ sites. In each instance, the diversity of abnormally structured tissues is incompatible with the notion of a simple dichotomy between normal and malignant tissue. Implicit in these observations is the idea that the individual cells that populate each of these aberrant growths have corresponding degrees of deviancy from their counterparts in fully normal tissue. This complexity contrasts starkly with the in vitro models of cell transformation, which portray cells as being either normal or transformed in their growth properties.

The various histopathologic entities seen in the colon can be arrayed in stages of increasing abnormalcy. Such alignments range from mildly hyperplastic tissue, to dysplastic tissue, and finally to frankly neoplastic growths. This arrangement is compatible with a process in which initially normal cell populations pass through a succession of increasingly abnormal stages on their way to becoming fully neoplastic. Importantly, these observations do not prove the existence of such a multistep model of tumorigenesis, being equally compatible with an alternative model in which normal cells can be transformed into a variety of abnormal states in single steps. For example, the histopathologic observations in the colon might also suggest the ability of some normal epithelial cells to convert themselves in a single step into cells that are capable of forming an adenomatous polyp, whereas other previously normal cells might undergo transformation directly into highly malignant carcinoma cells.

Epidemiology and Multistep Cancer Pathogenesis

Because histopathology has a limited ability to prove the concept of multistep tumorigenesis, one must look elsewhere for such evidence. Epidemiology provides some compelling evidence, albeit indirect, on this point. This evidence comes from analysis of the age-related risks of contracting various types of tumors. The risk of contracting most cancers increases steeply with age. In the case of colon cancer, this risk is as much as 1,000 times higher in a 70-year-old person than in a 20-year-old person [see Figure 1].

This example can be generalized: precise analysis of the age-dependent onset of many types of adult cancers indicates that tumor incidence increases with the 4th to 6th power of elapsed lifetime.[1] Such kinetics imply that tumor formation depends on a succession of four to six rate-limiting steps, each of which occurs with relatively low probability per year, and all of which must occur for a tumor to become clinically apparent. However,

a

b

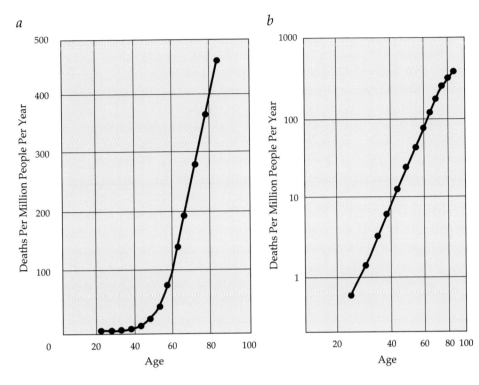

Figure 1 *Annual United States death rate from cancer of the large intestine in relation to age. (a) Linear scales. (b) Logarithmic scales.*

such analyses have substantial limitations, in that they reveal nothing about the nature of these steps, whether they must occur in a defined order, and whether the rate-limiting steps involve a succession of changes in the cells that are evolving toward malignancy or changes in the host that harbors the developing premalignant cell population. Moreover, only slowly occurring rate-limiting steps register in these kinetic analyses; yet other steps may occur rapidly and therefore do not significantly influence the time at which the end point is reached. For this reason, epidemiologic analysis may actually underestimate the number of steps involved in the process as a whole.

Nonetheless, epidemiology does provide clear indications that tumorigenesis in humans is a process of multiple steps, each of which requires years to reach completion. The extended time of tumor development implied by this model is reflected by the long duration between the initial cancer-provoking experiences and the ultimate appearance of tumors. For example, the great increase in female smoking rates in the United States in the years after World War II manifested itself in dramatically increased lung cancer frequency only after an interval of 25 to 30 years.[2] Similarly, shipyard workers exposed to heavy concentrations of asbestos often succumbed to mesothelioma many decades after their occupational exposure had ceased.[3]

Oncogene Collaboration

Many, and perhaps all, of the slow, rate-limiting steps that constitute tumor progression are mutations sustained in the genomes of evolving premalignant cell populations. This notion was first suggested from work on experimentally induced mouse skin tumors that were created by treatments involving combinations of initiating agents, such as the coal tar compound, 3-methyl-cholanthrene, and promoting agents, such as tetradecanoyl phorbol acetate.[4,5] The results of this work provided strong, albeit indirect, evidence that at least two genetic alterations were required for conversion of normal skin keratinocytes into those capable of forming squamous cell carcinomas.

A more direct demonstration of the importance of multiple genetic alterations in tumorigenesis came from the experimental manipulation of cloned oncogenes. For example, introduction of a *ras* oncogene into NIH3T3 mouse cells resulted in the malignant transformation of these cells. However, transformation was not observed when this oncogene was transfected into rat embryo cells that had been cultured for only a small number of passages after explantation from the embryo.[6] The responsiveness of the NIH3T3 cells was traced to their extended passage and establishment in vitro. This establishment, which included their acquisition of unlimited replicative ability (immortalization), enabled these cells to become transformed by a single oncogene. Hence, the act of establishment/immortalization, which itself appears to involve genetic alteration, represented a change in these cells that was essential to their ability to respond to an introduced *ras* oncogene by undergoing transformation. In effect, the genetic event or events that immortalized these cells collaborated with the *ras* oncogene in the process of creating the transformed cell phenotype.

Even more compelling were experiments in which multiple oncogenes were introduced directly into fully normal rat embryo fibroblast or kidney cells. These experiments revealed that certain pairs of oncogenes, such as *ras* and *myc,* could collaborate efficiently to transform these embryo cells [*see Figure 2*].[6] Indeed, almost 20 such pairs of collaborating oncogenes have been documented in the dozen years since this observation was first made [*see Table 1*]. In each instance, neither of the participating oncogenes could elicit malignant transformation when working alone.

This oncogene collaboration yielded one conceptual model through

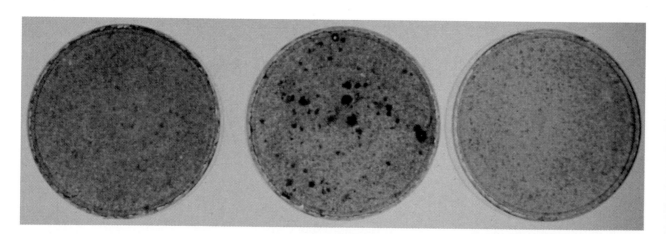

Figure 2 *Rat embryo fibroblasts into which a* ras *oncogene (left), a* myc *oncogene (right), or both oncogenes (center) have been introduced by gene transfer (transfection). Only the two oncogenes together induce foci of transformed cells.*

Table 1   Oncogenes Found to Collaborate
in Transformation of Fibroblasts

Nuclear Oncogene	Cytoplasmic Oncogene
Polyoma large T	Polyoma middle T
myc	ras
N-myc	ras
L-myc	ras
p53	ras
Adenovirus E1A	ras
SV40, polyoma large T	ras
HPV E7	ras
myc	bcr-abl
tax	ras
myc	src

which multistep tumorigenesis could be understood. Thus, the individual, rate-limiting steps of tumorigenesis might represent the successive mutation of an array of growth-controlling genes, notably proto-oncogenes. Any one of these mutated genes would be unable to elicit the phenotype of tumorigenicity on its own. Rather, the collaborative workings of two and perhaps more mutant genes seemed essential to produce the tumorigenic phenotype.

Manipulations of cloned oncogenes in vivo sustained and extended this conclusion. These experiments depended on the introduction of oncogene clones into the germ line of the mouse. Almost always, expression of the resulting transgenes has been governed by a tissue-specific transcriptional promoter. Hence, expression of the oncogene is confined to a narrow range of tissues, often in a well-defined window of time during development. In these transgenic models of tumorigenesis, the presence of an activated oncogene in a tissue is preordained rather than dependent on some stochastic somatic mutation. Mice bearing such transgenes demonstrate tumors at very high frequency and usually at tissue sites predicted by the promoter that is driving transgene expression.

With rare exception, tumors develop in these transgenic mice only after several months of life. One observation showed, for example, that mice bearing a *myc* oncogene under the control of a mouse mammary tumor virus promoter yielded mammary tumors beginning when the mice were three to four months of age.[7] These tumors appeared as discrete, focal outgrowths. Such a focal development contrasted starkly with the uniform expression of the oncogene in virtually all the cells of the mammary epithelium with attendant widespread hyperplasia.

Clearly the *myc* transgene, although strongly predisposing this tissue to the development of mammary carcinomas, could not create these tumors on its own. Moreover, the carcinomas appeared only after great delay, after many months of constant, high-level *myc* expression throughout the mammary tissue. Thus, a second, slowly occurring, rate-limiting event was required for the final conversion to malignant growth.

Such evidence indicated that the presence of the *myc* oncogene, although necessary for triggering carcinomas in these transgenic mice, was not sufficient. Rather, it predisposed mammary epithelial cells to undergo malignant transformation. This transformation appeared to depend on relatively rare stochastic events, likely somatic mutations, which conspired with the transgene to induce tumorigenic growth. The low probability of occurrence of these somatic mutations seemed to explain why a small number of focal outgrowths of neoplastic cells appeared amid large fields of hyperplastic precursors.

Other experiments with transgenic mice support the notion that these slowly occurring, stochastic events are indeed somatic mutations in the cells that already bear an oncogenic transgene. In this other work, somatic mutations were actively promoted in an attempt to ascertain whether they could accelerate the normally slow accretion of tumors in transgenic mice. These mutations were induced by infecting transgenic mice early in life with a murine leukemia virus (MLV). This retrovirus acts as a potent mutagen through its ability to insert its proviral genome randomly into millions of different sites in the genomes of infected host cells. Occasionally, the chromosomal integration of an MLV provirus may act as an "insertional mutagen" by perturbing the activity of genes that happen to lie next to its site of chromosomal integration.

Murine leukemia virus infection in mice bearing transgenic oncogenes invariably accelerates the pace of tumorigenesis. The precise mechanism of this acceleration can be determined by molecular cloning of the integrated proviruses in these tumors together with the adjacently located chromosomal domains. Often, the MLV proviruses are found to have inserted themselves adjacent to proto-oncogenes whose expression is now deregulated and greatly enhanced. Thus, in one case of mice bearing a *myc* transgenic oncogene, the MLV proviruses were found to have activated the *pim*-1 proto-oncogene.[8,9]

One can conclude that a somatically activated oncogene collaborated with the germ line transgene to trigger tumor formation. In a more general sense, it is apparent that the somatic events that collaborate with transgenic oncogenes are indeed mutations that activate yet other oncogenes.

The same theme of oncogene collaboration emerges from interbreeding of two strains of transgenic mice, each of which bears a transgenic oncogene. When MMTV-*myc* mice are bred with MMTV-*ras* mice, the rate of breast tumor formation in the F1 hybrids is greatly accelerated over that seen in either of the parental transgenic strains [*see Figure 3*].[10] This finding suggests that the complementary activities of two distinct oncogenes function collaboratively to create fully tumorigenic cells.

Mechanisms of Oncogene Collaboration

The observed need to introduce multiple oncogenes into cells so that malignant transformation can be achieved suggests the existence of a powerful antineoplastic mechanism that likely operates in all cells. Thus, the cellular growth-controlling machinery appears to be organized in a fashion that resists full deregulation by one or another mutant gene. Only when multiple control points are disrupted through multiple gene mutations is this machinery overwhelmed; only then does the cell respond by launching a neoplastic growth program.

Unexplained by this model are the precise mechanisms by which oncogenes collaborate to effect cell transformation. Various cell physiologic mechanisms have been invoked as explanations for the synergistic effects of these genes. For example, oncogenes like *ras* are seen to be particularly potent in inducing the phenotypes of morphological transformation and anchorage independence (the ability to grow without direct attachment to substrate) while being unable to affect the process of cell immortalization. Conversely, oncogenes like *myc*, which are relatively weak in inducing anchorage independence, are able to facilitate the processes that lead to cell immortalization. Together, these two complementary activities would seem to contribute vital components of the neoplastic growth program.

An alternative physiologic model of oncogene collaboration is derived from observations that several oncogenes, including *myc* and *E1A*, render cells susceptible to the process of programmed cell death, or apoptosis.[11,12] This cellular response appears to be somewhat paradoxical, given the implied role of these genes in the induction of transformation. However, this apoptosis can be easily rationalized: cells and tissues are organized to resist the process of transformation. For this reason, the first response of cells to the presence of an activated oncogene may often be a triggering of the pro-

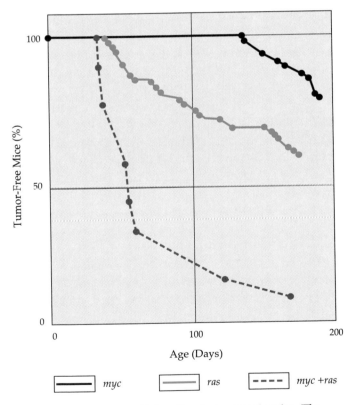

Figure 3   *Oncogene collaboration in transgenic mice. The graphs show the incidence of tumors in three types of transgenic mice, one carrying a* myc *oncogene, one carrying a* ras *oncogene, and one carrying both oncogenes.*

grammed cell death program. This response would appear to serve as a mechanism through which the body eliminates oncogene-bearing cells from its midst.

Viewed in this way, apoptotic death represents a major obstacle to the proliferative potential of the oncogene-bearing cell. A second, complementing oncogene arising in such a cell may save this cell from apoptotic death, enabling it to survive and proliferate into a tumorigenic cell clone. Only then can the growth-promoting effects of the first oncogene become manifest. For example, cells bearing only a *myc* or an *E1A* oncogene are highly susceptible to entering into apoptotic death; however, when other oncogenes such as *ras* are introduced into these cells, this tendency toward apoptosis is reversed.[13,14] As a consequence, cell growth and division can now benefit from the strong mitogenic impetus provided by the initially introduced oncogene.

Evidence from Human Tumors

Taken together, these various lines of experimentation lead to a general model of tumorigenesis in which the process of tumor progression is driven by a succession of somatic mutations sustained in the genome of premalignant populations of cells. Each of these mutations represents a rate-limiting event in this process. However, none of these mutations on its own suffices to achieve the end result of full tumorigenic conversion.

Such thinking is formally similar to models of darwinian evolution, in which a succession of mutations in the genome of an evolving population of organisms renders individuals in this population increasingly able to compete under conditions of natural selection. In tumorigenesis, the units undergoing selection are single cells; the succession of mutations would seem to allow premalignant cells to reproduce more effectively than their neighbors in the tissue.

Conceptual models like these are largely inspired by experiments involving the manipulation of cultured cells and mice. However, the relevance of these experiments to the natural process of tumor progression in humans is not immediately obvious. For example, tissues bearing transgenic oncogenes may not behave like those in which oncogenes arise through random somatic mutations. Moreover, the addition of specific oncogenes to the genomes of mouse strains prejudges the identities of the genes that actually participate in the formation of human tumors. In reality, relatively few human tumors have been found to carry more than a single activated oncogene, even though all are known or suspected to have undergone multiple genetic changes during tumorigenesis. Such observations suggest that other types of genes besides the proto-oncogenes are important targets of mutation during multistep tumor progression.

Evidence implicating these other genes in tumor pathogenesis has been obtained by careful genetic analysis of premalignant and malignant cell populations in numerous organ sites. This analysis has been most extensive in the case of tumorigenesis occurring in the colon. These studies were facilitated by the large number of individuals who were routinely studied by colonoscopy and by the ease of obtaining biopsies of colonic tissue.

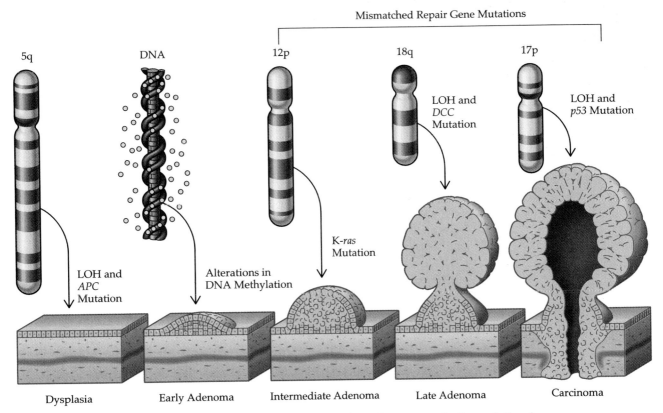

Figure 4 *A series of at least five molecular events has been proposed to account for the evolution (or transformation) of normal bowel mucosa first into an adenomatous polyp, then into carcinoma in situ, and finally into invasive cancer.*

As demonstrated by Vogelstein and Kinzler,[15] the increasing histopathologic abnormality of the colonic epithelium is accompanied by an increased number of mutations that are accumulated at defined genetic loci. Thus, cells of early colonic polyps carry mutations in the *APC* gene, whereas those in more advanced polyps carry mutations in this gene and in addition often carry a mutated *ras* oncogene. Yet more advanced polyps appear to have undergone changes at a locus close to and perhaps identical with the *DCC* gene. Finally, the conversion of an advanced adenomatous polyp to a frank carcinoma is often accompanied by mutation of the *p53* gene [*see Figure 4*].

On several occasions, such studies have analyzed carcinomas that appear to be growing directly out of advanced polyps. The two histologically distinct lesions were found to contain identical genetic lesions (e.g., the same unique point mutation in a *ras* oncogene).[16] This correlation provides the most direct evidence to date of the notion that more malignant cells derive directly from precursors that are themselves already aberrant in phenotype and genotype.

Significantly, only one of the four genes that have been implicated by these workers in colon tumorigenesis is an oncogene—*ras*. The other three genes are classified as tumor suppressor genes. As expected of tumor suppressor genes, the mutations that involve these genes in tumorigenesis result in their inactivation rather than in their potentiation. This characteristic creates a new dimension of complexity, in that it suggests that the mutations that collaborate to create a tumor may target both proto-oncogenes and tumor suppressor genes. Indeed, the involvement of yet other types of genes is possible, although not indicated directly by this work. Thus, although the mutation of these two classes of genes may suffice to create a deregulated growth state characteristic of a carcinoma in situ, such mutant genes may not explain other phenotypes of tumor cells, including their ability to invade and to metastasize.

The mutations affecting these genes would seem to represent the rare, rate-limiting events in tumorigenesis postulated by the epidemiologists. As such, each of these mutations appears to be an important milestone in the development of a fully malignant tumor. Although this assumption is unproved, it seems likely that these various mutations represent the molecular processes that underlie the successive histopathologic conversions that accompany tumor progression.

These observations and others appear to suggest a fixed and ordered sequence of mutations that convert normal colonic epithelial cells into malignant derivatives. In fact, none of the aforementioned genetic changes is found in all colonic tumors. For example, mutant alleles of the *ras* gene are seen in only about half of colon tumors; a slightly higher fraction of tumors carry mutant *p53* genes. Therefore, the sequence of mutations involving *APC*, *ras*, *DCC*, and *p53* represents only one genetic pathway of many that may be chosen by a colonic epithelial cell population that is progressing to malignancy. A series of alternative pathways involving other genes is implied; in colon cancers, the identities of these other genetic targets remain elusive.

The discovery that human cancer cells, particularly colon carcinoma cells, carry numerous mutant genes in their genomes suggests a simple model by which the complex spectrum of cancer-specific traits is induced: each cell or tumor-specific trait can be traced back to the actions of a distinct mutant gene carried in the genome of the tumor cell. This implies that the overall phenotype of the malignantly transformed cell is no more than the sum of the activities of the mutant genes that this cell carries. Because many genes, including oncogenes, act pleiotropically—being able to elicit many different traits simultaneously—the number of cancer-specific cell changes may be far larger than the number of mutant genes that are orchestrating these changes.

The particular scenario associated with colon carcinoma progression suggests that similar processes of tumorigenesis may occur in tissue sites throughout the body. To date, however, the genetic histories of other types of tumors have been less extensively documented. Over the next decade, catalogues will likely be developed of the genes that participate in multistep tumorigenesis in various organ sites throughout the body.

Sporadic and Familial Cancers

The initially mutated gene in most sporadic colon carcinomas, the *APC* tumor suppressor gene, also plays a prominent role in the familial adenomatous polyposis (FAP) syndrome. In particular, hundreds to thousands of adenomatous polyps often develop in the colons of individuals inheriting a defective alleles of *APC*; some of these polyps then progress to carcinomas.[17] Indeed, this progression provides yet another proof of the role of dysplastic growths as the direct (and apparently obligate) precursors of neoplasias.

This close genetic connection between sporadic and familial tumors is easily rationalized in terms of the multistep model of tumorigenesis. Thus, if a mutant allele of *APC* is inherited from one or another parent, this allele is present in all cells of the colonic epithelium. Its presence in an already mutated form in these cells obviates the normally required somatic mutation of this gene, thus hastening the entire process of tumorigenesis by circumventing an early, rate-limiting step. In effect, all the intestinal epithelial cells in the colon of a patient with FAP have been catapulted directly to the second genetic step in tumorigenesis, thus ensuring that many of them develop into cells that are capable of forming adenomatous polyps in several decades. In normal individuals, in contrast, the process of polyp formation is extremely slow and depends on rare, stochastic events that result in the appearance of few if any polyps during the course an average human life span.

The FAP syndrome is an example of an important general principle of familial cancers that affect other organ sites. In these other instances, a gene that is mutated somatically and participates in sporadic forms of a particular cancer may also be carried in mutant form in the germ line, yielding an inborn susceptibility to the same tumor. Retinoblastoma provides a highly illustrative example of this principle [*see Chapter 6*].

In truth, the relationships between sporadic and familial tumors may be more complex. For example, the *p53* gene is mutated as a relatively late event in sporadic colon tumor progression. Mutant germ line alleles of this tumor suppressor gene result in Li-Fraumeni syndrome, in which numerous organs are placed at high risk as sites for tumorigenesis; the colon does not figure prominently among these sites.[18] This discordance can be rationalized in several ways. Most attractive is the proposition that only those genes that are mutated as an early, initiating step in the genesis of a sporadic tumor yield familial forms of the same tumor when these genes are carried as mutant alleles in the germ line.

Other Mechanisms of Inborn Cancer Susceptibility

In the past several years, the genetic bases of another type of familial colon cancer has been uncovered. This other syndrome—hereditary nonpolyposis colon cancer (HNPCC)—involves a class of genes that is not directly connected to the regulation of cell proliferation. The study of HNPCC has opened a new vista on multistep tumorigenesis. Traditionally, growth-controlling genes—proto-oncogenes and tumor suppressor genes—have been considered the sole targets of mutational change during tumorigenesis. Now, when describing HNPCC, we recognize that the alteration of other classes of genes may be equally beneficial for the proliferative potential of cell clones.

Mutant alleles of at least four distinct genes (*MSH2*, *MLH*1, *PMS*1, and *PMS*2) have been implicated in the HNPCC syndrome.[19,20] The common feature of these genes is that they encode components of the cellular machinery that is responsible for maintaining the integrity of the cell genome, specifically the apparatus dedicated to repair of DNA mismatches. The products of each of the four distinct genes appear to be essential to the cell's ability to recognize and repair errors that occur as a consequence of the normal process of DNA replication.

As would be predicted from the known biochemical functions of the products of these four genes, cells that lack the ability to repair their genomes do indeed accumulate genetic damage at very high rates. Detailed examination of the tumor cells from individuals suffering from HNPCC reveals a high degree of genetic disorder throughout their genomes. This high mutability, in turn, seems to favor colon tumorigenesis. Unexplained by these observations are the reasons why deficiencies in DNA repair, which would seem prone to affect tissues throughout the body, have such profound and focused effects on the colon.

The HNPCC syndrome echoes a theme suggested by the study of the *APC* gene and FAP. In both instances, the complex process of multistep tumorigenesis is accelerated by alterations in the schedule with which the rate-limiting steps take place. In FAP, this acceleration occurs because an early, initiating step in tumor progression is obviated. In HNPCC, the increased mutability of the genome would seem to quicken the pace with which all of the normally slow, rate-limiting mutational steps occur [*see Figure 4*]. The same model can be extended to many other cancer susceptibility syndromes that stem from inborn deficiencies in the maintenance of genomic integrity.

Mechanisms Controlling Tumor Cell Proliferation

The mutations accumulated by tumor cells as they evolve toward malignancy must ultimately be explained in terms of cell physiology. More specifically, the question of how each of these genes, once mutated, confer increased proliferative advantage on clones of premalignant cells must be answered. The responses to this question are numerous.

Perhaps the most salient feature of cancer cells is their proliferative drive—their tendency to multiply continuously, in contrast to the behavior of normal cells, which do so only intermittently. This profound difference can be related to the interactions of these various cells with their surroundings. The growth of normal cells is strongly dependent on stimulation by external mitogenic signals conveyed to these cells by polypeptide growth factors; cancer cells, in contrast, have profoundly reduced requirements for such stimulation, which is manifested by the greatly reduced dependence on serum mitogens displayed by many kinds of cancer cells growing in culture. Such acquired independence from exogenous stimulation leaves the impression that the impetus for the growth of cancer cells comes from internal sources within these cells.

Reduced or absent requirements for external mitogenic stimulation are often associated with the actions of specific oncogenes. Significantly, many oncogene-encoded proteins sit astride the signal transduction pathways in the cell that normally receive and process signals initiated by external mitogens.[21] For example, oncogenes like *erb*-B and *erb*-B2, which are often overexpressed in human tumors, encode cell surface growth factor receptors.

The Ras oncoprotein functions downstream to transmit signals from these receptors to effectors inside the cell.

These oncoproteins release continuous streams of growth-stimulatory signals into the cell in the absence of exogenous growth factors, thereby eliminating the need for these factors. Oncogenes like *ras* also cause cells to release mitogenic growth factors to which these cells can also respond, resulting in an autostimulatory (autocrine) mitogenic signaling loop [*see Figure 5*]. In sum, these oncogenes liberate cells from their normal dependence on external mitogens that are supplied by neighbors by generating mitogenic signals within these cells.

Cells growing in the context of a complex tissue are also bombarded with a multitude of growth-inhibitory signals. For various experimental reasons, these negative signals are less well understand than those favoring proliferation. One such inhibitory signal is represented by the in vitro phenomenon of contact inhibition. Another type of growth-antagonizing signals is conveyed by diffusible polypeptide factors, such as the well-studied tumor growth factor–β (TGF-β).

The outgrowth of a tumor cell clone requires an escape from these inhibitory signals. In the case of TGF-β, this escape is often achieved by elimination of one or more of the cell surface receptors that allow cells to detect and respond to this factor. This phenomenon occurs through unknown mechanisms in many retinoblastoma tumors.[22] In HNPCC, one of the genes specifying a TGF-β receptor is often inactivated by mutations resulting from the DNA repair defect present in cells of patients suffering from this syndrome.[23] This defect, observed in the colon carcinoma cells of these individuals, allows these cells to escape inhibition by this important growth antagonist.

This escape suggests a larger theme, in that the *TGF-β* receptor gene operates in these cancer cells as a tumor suppressor gene that must be inactivated before neoplastic growth is fully developed. By extension, the products of many tumor suppressor genes appear to be components of the cellular signaling machinery that allows cells to receive and process growth-inhibitory signals received from their surroundings [*see Table 2*]. Inactivation of certain tumor suppressor genes may lead directly to a loss of responsiveness to these growth-inhibitory signals, a process that may be as important as the liberation from growth factor dependency conferred by oncogene activation. For example, inactivation of the *Rb* (retinoblastoma) gene causes some types of cells to lose responsiveness to TGF-β, even though such cells may continue to display functional TGF-β receptors.[24]

In recent years, yet another, equally important mandate of tumor cells has become apparent: they must escape the mechanisms that eliminate normal and neoplastic cells from the body. Without such avoidance, any proliferative advantage gained through the actions of oncogenes or the inactivation of tumor suppressor genes may be nullified by equal or even greater rates of cell death. Examples of these physiologic mechanisms of elimination abound. In the normal colonic epithelium, most cells are born and then die after three to four days, being lost through a process that involves movement down the colonic villi, terminal differentiation, and sloughing off into the colonic lumen. In the skin, keratinocytes similarly

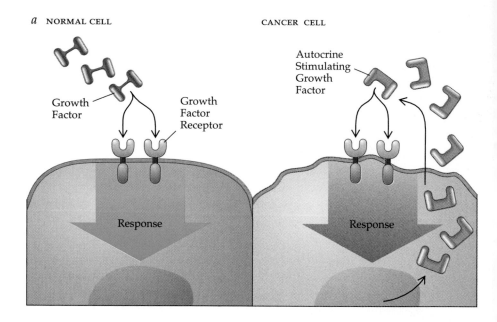

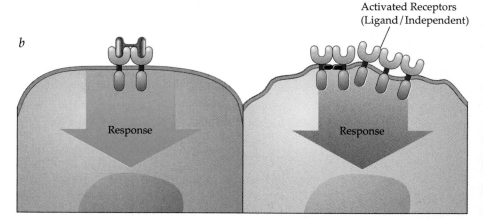

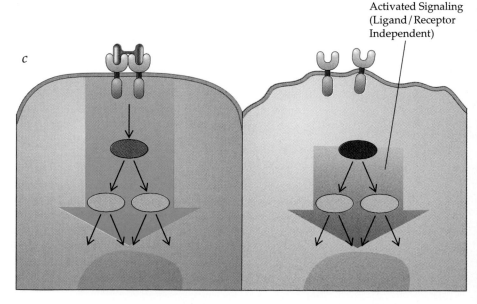

Figure 5 *Three ways by which oncogenes can allow cells to grow without stimulation by extracellular growth factors. (a) A normal cell requires extracellular growth factors to activate its growth factor receptors; a cancer cell often makes and secretes growth factors that stimulate the cell's own growth (autocrine stimulation). (b) Normal growth factor receptors require binding of growth factors to trigger signal release; aberrant (or overexpressed) receptors release signals into cells even without growth factor binding. (c) growth factor–activated receptors normally activate a cascade of signal transducers in the cytoplasm; in cancer cells, abnormal transducers in such a cascade may release growth-stimulating signals even without prompting by a growth factor–activated receptor.*

undergo differentiation into a postmitotic state, programmed death, keratinization, and sloughing. In lymphoid organs, large numbers of lymphoid cells are continually eliminated through apoptosis.

Escape from such programmed elimination appears to represent an early step in the evolution of many types of tumors. Thus, an initial step in the formation of a colonic adenomatous polyp would seem to involve the acquired ability of colonic epithelial cells to avoid migration from the colonic crypts to the tips of villi and subsequent sloughing into the colonic lumen. This avoidance may be achieved by mutation of the *APC* gene.[25] Analogous changes are seen in the phenotype of basal keratinocytes, which may acquire the ability to resist end-stage differentiation, including keratinization and cell death; the genetic basis of this particular avoidance is unclear. In lymphoid tissues, overexpression of the *bcl*-2 oncogene confers on lymphocytes an ability to avoid programmed cell death.[26,27] In each organ, these physiologic changes lay the groundwork for subsequent steps in tumor progression by creating hyperplastic but otherwise normal cell populations.

The activation of an oncogene or the inactivation of a tumor suppressor gene early in tumor progression may provide some mitogenic impetus to the cell; however, as mentioned earlier, cells bearing these lesions are often especially susceptible to apoptosis. This latter tendency must be neutralized for the cell to reap the full advantage of the initial gene alteration.

The importance of these antiapoptotic responses has been highlighted by observations derived from mouse models of tumorigenesis. In one case, germ line inactivation of the *Rb* tumor suppressor gene causes cells in the brain of an embryo to exhibit high rates of apoptosis; this response precludes the outgrowth of malignant cells in this tissue.[28] In another, a transgenic mouse model of cancer, pancreatic islet cell tumors appear in re-

Table 2 Known and Proposed Tumor Suppressor Genes

Gene	Chromosome	Inherited Tumors	Proposed Functions
Rb	13q14	Retinoblastoma, osteosarcoma	Regulates transcription factors (E2F-DP1), regulates the cell cycle
p53	17p13	Osteosarcoma, breast, brain, Li-Fraumeni syndrome	Transcription factor, regulates the cell cycle and apoptosis
APC	5q21	Familial adenomatous polyposis	Communicates between cell surface proteins and cytoskeleton
WT-1	11p13	Wilms' tumor, nephroblastoma	Transcription factor important for kidney development
NF-1	17q11.2	von Recklinghausen neurofibromatosis	GTPase-activating protein for *ras* from neural crest–derived cells
NF-2	22q11.1	Acoustic neuroma, bilateral meningiomas	A cytoskeletal protein termed merlin
DCC	18q21	None demonstrated (only somatic mutations so far)	Membrane receptor–like protein
*MTS*1	9p21	Medullary blastomas, some melanomas, pancreatic cancers; deleted in many tissue culture cell lines	A 16-kd protein that blocks the activity of Cdk4
*MTS*2	9p21	Unknown	A 15-kd protein that blocks the activity of Cdk's

sponse to the tissue-specific activation of a germ line–borne SV40 *LT* oncogene. The expansion of early nests of tumor cells depends strongly on their
ability to elaborate insulinlike growth factor–II; it operates as a survival factor that enables the cells to circumvent the apoptosis occurring as a specific
response to SV40 *LT* oncogene expression.[29]

Apoptosis may also occur as a specific response to genomic damage sustained by a cell. In the case of evolving populations of premalignant cells,
this issue assumes great importance because apoptosis effectively blocks
the ability of these cells to create the genetic plasticity that favors rapid tumor progression. Many types of cells enter apoptosis in response to DNA
damage through a process that is dependent on the p53 tumor suppressor
protein.[30,31] This response suggests that the mutant *p53* genes found in
more than half of all human cancers have contributed to the outgrowth of
these tumors by uncoupling genomic damage from the apoptotic response. These examples represent only a small sampling of the cases in
which escape from apoptosis has been found to be vital to the process of
tumor progression.

Cell Immortalization and Tumor Progression

The foregoing discussions imply that the proliferative advantage of cancer
cells is governed by the activities of genes that favor proliferation or help to
avoid cell death. A set of DNA repair genes was also cited that can affect the
rates at which proto-oncogenes and tumor suppressor genes become recruited into the process of tumorigenesis. Recent work has shed light on yet
another type of growth-controlling mechanism and the genes that underlie
it. This mechanism, which involves cell immortalization, is likely to be as
important for tumor progression as are the proliferative controls governed
by the well-studied oncogenes and tumor suppressor genes.

Research over several decades has revealed that the ability of embryo cells
to multiply in culture is limited to a fixed number of doublings. For example, populations of human embryo fibroblasts typically expand exponentially in culture for about 50 doublings. Having passed through this number
of cell generations, these populations slow their growth and enter into a
nongrowing but viable state called senescence. Cells may subsequently
emerge from senescence and pass through 10 to 20 more doublings, after
which the cell population as a whole begins a massive die-off known as crisis. A rare variant cell (one in 10^7) may emerge from this population and
once again begin to grow exponentially. The descendants of this cell now
enjoy unlimited replicative ability and thus are said to be immortalized.[32]

These phenomena point to the workings of a clocking device that is carried by cells and tallies the number of generational doublings that separates
them from their ancestors in the early embryo. Further evidence for the existence of such a generational clock comes from observations indicating
that cells from young mammals, including humans, invariably pass
through a greater number of doublings in vitro than do cells from older
individuals.

Malignant tumor cells generally appear to have unlimited replicative potential when their growth is gauged in culture. Thus, acquisition of the im-

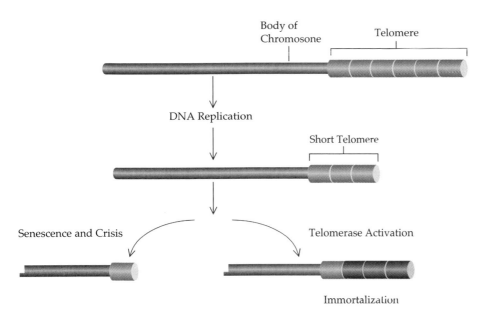

Figure 6   *Activation of telomerase avoids telomere length reduction and consequent senescence to allow continuous cell proliferation. The telomeric repeat structures on the ends of chromosomes are shortened by DNA replication. When a critical limiting telomere length is reached, most cells exit the cell division cycle and become terminally senescent. An enzyme, telomerase, adds telomeric repeats onto the ends of chromosomes, maintaining the capability to divide without reaching the critical minimal telomere length. Germ cells, certain normal stem and progenitor cells, most immortal cells in culture, and most malignant cancer cells are known to express telomerase, thereby maintaining telomere length and preserving the capability for continuing cell proliferation.*

mortalized phenotype should be added to the many other novel traits accumulated by cell clones as they advance through the process of tumor progression. This immortalization also points to an important antineoplastic defense mechanism that operates in normal tissues and, by extension, a barrier that must be breached by all evolving populations of premalignant cells. In particular, the replicative potential of normal cell populations is limited by the generational clock carried by all the member cells of these populations. Most evolving premalignant cell clones may exhaust their preprogrammed allotment of generational doublings at some time during tumor progression, resulting in the senescence of these clones. This scenario implies that successful progression to a fully malignant state requires an escape from senescence and crisis; such escape is achieved by overriding the control imposed by the generational clock.

A large body of evidence, much of it recent, has revealed the molecular apparatus that serves as the generational clock.[33] The progressive decline of proliferative potential demonstrated by aging cell clones is directly correlated with the progressive shortening of the telomeres, the DNA structures that form the protective ends of their chromosomes [*see Figure 6*]. Telomeres undergo incremental shortening as a natural result of each round of DNA replication. As a consequence, telomeres of cells prepared from older individuals are shorter than those prepared from newborns. If this progressive shortening is unopposed, telomeres shrink to a small size that triggers entrance of a cell into the senescent state. Should cells succeed in passing through senescence, telomeres may eventually collapse to a size that is too small to stabilize the ends of the chromosomes. The resulting unprotected chromosomal ends precipitate fusions with other chromosomes, the resulting formation of dicentric chromosomes, and the karyotypic disarray seen in populations of cells in crisis.

Most cancer cells have acquired the ability to ward off telomeric collapse. More than 90 percent of cancer cells tested to date have been found to accomplish this by expressing telomerase, an enzyme that is able to compensate for the normal telomeric shortening associated with DNA replication by adding nucleotide segments onto recently replicated chromosomal ends.[34] Accordingly, in the presence of telomerase, cancer cells are able to maintain stable telomere length, thereby ensuring chromosomal integrity and avoidance of crisis and cell death.

During the course of normal development, telomerase is an enzyme that is expressed early in the embryo and then repressed in all cell lineages except the germ line.[35] As such, the appearance of telomerase in tumor cell clones represents the resurrection of an enzyme activity that has been absent from somatic cells for many cell generations. This resurrection appears to occur when rare variant cells escape from crisis and acquire an immortalized phenotype.

Taken together, these data indicate that the acquisition of cell immortality through the resurrection of telomerase is a step executed by most, and perhaps all, populations of malignant cells. This step would seem to occur relatively late in tumor progression, when cell populations have begun to exhaust their allotment of doublings. However, direct evidence on this point is lacking. For example, it is still unclear when telomerase activation occurs during tumor progression in the colon.

Importantly, observations made to date indicate that the repression of telomerase and its activation during tumorigenesis is not under the control of oncogenes and tumor suppressor genes. This central step, which appears to be vital to the development of many types of malignant tumors, must be directed by alteration of another, novel class of genes. The nature of these genes is elusive.

Angiogenesis

These discussions of tumor progression have suggested that the proliferative potential of incipient tumor cell clones is determined exclusively by the growth-regulating genes carried by the tumor cells themselves. In particular, some of these mutant cancer-causing genes affect the responses of tumor cells to signals received from their environment. Yet others, notably the genes controlling DNA repair and immortalization, affect only the intracellular, domestic housekeeping machinery of these cells.

However, the successes of tumor cell clones are also governed by a complex interplay between tumor cells and the normal tissues that surround them. Signals must be exchanged bidirectionally between the tumor mass and the normal adjacent tissues. The most vivid example of these interac-

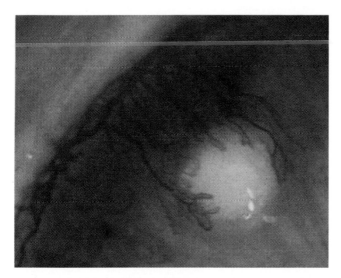

Figure 7 *Partially purified angiogenic activity is released from a polymer capsule (white ball) implanted in the rabbit cornea. New capillaries have grown around it, being attracted by fibroblast growth factor responsible for the activity.*

tions is revealed by the process of neovascularization that occurs during the formation of many types of cancers.[36]

As is the case with normal developing tissues, the proliferation of tumor masses depends on access to nutrients and oxygen and on elimination of metabolic wastes and carbon dioxide. In tumor masses that are less than 0.5 mm in diameter, these requirements can be addressed by the process of diffusion. However, in masses of greater size, diffusion no longer suffices, and nests of tumor cells require direct access to the circulatory system for the supply of nutrients and removal of waste.

This access is secured through the process of angiogenesis, in which tumor cells encourage the in-growth of capillaries and larger vessels from adjacent normal tissue. The tumor cells succeed in recruiting these vessels through their release of angiogenic factors. Once released, these factors impinge on endothelial cells present in nearby tissues and induce their proliferation, causing them to extend capillaries into the tumor mass [*see Figure 7*]. In the absence of this angiogenesis, cell proliferation within a small tumor cell nest may continue unabated but is accompanied by an equal and compensating rate of cell death caused by anoxia, starvation, and metabolic poisoning.

Tumor cells have been found to release numerous angiogenic factors, including notably basic fibroblast growth factor and vascular endothelial growth factor.[37-39] TGF-β may also play an important role in angiogenesis. Although not yet proved, it seems likely that these and other angiogenic factors are released by cells during development and tissue repair as part of the mechanisms that lead to the vascularization of normal tissues. Virtually all tumors are highly vascularized and have abundant new capillaries, suggesting that tumor cells release these factors in especially large amounts. This active angiogenesis contrasts with the state of normal tissues, in which the capillary beds are relatively static, reflecting the long lifetime (1,000 to 3,000 days) of the endothelial cells. In tumor masses, anoxia may be the stimulus that causes individual tumor cells to release the factors.[40]

The capillary beds in a tumor mass can be visualized by immunostaining with antibodies that recognize proteins that are expressed specifically by endothelial cells; these proteins include von Willebrand's factor and CD31. The use of immunostaining provides a measure of the density of capillaries in that tumor and yields an "angiogenic index" of the tumor. This method reveals that solid tumors contain various densities of capillaries; those that are highly vascularized typically show fewer necrotic regions than those that are less densely vascularized. Moreover, in studies of human breast and prostate cancers, a higher density of vascularization of invasive primary tumors was closely correlated with their tendency to have spawned metastases, a finding that is consistent with the causal role played by angiogenesis in this later step of tumor progression [*see Figure 8*].[41,42]

This theme is echoed in several experimental models of tumor progression. In the transgenic mouse model of islet cell tumors, a large number of islet cells are seen initially to express the SV40 *LT* oncogene, although they form only small, dysplastic clumps. After some weeks, however, some of these dysplastic nests begin to expand into obvious neoplastic masses. Importantly, the induction of angiogenesis precedes this neoplas-

a

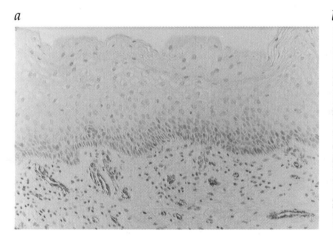

b

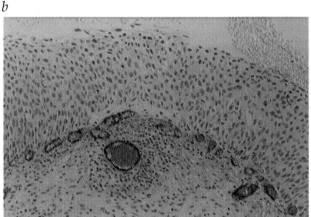

c

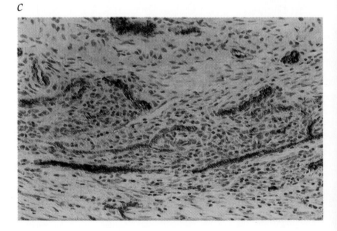

Figure 8   *(a) In a normal cervix, capillaries are evident in the stroma underlying the squamous epithelium. In a cervical intraepithelial neoplasia–III (CIN-III) lesion (b), there is abundant new blood vessel growth, with a dense accumulation of new capillaries along the basement membrane below the transformed epithelium. (c) The neovascularization persists in an invasive cancer, which has breached the basement membrane and is invading through the stroma.*

a CARCINOMA IN SITU

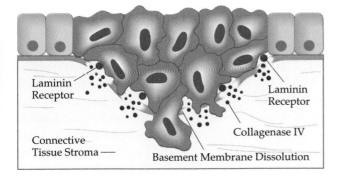

b MICROINVASION

c STROMAL INVASION

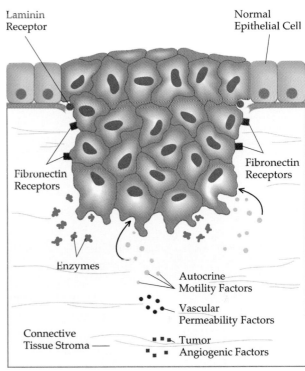

Figure 9 *Invasion into the underlying connective tissue by the primary tumor proceeds in stages and is facilitated by various mediators produced by the tumor cells. Tumor cells that have not invaded the basement membrane and remain confined within the epithelium are termed carcinoma in situ (a). Release of collagenase IV by these cells dissolves the collagen in the basement membrane and allows the tumor to penetrate the subjacent stroma (b). Invasive tumor cells carry membrane receptors for laminin and fibronectin, large glycoprotein components of the basement membrane and connective tissue stroma, respectively; binding to these elements provides the tumor cells with a lattice for anchorage and advancement (b, c). Enzymes released by tumor cells, such as plasminogen activators, collagenases I, II, and III, cathepsins, heparanase, and hyaluronidase, destroy matrix constituents, including fibrin, glycoproteins, proteoglycans, and hyaluronic acid, thus enabling the cells to advance further into the connective tissue. Tumors also secrete autocrine motility factors, which direct the motion of the advancing tumor; vascular permeability factors, which allow plasma proteins to accumulate in the tumor; and angiogenic factors, which increase the vascularity of the tumor (c). Tumor cells preferentially invade along pathways that provide the least resistance, such as the connective tissue stroma.*

tic conversion and provides evidence that neovascularization is a prerequisite for tumor formation.[43] In a transgenic mouse model of fibrosarcoma tumor progression, the onset of basic fibroblast growth factor secretion by tumor cells is closely associated with the development of angiogenic capacity.[44]

The activation of angiogenesis at an intermediate stage of tumor progression has also been detected in a third transgenic mouse model of cancer, involving epidermal squamous cell carcinoma. Evidence of a discrete angiogenic stage in human cervical, melanocyte, and glial cell cancers has also been obtained. These and other lines of evidence suggest that acquisition of angiogenic capacity is essential for the successful expansion of all types of neoplastic cell clones.

Invasion and Metastasis

The escape of a tumor mass from confinement by surrounding capsule or basement membrane signals its progression from a benign to an actively malignant growth state [*see Figure 9*]. In the case of epithelial cells, this escape begins with dissolution of the basement membrane that normally underlies the epithelium. This invasiveness is often accompanied by the ability to degrade the stroma as well. These capabilities are provided in part by secreted proteases, such as type IV collagenase, which degrades basement membranes; type I collagenase, which degrades the collagenous stromal architecture; and urokinase-type plasminogen activator (uPA). Degradation of adjacent tissue also serves to create space for the expanding tumor cell mass.[45]

Urokinase-type plasminogen activator is frequently found in greatly elevated amounts in invasive tissues, including most carcinomas; it functions to convert plasminogen to plasmin, which is a protease of broad substrate specificity.[45] The latter enzyme may be the direct mediator of much of the proteolysis observed adjacent to invasive tumor masses. In multistep tumor progression in the colon, uPA is found in increased amounts in carcinomas but not in the normal intestinal mucosa or in adenomatous polyps.[46]

The production of plasmin involves a tight collaboration between carcinoma cells and nearby stromal cells. Thus, the carcinoma cells induce cells of the stroma to release uPA, which then adsorbs to uPA receptors displayed by the carcinoma cells.[47] These cells then wield the uPA tethered to their surfaces to activate plasminogen in the surrounding extracellular fluid. Once activated in the extracellular fluid, matrix-degrading proteases have numerous effects. They can degrade not only the extracellular matrix but also the sheaths surrounding the lymphatics and the blood vessels, thereby providing tumor cells with direct access to the vessel walls. Subsequent erosion through these walls then allows clumps of tumor cells to pass to distant sites in the body, the first step in the process of metastasis. In addition, these proteases can activate latent growth factors present in the extracellular space, including notably insulinlike growth factor–I (IGF-I), basic fibroblast growth factor (bFGF), and hepatocyte growth factor/scatter factor (HGF).[48-50] Basic fibroblast growth factor plays a prominent role in the promotion of angiogenesis. Hepatocyte growth factor/scatter factor takes on special importance in the process of metastasis because it is a potent inducer of cell motility and hence migration.

As is the case with angiogenesis, the release of factors seems to reflect closely the mechanisms used by normal cells to remodel their immediate surroundings as part of the processes of tissue growth and wound repair. The identity of the genes responsible for orchestrating the exaggerated release of these proteases and the resulting invasive phenotype remains unclear.

Most insidious is the capability that develops in many cancers to migrate to distant sites in the body and establish new tumor masses at those sites. The process of metastasis is likely related in part to natural cell migrations that occur during development and often depends on the access of tumor cells to capillaries, larger blood vessels, and lymphatics.

The process of metastasis can be divided into several distinct components. Initially, cancer cells enter the lumina of blood or lymphatic channels (intravasation). Once in these vessel systems, they may be carried passively to distant sites. Alternatively, they may attach to other, normally circulating cell types, riding with them to distant sites. For example, metastasizing melanoma cells often express the ICAM-1 cell adhesion molecule on their surfaces, which allows them to attach to leukocytes, specifically granulocytes and macrophages that express the LFA-1 and MAC-1 proteins.[51]

After they are transported, cancer cells must become tethered to specific sites that are exposed in the lumina of these vessels. These attachments are also mediated by cell surface adhesion molecules (integrins). In highly progressed melanoma cells, the $\alpha_v\beta_3$ integrin expressed by these cells allows them to attach to many types of extracellular matrix elements, including collagen, vitronectin, fibrinogen, von Willebrand factor, and laminin.[52,53] The fibrinogen interaction in particular may allow these cells to attach to thrombi, thereby facilitating association with the endothelial wall. Thereafter, metastasizing cells must escape from these vessels (extravasate) by moving through the wall of the vessel and burrowing into the adjacent stroma or parenchyma. Having penetrated these tissues, these cells must be able to proliferate in a foreign environment that contains growth-stimulatory and growth-inhibitory signals not previously encountered at the site of primary tumorigenesis. As is the case with invasiveness, the genes that serve as templates for the metastatic phenotype are poorly understood.

These descriptions of invasiveness and metastasis, which are necessarily superficial, indicate that the two processes are extremely complex. Indeed, the degree of complexity suggests that each process may depend on the actions of several genes that undergo mutation during tumor progression. For example, an activated *ras* oncogene induces increased expression of vascular endothelial growth factor, a potent angiogenic factor, by the oncogene-bearing cell.[54,55] Moreover, the *p53* tumor suppressor gene, which is inactivated in about one half of human cancers has been shown to induce the expression of thrombospondin, a potent antiangiogenic factor,[56-58] thus presenting further impetus to the tumor cell to inactivate its *p53* gene.

The processes of angiogenesis, invasion, and metastasis are currently the subjects of intensive investigations that should reveal their genetic and biochemical bases. With such information in hand, we will be able to write the complete biography of a human tumor from its inception to its acquired ability, decades later, to threaten life through the aggressive invasion of adjacent tissues and distant organ sites.

References

1. Peto R: Epidemiology, multistage models and short-term mutagenicity tests. *Origins of Human Cancer Book C: Human Risk Assessment.* Hiatt HH, Watson JD, Winsten JA, Eds. Cold Spring Harbor Conferences, Vol. 4, Cold Spring Harbor Press, Cold Spring Harbor, NY, 1977, p 1403

2. Pike MC, Forman D: Epidemiology of cancer. *Introduction to the Cellular and Molecular Biology of Cancer.* Franks LM, Teich NM, Eds. Oxford University Press, New York,1991, p 49

3. Selikoff IJ: Cancer risk of asbestos exposure. *Origins of Human Cancer Book C: Human Risk*

Assessment. Hiatt HH, Watson JD, Winsten JA, Eds. Cold Spring Harbor Conferences, Vol. 4, Cold Spring Harbor Press, Cold Spring Harbor, NY, 1977, p 1765

4. Bickers DR, Lowy DR: Carcinogenesis: a fifty-year historical perspective. *J Invest Dermatol* 92 (4 suppl):121S, 1989

5. Brown K, Balmain A: Transgenic mice and squamous multistage skin carcinogenesis. *Cancer Metastasis Rev* 14 :113, 1995

6. Land H, Parada LF, Weinberg RA: Tumorigenic conversion of primary embryo fibroblasts requires at least two cooperating oncogenes. *Nature* 304:596, 1983

7. Stewart TA, Pattengale PK, Leder P: Spontaneous mammary adenocarcinomas in transgenic mice that carry and express MTV/*myc* fusion genes. *Cell* 38:627, 1984

8. Selten G, Cuypers HT, Berns A: Proviral activation of the putative oncogene Pim-1 in MuLV induced T-cell lymphomas. *EMBO J* 4 :1793, 1985

9. Berns A: Tumorigenesis in transgenic mice: identification and characterization of synergizing oncogenes. *J Cell Biochem* 47:130, 1991

10. Sinn E, Muller W, Pattengale P, et al: Coexpression of MMTV/v-Ha-*ras* and MMTV/c-*myc* genes in transgenic mice: synergistic action of oncogenes in vivo. *Cell* 49:465, 1987

11. Evan GI, Wyllie AH, Gilbert CS, et al: Induction of apoptosis in fibroblasts by c-myc protein. *Cell* 69:119, 1992

12. Harrington EA, Fanidi A, Evan GI: Oncogenes and cell death. *Curr Opin Genet Dev* 4 : 120, 1994

13. Arends MJ, McGregor AH, Toft NJ, et al: Susceptibility of apoptosis is differentially regulated by c-myc and mutated H-ras oncogenes and is associated with endonuclease availability. *Br J Cancer* 68:1127, 1993

14. Lin HJ, Eviner V, Prendergast GC, at el: Activated H-ras rescues E1A-induced apoptosis and cooperates with E1A to overcome P53-dependent growth arrest. *Mol Cell Biol* 15:4536, 1995

15. Vogelstein B, Kinzler KW: The multistep nature of cancer. *Trends Genet* 9:138, 1993

16. Vogelstein B, Fearon ER, Hamilton SR, et al: Genetic alterations during colorectal-tumor development. *N Engl J Med* 319:525, 1988

17. Hamilton S: Histopathologic considerations in the adenoma-carcinoma sequence. *Familial Polyposis.* Herrera L, Ed. Alan R. Liss, New York, 1989, p 35

18. Malkin D, Li FP, Strong LC, et al: Germ line p53 mutations in a familial syndrome of breast cancer, sarcomas, and other neoplasms. *Science* 250:1233, 1990

19. Fishel R, Kolodner RD: Identification of mismatch repair genes and their role in the development of cancer. *Curr Opin Genet Dev* 5:382, 1995

20. de Wind N, Dekker M, Berns A, et al: Inactivation of the mouse Msh2 gene results in mismatch repair deficiency, methylation tolerance, hyperrecombination and predisposition to cancer. *Cell* 82 :321, 1995

21. Cantley LC, Auger KR, Carpenter C, et al: Oncogenes and signal transduction. *Cell* 64:281, 1991

22. Kimchi A, Wang X-F, Weinberg RA, et al: Absence of transforming growth factor-β receptors and growth inhibitory responses in retinoblastoma cells. *Science* 240:196, 1987

23. Wang J, Sun L, Myeroff L, et al: Demonstration that mutation of the type II transforming growth factor beta receptor inactivates its tumor suppressor activity in replication error-positive colon carcinoma cells. *J Biol Chem* 270:22044, 1995

24. Pietenpol JA, Stein RW, Moan E, et al: TGF-β1 inhibition of c-myc transcription and growth in keratinocytes is abrogated by viral transforming proteins with pRB binding domains. *Cell* 61:777, 1990

25. Polakis P: Mutations in the APC gene and their implications for protein structure and function. *Curr Opin Genet Dev* 5 :66, 1995

26. Osborne BA: Induction of genes during apoptosis: examples from the immune system. *Semin Cancer Biol* 6:27, 1995

27. Boise LH, Gottschalk AR, Quintans J, et al: Bcl-2 and Bcl-2-related proteins in apoptosis regulation. *Curr Top Microbiol Immunol* 200:107, 1995

28. Jacks T, Fazeli A, Schmitt EM, et al: Effects of an Rb mutation in the mouse. *Nature* 359:295, 1992

29. Naik P, Christofori G, Hanahan D: IGF-II is focally up-regulated and functionally involved as a second signal for oncogene-induced tumorigenesis. *Cold Spring Harb Symp Quant Biol* 59:459, 1995

30. Lee JM, Bernstein A: Apoptosis, cancer and the p53 tumour suppressor gene. *Cancer Metastasis Rev* 14:149, 1995

31. Morgenbesser SD, Williams BO, Jacks T, et al: p53-dependent apoptosis produced by Rb-deficiency in the developing mouse lens. *Nature* 371:72, 1994

32. Harley CB, Kim NW, Prowse, KR, et al: Telomerase, cell immortality and cancer. *Cold Spring Harb Symp Quant Biol* 59 :307, 1994

33. Kim NW, Piatyszek MA, Prowse KR, et al: Specific association of human telomerase activity with immortal cells and cancer. *Science* 266:2011, 1994

34. Blasco MA, Funk W, Villeponteau B, et al: Functional characterization and developmental regulation of mouse telomerase RNA. *Science* 269:1267, 1995

35. Wright WE, Piatyszek MA, Rainey WE, et al: Telomerase activity in human germline and embryonic tissues and cells. *Dev Genet* (in press)

36. Folkman J: What is the evidence that tumors are angiogenesis-dependent? *J Natl Cancer Inst* 82:4, 1990

37. Folkman J: Tumor angiogenesis. *The Molecular Basis of Cancer.* Mendelsohn J, Howley PM, Israel MA, Liotta LA, Eds. WB Saunders, Philadelphia, 1995, p 206

38. Rak JN, St. Croix B, Kerbel RS: Consequences of angiogenesis for tumor progression, metastasis and cancer therapy. *Anticancer Drugs* 6:3, 1995

39. Dvorak H: VPF/VEGF. *Control of Angiogenesis.* Goldberg ID, Rosen E. Birkhauser Verlag, (in press)

40. Shweiki D, Neeman M, Itin A, et al: Induction of vascular endothelial growth factor expression by hypoxia and by glucose deficiency in multicell spheroids: implications for tumor angiogenesis. *Proc Natl Acad Sci USA* 92:768, 1995

41. Weidner N, Semple JP, Welch WR, et al: Tumor angiogenesis and metastasis: correlation in invasive breast carcinoma. *N Engl J Med* 324:1, 1991

42. Weidner N, Carroll PR, Flax J, et al: Tumor angiogenesis correlates with metastasis in invasive prostate carcinoma. *Am J Pathol* 143:401, 1993

43. Folkman J, Watson K, Ingber D, et al: Induction of angiogenesis during the transition from hyperplasia to neoplasia. *Nature* 339:58, 1989

44. Kandel J, Bossy-Wetzel E, Radvanyi F, et al: Neovascularization is associated with a switch to the export of bFGF in the multistep development of fibrosarcoma. *Cell* 66:1095, 1991

45. Mignatti P, Rifkin DB: Biology and biochemistry of proteinases in tumor invasion. *Physiol Rev* 73:161, 1993

46. de Bruin PAF, Griffoen G, Verspaget HW, et al: Plasminogen activator profiles in neoplastic tissue of the human colon. *Cancer Res* 48:4520, 1988

47. Puke C, Kristenson P, Raltkier E, et al: Urokinase-type plasminogen activator is expressed in stromal cells and its receptor in cancer cells at invasive foci in human colon adenocarcinomas. *Am J Pathol* 138:1059, 1991

48. Campbell PG, Novak JF, Yanosick TB, et al: Involvement of the plasmin system in dissociation of the insulin-like growth factor-binding protein complex. *Endocrinology* 130:1401, 1992

49. Vlodavsky I, Bar-Shavit R, Ishai-Michaeli R, et al: Extracellular sequestration and release of fibroblast growth factor: a regulatory mechanism? *Trends Biochem Sci* 16:268, 1991

50. Naldini L, Tamagnone L, Vigna E, et al: Extracellular proteolytic cleavage by urokinase is required for activation of hepatocyte growth factor/scatter factor *EMBO J* 11:4925, 1992

51. Si Z, Hersey P: Immunohistological examination of the relationship between metastatic potential and expression of adhesion molecules and "selectins" on melanoma cells. *Pathology* 26:6, 1994

52. Hart IR, Birch M, Marshall JF: Cell adhesion receptor expression during melanoma progression and metastasis. *Cancer Metastasis Rev* 10:115, 1991

53. Nesbit M, Herlyn M: Adhesion receptors in human melanoma progression. *Invasion Metastasis* 14:131, 1994-95

54. Grugel S, Finkenzeller G, Weindel K, et al: Both v-H-*ras* and v-raf stimulate expression of the vascular endothelial growth factor in NIH 3T3 cells. *J Biol Chem* 270:25915, 1995

55. Rak J, Mitsuhashi Y, Bayko L, et al: Mutant *ras* oncogenes upregulate VEGF/VPF expression: implications for induction and inhibition of tumor angiogenesis. *Cancer Res* 55:4575, 1995

56. Bouck N, Stellmach V, Hsu S: How tumors become angiogenic. *Adv Cancer Res* (in press)

57. Dameron KM, Volpert OV, Tainsky MA, et al: Control of angiogenesis in fibroblasts by p53 regulation of thrombospondin-1. *Science* 265:1582, 1994

58. Van Meir EG, Polverini PJ, Chazin VR, et al: Release of an inhibitor of angiogenesis upon induction of wild type p53 expression in glioblastoma cells. *Nature Genet* 8:171

Acknowledgments

Figure 1   Marcia Kammerer. Adapted from *Cancer: Science and Society*, by J. Cairns, W.H. Freeman and Company, San Francisco, 1978.

Figure 2   From *Genes and the Biology of Cancer*, by H. Varmus and R.A. Weinberg, Scientific American Library, New York, 1993

Figure 3   Marcia Kammerer. Adapted from *Molecular Biology of the Cell*, by B. Alberts, D. Bray, J. Lewis, et al., Garland Publishing Inc., New York, 1983. Used by permission.

Figure 4   Jared Schneidman. Modified from "Gastrointestinal Cancer," by R.J. Mayer, in *Scientific American Medicine*, edited by D.C. Dale and D.D. Federman, Section 12, Subsection VIII. Scientific American, Inc., New York, 1996, All rights reserved.

Figure 5   Seward Hung.

Figure 6   Talar Agasyan. Adapted from an illustration Mike Rizen, University of California San Francisco.

Figure 7   From *Genes and the Biology of Cancer*, by H. Varmus and R.A. Weinberg, Scientific American Library, New York, 1993

Figure 8   vWF-stained tissues courtesy of K. Smith-McCune, University of California San Francisco. Photography by D. Hanahan.

Figure 9   Dana Burns-Pizer. From "Pathobiology of Cancer," by E. Frei, III, in *Scientific American Medicine*, edited by D.C. Dale and D.D. Federman, Section 12, Subsection III. Scientific American, Inc., New York, 1996. All rights reserved.

CHAPTER 9

Molecular Genetics in the Management of Patients with Cancer

Mark A. Israel, M.D.

Succcss in the control and treatment of cancer eludes our grasp. Despite the development of effective therapies for a few specific tumors, curative therapy for most common tumors remains elusive. Clearly, the lack of a comprehensive, integrated view of tumorigenesis and the attendant problems of tissue invasion and metastases have been major factors inhibiting a systematic approach to the treatment of cancer.

Cancer arises because of genetic alterations that confer properties on cells that allow them to grow inappropriately. Such cells must also escape both cellular and systemic defense mechanisms that normally protect against cells that acquire malignant characteristics. The genetic alterations responsible for these cellular changes occur both spontaneously, as the result of mistakes in DNA replication and repair, and after the exposure of cells to environmental mutagens. Importantly, the frequency of such mutations and their pathological implications for the development of cancer reflect host predispositions, some of which can now be defined as heritable disorders of known genes.

The fundamental insights into cell growth and tissue maturation detailed in previous chapters of this book provide a framework for an understanding of cancer and the development of improved strategies for its control and treatment. An understanding of the specific genetic alterations that cause cancer, the cellular pathways in which the products of these genes are active, and the biochemical and physiologic changes in function that result has evoked a panoply of strategies for cancer prevention and treatment. Research seeking to translate these insights into useful clinical practice has a solid foundation in cell biology and molecular biology and has already affected virtually all aspects of cancer medicine.

Epidemiology and Cancer Prevention

Novel Risk Determinants

Epidemiology identifies the causes of human cancer and the populations that are at high risk for developing cancer. Epidemiological studies have historically sought to measure the exposure of individuals to candidate carcinogens or known risk factors and to correlate this information with the occurrence of overt disease in populations of exposed individuals. Molecular epidemiology is an emerging area of investigation that seeks biomarkers for identifying environmental causes of cancer and for determining the risk of tumor development in individuals. Biomarkers are tumor-specific changes in DNA or other cellular components that can be assayed in patient specimens. Previous attempts to identify biomarkers of cancer risk have recognized the central role of mutations in the pathogenesis of tumors and have included such nonspecific measures of DNA damage as chromosomal aberrations and formation of micronuclei in peripheral blood cells. These measures of DNA damage have been too insensitive to be easily correlated with cancer predisposition or development of specific tumors, and they generally do not correlate well with cancer incidence. Identification of the cellular mechanisms that mediate malignant transformation provides an opportunity to seek correlations between environmental exposures and specific cellular alterations thought to play a significant role in tumorigenesis.

CANCER GENES AS BIOMARKERS

Based on the emerging view of cancer as a genetic disorder, it has been possible to identify biomarkers that play a role in malignant transformation. Activating mutations of dominantly acting genes and loss-of-function mutations of tumor suppressor genes are now known to play key roles in carcinogenesis, and genetic alterations are recognizable in virtually all commonly occurring tumors [*see Chapter 7, Tables 1 and 3*]. Studies seeking to determine the association between a particular environmental exposure and a specific genetic alteration in any type of tumor are now feasible. Tumor-associated genetic alterations that can be detected before a malignancy is otherwise recognizable are likely to emerge as important biomarkers that are useful for the epidemiological study of many tumor types. The use of tumor suppressor genes as biomarkers for risk assessment is more complex than the analysis of oncogenes because the use of tumor suppressor genes requires the detection of a loss of genetic material in specimens that may be contaminated with large amounts of normal cells. Such hurdles, however, are not encountered in the evaluation of activating mutations in proto-oncogenes.

The analysis of tissues for oncogene activation involves the identification of a novel genetic change not found in normal tissue. Assays based on polymerase chain reaction (PCR) amplification and sequence-specific DNA probes have enabled the identification of oncogene activation in premalignant lesions of healthy individuals who are known to be at high risk for the development of cancer [*see Figure 1*]. For example, adenomatous polyps of the large colon, which are generally regarded as premalignant lesions, carry a mutated *ras* gene that can be recognized in cells obtained from colonic

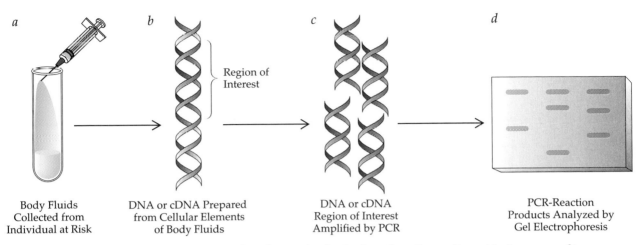

a Body Fluids Collected from Individual at Risk

b DNA or cDNA Prepared from Cellular Elements of Body Fluids

Region of Interest

c DNA or cDNA Region of Interest Amplified by PCR

d PCR-Reaction Products Analyzed by Gel Electrophoresis

Figure 1 *Polymerase chain reaction (PCR)–based strategies for the detection of premalignant lesions or occult tumors. From apparently well individuals, body fluids such as blood are collected (a), DNA or complementary DNA (cDNA) is prepared from the cellular elements present (b), PCR-based technologies are used to amplify DNA that corresponds to regions of genes or cDNA of interest (c), and the products of these amplification analyses are analyzed—most frequently by gel electrophoresis (d).*

washings.[1] PCR-based assays have enabled the detection of cells bearing oncogenetic mutations in cytologically negative sputum samples before lung cancer is diagnosed. Such assays that require premalignant or malignant tissue for evaluation are, however, of limited value. Many tissues in which tumors commonly occur are simply not available for screening, especially for the epidemiological evaluation of large populations of seemingly healthy individuals, and premalignant lesions have not yet been recognized for many of the most commonly occurring tumors.

Other approaches to the detection of oncogene activation in preclinical disease are therefore needed. Recently, it has also become feasible to assay blood and body fluids for circulating oncogene products and tumor-derived growth factors. For example, increased levels of several different proto-oncogene products, including p21[K-ras], p30[sis], and p60[src], and the HER-2/*neu* oncoprotein have been found in the urine and serum of cancer patients. Most importantly, elevated serum oncoprotein levels have been detected in asymptomatic individuals who were exposed to known pulmonary carcinogens and later developed lung cancer. Such observations suggest that it may be possible to identify individuals at risk for the development of cancer before it occurs.

TUMOR SUPPRESSOR GENES AS HERITABLE MARKERS OF CANCER RISK

The development of cancer is a reflection of both environmental and genetic factors, and recent studies of the mechanisms by which tumors arise have determined that tumor suppressor genes play a particularly important role in determining the genetic predisposition of individuals to many different kinds of tumors [*see Chapter 6*]. The inheritance of mutated tumor suppressor genes can play a critical role in determining an individual's predisposition for many different tumor types, including those arising in colon, breast, and connective tissues. The function of tumor suppressor genes is recognizable only when both alleles of the gene have been inactivated [*see Chapter 6*]. Heterozygous individuals who are at increased risk for tumor development carry one mutated allele, and an additional mutation in the second allele is found in tumors that arise in these individuals. Because these individuals carry the mutation in their germ line tissues, this predisposition is inherited by subsequent generations.

The primary manifestation of inherited cancer predisposition syndromes is sometimes the development of a tumor, and the syndrome may not be recognized clinically before a tumor develops [*see Table 1*]. Among the best known of these syndromes are familial retinoblastoma and the Li-Fraumeni syndrome. The examination of tissues from patients with familial retinoblastoma led to identification of the *Rb* (retinoblastoma) gene, the first tumor suppressor gene to be characterized. Individuals at risk for familial retinoblastoma are recognizable because of germ line mutations in one allele of their two *Rb* genes [*see Chapter 6*]. Once a heritable mutation has been characterized, PCR-based assays for the routine identification of that

Table 1 Selected Hereditary Cancer Syndromes

Syndrome	Gene	Chromosomal Location	Common Neoplastic Pathology
Breast/ovarian cancer syndrome*	BRCA1	17q12	Breast and ovarian carcinoma
Familial adenomatous polyposis coli	APC	5q21	Colorectal carcinoma
Gardner's syndrome*	APC	5q21	Intestinal polyps; osteomas; fibromas; sebaceous cysts; carcinoma of the colon, ampulla of Vater, pancreas, thyroid, and adrenal glands; colorectal cancer
Hereditary nonpolyposis colon cancer	MLH1 MSH2	3p21 2p22	Colorectal carcinoma Colorectal carcinoma
Li-Fraumeni syndrome*	p53	17p13	Sarcomas, breast carcinoma, brain tumors
Multiple endocrine neoplasia type II* (Sipple's syndrome; MEN II)	ret	10q11	Medullary carcinoma of the thyroid, parathyroid adenoma, pheochromocytoma
Multiple endocrine neoplasia type I* (Wermer's syndrome; MEN I)	Not known	11q13	Adenomas of islet cells, parathyroid, pituitary, and adrenal glands; malignant schwannoma; nonappendiceal carcinoid
Multiple mucosal neuroma syndrome			Pheochromocytoma, medullary carcinoma of the thyroid, neurofibroma, submucosal neuromas of the tongue, lips, and eyelids
Nevoid basal cell carcinoma syndrome (Gorlin's syndrome)			Basal cell carcinoma, ovarian fibroma
Retinoblastoma*	Rb	13q14	Sarcoma, pinealoblastoma, carcinoma
Wilms' tumor	WT-1	11p13	Embryonal kidney tumors

*Genetic testing possible.

mutation can be developed, or other techniques, such as linkage analysis using restriction enzyme fragment length polymorphisms or other chromosome specific structural markers (such as microsatellite DNA), can be used to detect the specific allele associated with tumor development.[2] These easily conducted tests can evaluate the DNA of family members who are at risk for the development of cancer; for example, the analyses can determine which individuals carry a mutant allele of *Rb* and are therefore at increased risk for the development of retinoblastoma. These tests can also be used to examine fetal tissue, thereby providing prenatal evidence of a predisposition for cancer.[3]

Germ line mutation of the *p53* gene occurs in families with the Li-Fraumeni syndrome. In contrast to families affected by hereditary retinoblastoma, Li-Fraumeni syndrome family members carry a predisposition to a large number of different tumor types, the most common of which are sarcomas, breast cancer, and brain tumors. The analysis of *p53*, like that of *Rb* and other more recently identified tumor suppressor genes associated with increased cancer risk, has been proposed for screening large populations and for evaluating individuals at risk for the development of specific tumors. Our inability to develop tests that recognize the entire spectrum of possible mutations, as well as the rarity of these cancer syndromes, makes such programs unlikely in the foreseeable future. Also, it has not yet been possible to develop cancer prevention strategies based on known genetic alterations that confer a cancer predisposition, although knowledge of such an enhanced predisposition generally leads to increased medical surveillance of individuals at risk, with the goal of intervening earlier in the disease process.

In contrast to cancer syndromes such as hereditary retinoblastoma and the Li-Fraumeni syndrome, in most familial syndromes associated with enhanced tumor predisposition, tumors are only one manifestation of an otherwise complex syndrome associated with multiple nonmalignant, although often disabling, clinical disorders [*see Table 2*]. These complex tumor syndromes include chromosomal disorders, such as Down's syndrome (trisomy 21) and Klinefelter's syndrome (XXY), which predispose to leukemia. Identification of the genetic alterations underlying each of these disorders will contribute substantially to the development of precise, measurable criteria of an individual's cancer predisposition.

VIRUS INFECTION AS A BIOMARKER

Recognition of the role of viruses in the development of many human cancers has led to other approaches for identifying and monitoring individuals at high risk for the development of cancer [*see Table 3*], including anogenital carcinomas, hepatocellular carcinoma, and adult T cell leukemia [*see Chapter 8*]. The development of molecular probes and assays for the detection of virus infection can be used in epidemiological studies to better characterize the incidence and pathogenesis of these tumors and to seek associations between tumor viruses and other tumors. This theme is well illustrated in studies that have evaluated the role of human papillomaviruses (HPV) in the etiology of many different types of cancer, including poorly understood tumors, such as bowenoid papulosis of the penis, a preneoplastic le-

Table 2 Selected Hereditary Syndromes in Which Malignant Tumors Occur

Syndrome	Gene	Chromosomal Location	Neoplastic Pathology
Agammaglobulinemia		X	Leukemia, gastrointestinal
Ataxia-telangiectasia	ATM		Lymphoreticular, leukemia, carcinoma of the stomach, brain tumors (chromosomal breaks)
Beckwith-Wiedemann syndrome	WT-1	11p13	Visceromegaly, cytomegaly, macroglossia, adrenocortical neoplasia, Wilms' tumor, hepatoma
Fanconi's pancytopenia	M†		Acute monomyelogenous leukemia, squamous cell carcinoma of mucocutaneous junctions, hepatic carcinoma and adenoma (chromosomal breaks)
Hemochromatosis		6p	Hepatocellular carcinoma
Neurofibromatosis type 2*	NF-2	22q12	Adenoma sebaceum, periungual fibroma, glial tumors, rhabdomyoma of the heart, renal tumor, lung cysts
Tuberous sclerosis	TSC1 TSC2	9q 16p13	Astrocytoma
Turcot's syndrome	APC	5q21	Brain tumor, intestinal polyposis
von Hippel–Lindau syndrome*	VHL		Retinal angioma, cerebellar hemangioblastoma, other hemangiomas, pheochromocytoma, hypernephroma, cysts
von Recklinghausen's disease (neurofibromatosis type 1)*	NF-1	17q	Sarcoma, neuroma, schwannoma, meningioma, optic glioma, pheochromocytoma, leukemia
Wiskott-Aldrich syndrome	WASP	Xp11.23	Lymphoreticular
Xeroderma pigmentosum	M†		Skin cancer

*Genetic testing possible.
†M indicates multiple complementation groups identified.

sion that can now be recognized as the counterpart of carcinoma in situ when it occurs in the female genital tract.

Only a few subtypes of papillomavirus are associated with cancer induction; these high-risk subtypes include HPV-16, HPV-18, and HPV-31. Because viral infection can be documented in premalignant, dysplastic lesions, assays to identify viral infection can be used as epidemiological tools to evaluate individuals at high risk for the development of malignant tumors.[4] A particularly well-characterized example of such a dysplastic lesion is cervical intraepithelial neoplasia, which is often a precursor of cervical carcinoma. The cellular changes associated with such dysplasia are the basis of the Papanicolaou test for cervical cancer, perhaps the most widely used cancer screening strategy. Studies identifying the importance of HPV in causing dysplastic lesions have led to the identification of HPV as a biomarker of cervical cancer risk, and they have identified an etiologic agent against which cancer prevention attempts can be targeted. Recognition of the role for the HPV-encoded oncogenes *E6* and *E7* in the development of anogenital cancers and some upper airway neoplasms means that evaluation of HPV infection patterns may provide further insight into these tumors.

Hepatitis virus is another infectious agent of considerable oncologic importance. The incidence of hepatic carcinoma is closely correlated with the prevalence of viral hepatitis, and it has been suggested that hepatitis B infection contributes to the development of 75 to 90 percent of hepatic carcinomas worldwide. The recognition of hepatitis B infection as a risk determinant for hepatic carcinoma has important implications for cancer prevention, and the use of assays to detect hepatitis B infection can be expected to play an expanded future role in the identification of populations with an increased risk for liver cancer.

Cancer Prevention

RISK AVOIDANCE AND CHEMOPROVENTION

For many of the most common tumors, decreasing exposure to known risk factors can have tremendous effects on cancer incidence. The precise identification of etiologic agents is critical for the success of these efforts. A particularly good example of the interplay between epidemiological studies, molecular analysis, and cancer prevention can be seen in viral carcinogenesis. Papillomaviruses associated with anogenital cancer are spread largely as a venereal infection. More than 70 percent of such infections, however, occur without associated symptomatology. Public health efforts using HPV as a biomarker for identifying individuals at high risk for the development of cancer and prevention programs targeted at reducing the spread of infection hold great promise for the control of genital tract malignancies, such as cervical carcinomas in women and penile cancer in men. Ongoing efforts are also focused on the development of more effective and less toxic antiviral agents for the treatment of papillomavirus infection. The public health implications of such strategies are significant because more than 90 percent of women with cervical cancer have evidence of HPV infection, and because

Table 3 Viruses Associated with Human Tumors

Virus	Human Tumor
Epstein-Barr	Burkitt's lymphoma, nasopharyngeal carcinoma
Hepatitis B	Hepatocellular carcinoma
Hepatitis C	Hepatocellular carcinoma
HPV-16, HPV-18, HPV-31, HPV-39	Anogenital cancers, upper airway cancers
HPV-5, HPV-8, HPV-17	Skin cancer
HTLV-I	Adult T cell leukemia/lymphoma
HTLV-II	Hairy cell leukemia

HPV—human papillomavirus; HTLV—human T cell lymphotropic virus.

the cost of managing cervical dysplasia by conventional means was estimated to exceed $6 billion in 1992.[5]

The development of vaccines against virion proteins of common papillomavirus subtypes is another active area of investigation. Furthermore, viral oncoproteins are invariably expressed in HPV-induced tumors, and one, *E7*, has been demonstrated to be immunogenic.[6] This observation suggests that it may be possible to immunize individuals against the oncoprotein itself with the intention of providing protection from transformed cells. Similarly, the development of vaccines to decrease hepatitis infection rates and the use of antiviral agents to treat this infection after it occurs could have a dramatic impact on the incidence of hepatic carcinoma. Vaccination against hepatitis B has been available for almost a decade in some areas where infection is very common, and it should soon be possible to evaluate the effectiveness of such a strategy in decreasing the incidence of hepatic cancer.

Epidemiological studies have also provided preliminary evidence that some dietary components and drugs may prevent the development of tumors. An understanding of the molecular events that are important for carcinogenesis provides an opportunity to enhance the therapeutic activities of such agents. Chemopreventive agents that have attracted the greatest attention include retinoic acid, a known regulator of gene expression, and β-carotene, which is thought to be an electron-scavenging antioxidant. Although no chemopreventive agents have been identified that inhibit the alteration of specific genes known to be important in the development of common human tumors, important targets for prevention efforts should be modification of the genetic alterations that mediate tumorigenesis and the cellular processes in which they are active. Trials are presently underway to assess the value of several chemopreventive agents and dietary measures.

EARLY INTERVENTION AND GENETIC COUNSELING

Just as genetic alterations may serve as a basis for identifying individuals with an increased cancer risk, knowledge of the genetic basis for tumor development affects the treatment of individuals thought to be at increased risk because of their family history. A key strategy for cancer prevention has been enhanced surveillance and early intervention to eradicate premalignant lesions or to treat tumors early, before they metastasize to distant locations. Early preventive interventions based on a patient's family history or the presence of premalignant lesions can be life saving. However, the need for a more accurate means of predicting inherited predispositions and for the development of more effective prevention strategies is obvious. For example, current clinical practice includes removal of the colon in patients with familial adenomatous polyposis and bilateral mastectomy in some patients with hereditary breast cancer. In contrast to familial adenomatous polyposis, in which precancerous polyps occur, in hereditary breast cancer, no premalignant lesion is known. Hereditary breast cancer, which is frequently bilateral, is currently suspected to be present when a high number of first-degree relatives have breast cancer that occurs at a young age. Although the risk of hereditary breast cancer development in such families rarely exceeds 25 percent, prophylactic mastectomy has been (and is currently) one approach to the treatment of these patients. Although linkage analysis using conventional chromosomal markers can help identify patients at risk when the DNA from many different family members is available, this situation arises only infrequently. The identification of breast cancer predisposition genes, such as *BRCA*1 should make it possible to pursue more effective prevention strategies by allowing the precise identification of family members at increased risk for tumor development. In this regard, *BRCA*1 is likely to be of particular importance because it may be responsible for as much as half of early-onset familial breast cancer and for most of the familial breast/ovarian cancer syndrome.

Knowledge of the specific genetic alterations involved in many heritable cancer predispositions [*see Tables 1 and 2*] should provide an opportunity to more accurately assess an individual's risk of cancer development decades before tumors might occur. The economic, psychosocial, personal, and ethical issues surrounding such undertakings are still emerging, yet the complexity of these issues is already recognizable.[7] Screening for enhanced cancer predisposition is further complicated by the fact that in only a very few cases are the incidences or implications of mutations in cancer susceptibility genes known. In most cases, only preliminary information exists on such diverse but critical clinical parameters as the sites at greatest risk for the development of tumors or the optimal intervention once a specific predisposition is recognized. Furthermore, the development of functional assays for cancer predisposition genes that may provide a more accurate assessment of the pathological implications of specific mutations is in its infancy. Converting the knowledge of specific risk factors into prevention strategies that are both effective and acceptable to individuals at increased risk is a key challenge for future cancer research.

Oncologic Pathology

Knowledge of tumor-specific genetic alterations has influenced the manner in which tumors are pathologically classified. A fundamental tenet of clinical medicine is that a specific diagnosis is required so that a specific treatment can be administered, and patients with a single disorder must be grouped together for optimal patient management and development and evaluation of new therapies. In this regard, oncology has faced a particularly distressing situation in that it has not been possible to define pathologically homogeneous groups of patients. Nonetheless, oncologic pathology has sought to classify tumors in a manner that facilitates their recognition and provides an organizational structure through which clinicians can develop and use optimal treatment regimens. The oncogenetic changes found in specific tumors or the biochemical changes they cause may be useful for tumor classification and prognostication. The need for a revised classification system based on pathogenesis will become even more important as additional tumor-specific, targeted therapies are developed.

Molecular Pathology of Hematopoietic Tumors

The greatest progress toward a molecular nosology for tumors has been achieved in the hematopoietic tumors, particularly lymphoid neoplasms. Study of cell surface antigens whose expression changes over the course of lymphocyte maturation and the association of these changes with developmentally regulated rearrangements of immunoglobulin and T cell receptor genes has revealed that different lymphoid tumors correspond to microscopically indistinguishable [*see Figure 2*] normal cell types that appear during lymphoid cell differentiation.[8] These tumors, which have characteristic clinical behaviors and biologic features, are each associated with a limited number of distinctive cytogenetic alterations known to mark the location of specific oncogenes that contribute to tumor development.[9] As a result, the categorization of lymphoid tumors has been modified to include the expansive cytogenetic and molecular genetic data that characterize them [*see Table 4*].

Hematopoietic tumors of many different cell lineages possess different chromosomal rearrangements, and these rearrangements can mark distinctive biologic and pathological entities. These genetic alterations provide a unique framework for the development of tumor classification schema based not only on the appearance of a tumor or a particular biologic property but also on a pathological characteristic of etiologic importance. Such classification schema will be of increasing importance as therapies targeted to specific biochemical alterations or tumor-specific gene products emerge. For the present, however, it should be possible to define more homogenous groups of patients so that even the nonspecific antineoplastic agents currently available can be more effectively used.

An important example of the usefulness of such a genetically oriented approach to the stratification of patients for treatment is children with acute lymphoblastic leukemia. Although many such patients have leukemias that can be morphologically classified as being pre–B cell tumors, the biologic behavior and response of these tumors to conventional therapies remains unpredictable. The use of cytogenetics to classify patients with these tumors has resulted in the stratification of patients into more homogeneous treat-

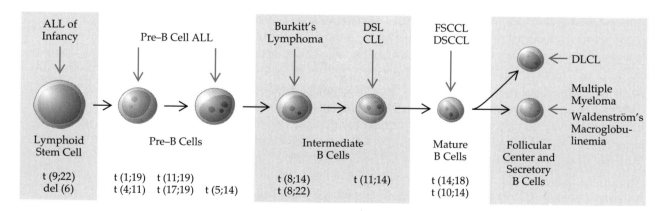

Figure 2 *Lymphoid malignancies that correspond to recognizable cell types seen during normal B cell ontogeny. The degree of B cell differentiation is defined by the extent of immunoglobulin gene rearrangement and the expression of various cell surface markers. The genetic alterations found in these cell types and their corresponding malignancies are indicated: acute lymphocytic leukemia of infancy (ALL of infancy); pre–B cell acute lymphocytic leukemia (pre–B cell ALL); diffuse small-cell lymphoma (DSL), chronic lymphocytic leukemia (CLL); follicular, small cleaved cell lymphoma (FSCCL); diffuse, small cleaved cell lymphoma (DSCCL); and diffuse large-cell lymphoma (DLCL).*

Table 4 Genetic Alterations in Lymphoid Malignancies

Tumor Type	Chromosomal Abnormality	Gene Affected
Early pre–B cell ALL, pre–B cell ALL, infant ALL	t(1;19)(q23;p13)	*E2A-pbx*1
	t(4;11)(q21;q23)	*ALL1/hrx-AF4*
	t(11;19)(q23;23)	*ALL1/hrx-ENL*
	t(17;19)(q22;p13)	*E1A-Hlf*
	t(9;22)(q34;q11)	*bcr-abl*
Pre–B cell ALL	t(5;14)(q31;q32)	*IL-3*
BL, B cell ALL, diffuse B cell NHL, immunoblastic B cell NHL, AIDS-NHL	t(8;14)(q24;q32)	*c-myc*
	t(2;8)(p11;q24)	
	t(8;22)(q24;q11)	
Mantle zone B cell NHL	t(11;14)(q13;q32)	*bcl*-1
Follicular B cell NHL	t(14;18)(q32;q21)	*bcl*-2
Low-grade B cell NHL, CTCL	t(10;14)(q24;q11)	*lyt*-10
Diffuse B cell NHL	t(3;?)(q27)	*bcl*-6
T cell ALL	t(8;14)(q24;q11)	*c-myc*
T cell ALL	t(1;14)(p32;q11)	*tal*-1
T cell ALL	t(10;14)(q24;q11)	*hox*-11
T cell ALL	t(11;14)(p15;q11)	*ttg-1/Rhom*-1
T cell ALL	t(11;14)(p13;q11)	*ttg-2/Rhom*-2
T cell ALL	t(7;9)(q34;q32)	*tal*-2
T cell ALL	t(7;19)(q35;p13)	*lyl*-1
T cell ALL	t(1;7)(p34;q34)	*lck*
T cell ALL	t(7;9)(q34;q34.3)	*tan*-1

ALL—acute lymphocytic leukemia; BL—Burkitt's lymphoma; NHL—non-Hodgkin's lymphoma; AIDS-NHL—acquired immunodeficiency syndrome–associated non-Hodgkin's lymphoma; CTCL—cutaneous T cell lymphoma.

ment groups, a likely prelude to the development of the truly tumor-specific therapies.

Molecular Pathology of Tumors Arising in Solid Tissues

Although many tumors of nonhematopoietic, solid tissues have been identified as having characteristic cytogenetic alterations, tumors of solid tissues seem to be genetically less stable than hematopoietic tumors and are typically characterized by a large number of different genetic alterations [*see Table 5*]. Within a single tumor cell, important genetic rearrangements may involve many different chromosomal regions distributed throughout the entire genome. As a result of the cytogenetic alterations that are found in solid tumors, some evidence indicates the involvement of multiple oncogenes and tumor suppressor genes in the pathogenesis of these tumors. Although the large number of different genetic alterations in solid tumors that are available for evaluation provides many opportunities for solid tumor classification, it has complicated attempts at classifying solid tumors into pathologically and genetically homogeneous subgroups.

One instance in which the ability to recognize genetically defined subgroups of a solid tumor has proved particularly useful has been in the evaluation of neuroblastoma. In metastatic neuroblastomas, a subgroup of tumors exists that has a distinctive pattern of proto-oncogene expression.[10] This subgroup consists of peripheral nervous system tumors (peripheral neuroepitheliomas) arising in precursors of parasympathetic neurons; the

Table 5   Genetic Alterations in Common Solid Tumors

Tumor Type	Genetic Alteration	Gene
Breast Cancer	Gene amplification Inactivated by mutation	*c-myc, HER-2/neu, EGFR,* cyclin D
Colon and rectal cancer	Gene amplification Activated by mutation Inactivated by mutation	*HER-2/neu, c-myc, myb* *K-ras, N-ras* *p53, APC, DCC, MCC*
Lung cancer	Gene amplification Activated by mutation 3p chromosomal deletion Inactivated by mutation	*c-myc, L-myc, N-myc* *K-ras, H-ras* *p53, Rb*
Childhood solid tumors Rhabdomyosarcoma Wilms' tumor Ewing's sarcoma	Gene rearrangement Inactivated by mutation Gene rearrangement Gene amplification	*pax3-FKHR* *WT*-1 *EWS-FL*1 *c-myc*

group is distinctive from the larger group of neuroblastoma tumors, which arise in precursors of sympathetic neurons. Although histologically indistinguishable, these subgroups have different prognoses and, because they respond differently to antineoplastic therapy, require different treatment approaches. Because a cell's biologic characteristics that are regulated during normal differentiation may contribute to many of a tumor cell's pathological features, classifying tumors by their pattern of proto-oncogene expression has a strong rationale and may reveal other pathologically homogeneous groups of tumors.

Despite many attempts to identify specific genetic alterations that are closely associated with key pathological features of solid tumors, such as their metastatic potential or invasiveness, and despite occasionally promising preliminary data, such determinations have not yet been possible. The reason for this failure is unclear, but an understanding of the mechanisms by which such malignant characteristics of tumors are regulated will be an important future contribution to oncologic pathology.

Patient Management

Prognostication

The prognosis is the expected outcome of a disease, and accurately determining the prognoses of patients with cancer is of great importance. In addition to providing the patient with an opportunity to plan for the future, the patient's prognosis provides the physician with a guide for proper treatment and provides the cancer researcher with aid in designing and evaluating new therapies. The emergence of tumor classification schema based on pathological alterations that are critical for tumor development and malignant cell behavior has led to the development of more accurate prognostic markers. Numerous cytogenetic alterations in hematopoietic malignancies, such as translocations involving 11q23,[11] have already been identified as prognostic markers.[12] Such prognostic opportunities are of particular importance when they permit the identification of patients who are likely to have a poor therapeutic response to conventional strategies because they allow such patients to avoid the side effects of a useless therapy and provide patients with an opportunity to receive investigational, but potentially efficacious, therapies. In the future, prognostic evaluation is likely to have increasing clinical significance because intensification of therapy clearly enhances treatment efficacy for patients with tumors that are refractory to conventional therapies.

Tumor-specific chromosomal rearrangements and structural changes in specific oncogenes have also been defined as prognostic markers in solid tumors, although biologically significant alterations have not been as easily recognized as they were in hematopoietic tumors. Perhaps this difficulty is a reflection of the genetic instability of solid tumors. One solid tumor in which the activation of a specific oncogene is associated with a predictable outcome is neuroblastoma. N-*myc* amplification in neuroblastoma is associated with rapid tumor progression, and it is an important predictor of poor prognosis in children with this tumor.[13] Studies examining the expression of oncogenes in other solid tumors have also pointed to the likelihood that their expression can be of prognostic significance.[14] For example, HER-2/*neu* expression and codon 12 K-*ras* mutations are predictors for shortened survival of patients with adenocarcinoma of the lung, and HER-2/*neu* expression is of prognostic significance in patients with cervical adenocarcinoma. The HER-2/*neu* oncogene is amplified in 25 to 30 percent of breast cancers, and this amplification is associated with early relapse and shorter survival after diagnosis. Most studies have shown the amplification of HER-2/*neu* to be a predictor of aggressive clinical behavior (e.g., growth, invasion, angiogenic stimulation, metastatic potential, and therapeutic resistance) that is independent of other known prognostic factors for breast cancer. When considered together with another independent prognostic indicator, such as nuclear grade, the power and use of HER-2/*neu* as a prognostic marker is greatly enhanced, suggesting that such oncogenetic alterations are best considered within the overall biology of the particular tumor type being examined.[15] Patients with breast cancer who have no evidence of lymph node involvement at diagnosis but who nonetheless experience recurrence are likely to benefit from more intensive therapy at initial presentation. Unfortunately, HER-2/*neu* amplification is not useful in identifying this important subgroup.

At the present time, our inability to identify specific genetic alterations as reliable prognostic markers for most tumor types remains a conundrum. Perhaps more easily performed assays with enhanced sensitivity to detect proteins encoded by oncogenes in the serum of cancer patients will facilitate their evaluation. In breast cancer, evaluation of a soluble fragment of the protein encoded by HER-2/*neu* in serum has suggested an association between elevated serum HER-2/*neu* protein levels and poor clinical outcome.[16] The availability of such technologies should increase the feasibility of screening patients to define which molecular changes are of greatest prognostic significance.

Staging at Diagnosis and Monitoring Therapy

Cancer staging is an important adjunct to diagnosis because it is an assessment of the spread of tumor cells beyond the site of tumor origin. Such information also affects the choice of therapy. Even when genetic alterations found in tumors are not of diagnostic or prognostic significance, these markers are tumor specific, and their evaluation can facilitate the identification of tumor cells that are not otherwise detectable. Such assessments are making important contributions to tumor staging. Tumor-specific genetic alterations are now the target of strategies designed to identify malignant cells both at the time of diagnosis and during the course of therapy. For example, imaging technologies using monoclonal antibodies directed against tumor-specific antigens, which are sometimes encoded by unique genetic rearrangements, are being developed to enhance the visualization of such cells. One such strategy uses antibodies that recognize a truncated form of the epidermal growth factor (EGF) receptor (resulting from an in-frame deletion), but not the wild-type EGF receptor, to localize tumor xenografts that express mutant EGF receptor.[17] Serial evaluation of serum specimens for proteins encoded by mutated oncogenes may also improve the means by which patients' response to therapy and their clinical course can be monitored.

Polymerase chain reaction–based assays used to detect tumor-specific rearrangements are the most widely used approach for detecting rare tumor cells in patients' specimens. If a tumor-specific genetic alteration has been defined, PCR assays can be used to detect the presence of otherwise undetectable tumor cells in virtually any patient specimen.[18] This characteristic is especially important for the assessment of tissues that can be conveniently obtained, such as peripheral blood, sputum, and urine. Microscopic examination usually requires that greater than 1 percent of cells be malignant before the tumor cells are likely to be recognizable. When the DNA sequence of tumor-specific gene rearrangements, such as the chromosomal translocations found in hematopoietic tumors, are known, PCR-based strategies are sensitive enough to detect one tumor cell in 10^5 to 10^7 normal cells.[19] PCR-based assays enable a significant number of patients with lung, breast, and prostate tumors who appear to have localized disease by conventional technologies, such as x-ray study and histologic evaluation of tissue specimens, to be identified as having disease that has already disseminated at the time of diagnosis. PCR-based assays to detect point mutations in the H-*ras* and K-*ras* oncogenes have made it possible to detect otherwise occult malignant cells in the sputum of patients with lung cancer and in the urine of patients with bladder cancer. Mutations in the *p53* gene have similarly been detected in tumor cells shed into the saliva, sputum, and urine of patients with carcinomas of the head and neck, lung, and bladder, respectively.[20]

When informative oncogenetic mutations or rearrangements cannot be identified, malignant cells of some tumor types can nonetheless be detected, based on the presence of other tumor-specific markers, such as the antigen receptor rearrangements that characterize clonal B and T cell tumors. In solid tumors, the use of PCR to detect malignant cells expressing messenger RNA (mRNA) that encodes known tumor antigens can also reveal otherwise occult disease. By use of such an approach, tumor cells circulating in the blood or bone marrow have been detected by the evaluation of keratin 19 expression in patients with breast cancer, prostate-specific membrane antigen in patients with prostate cancer, and choriocarcinoma embryonic antigen in patients with carcinoma of many different abdominal organs. These genes are typically evaluated in tissues from sites where these tumors are known to metastasize when these sites do not physiologically express these tumor markers.

Because of the accessibility of peripheral blood and other body fluids, such PCR-based assays are likely to become important strategies for monitoring a patient's response to therapy, in addition to establishing the stage of the tumor at diagnosis [*see Figure 1*]. "Complete clinical remission" is the term used to designate a time during cancer therapy when patients have no evidence of identifiable disease by any of the conventional detection modalities. Most patients require additional therapy after a complete clinical remission is achieved because patients who do not receive this therapy often experience a relapse of their disease. Tumors that emerge during such relapses are typically marked by genetic alterations that are identical to those found in the original tumor, indicating that they arise as the result of residual disease. Although it is generally agreed that all or almost all neoplastic cells must be destroyed during therapy for cancer patients to be cured, it has not been possible to sensitively detect the presence of small numbers of tumor cells. The decision of when to stop therapy is typically made based on prior experience treating other patients rather than on knowledge of a particular patient's response to treatment. PCR-based strategies for detecting persistent tumor cells during therapy will provide opportunities to better assess the efficacy of therapy and the need for continued therapy. Although the need to treat patients until the number of cells decreases below the level of detection by sensitive PCR-based assays has not been critically evaluated, it seems likely that such treatment will be necessary. In patients who have received intensive chemotherapy and autologous bone marrow transplantation, detection in transplanted bone marrow of even very few malignant cells marked by an oncogenetic rearrangement is a strong indicator of impending relapse.[21]

Diagnostic Imaging

The availability of reagents that recognize molecules specifically expressed on the surface of tumor cells has provided an opportunity for the development of novel approaches to the diagnostic imaging of tumors. Tumor-specific cytogenetic alterations may rarely produce a tumor-specific cell surface molecule if the mutated gene encodes a membrane protein. Such molecules include antigen receptors, such as antibodies, T cell receptors, and growth factor receptors, such as the rearranged and amplified EGF receptor. More commonly, malignant cellular transformation results in the expression of a unique genetic program that determines the biologic behavior of malignant cells. This genetic program includes overexpressed proto-oncogenes that may contribute to the malignant behavior of the tumor cells and modify the expression of other cellular genes that are not physiologically expressed in growth-arrested, normal adult tissues. Many of these normal, yet tumor-specific, molecules were first detected by antibodies developed to recognize specific types of tumor cells. These molecules are generally known as oncofetal antigens because their expression, although not detectable in mature tissues of the adult, can frequently be found in fetal tissues that correspond to the mature tissue type in which specific tumors arise. These classes of molecules, activated proto-oncogenes and oncofetal antigens, include many specific molecules being evaluated as efficacious targets for antibody-mediated external tumor imaging and therapy.

Monoclonal antibodies, which recognize tumor-specific proteins, or ligands, that recognize receptors highly expressed in tumors, can be labeled with a variety of isotopes, such as indium-111 (^{111}In) and technetium-99m (^{99m}Tc). After they are administered to a patient, these labeled molecules can localize to tumor tissue and then be identified by external scintigraphy [*see Figure 3*].[22] Several such ligands and antibodies have been examined in cancer patients and have been found to detect tumors with excellent specificity and sensitivity. Although most monoclonal antibody imaging techniques use reactivity against oncofetal antigens, tumor-specific genetic alterations may also provide a satisfactory cell surface target for tumor localization.[23] For example, radiolabeled murine monoclonal antibodies directed against the EGF receptor or HER-2/*neu* produce good images of tumors in which the genes encoding those proteins are amplified.

Other radiolabeled monoclonal antibodies that recognize the cytoplasmic product of the *ras* proto-oncogene have also been used to effectively image human breast cancer xenografts in animal models.[24] This suggests that antibodies may be able to target intracellular proteins in areas of tumor necrosis, where such proteins are presumably exposed to the extracellular milieu. Although the finding that cytoplasmic proteins, such as p21^{K-ras}, can be targets for immunoscintigraphy must be critically assessed, this possibility increases the potential targets of such imaging modalities.

Another novel target that has been used to image human tumor xenografts in rodents is the transmembrane "P-glycoprotein" (p170), the product of the *mdr* gene. This protein acts as an effluent pump that removes cytotoxic molecules from the cell and is an important determinant of tumor cell resistance to antineoplastic agents. The protein p170 is expressed at high levels on the surface of many different types of tumor cells. Its use as an imaging target may prove efficacious not only for tumor localization but also for monitoring of the development of drug resistance.

The reactivity of radiolabeled monoclonal antibodies to tumor-specific antigens has opened other, unanticipated opportunities for identifying malignant tissues. For example, the availability of a hand-held gamma ray detection probe has made possible the intraoperative identification of sites of malignant lesions that might not otherwise have been detected.[25] Although the efficacy of tumor site detection has varied somewhat among the different studies that have evaluated this technology, after the administration of an iodine-125 (^{125}I)–labeled monoclonal antibody directed against an oncofetal antigen, an intraoperative probe was able to detect approximately 85

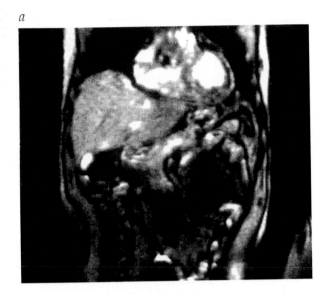

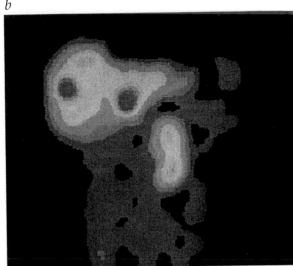

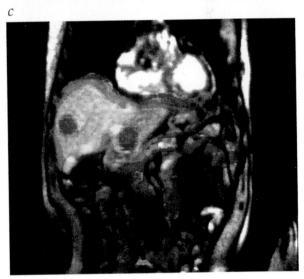

Figure 3 *Somatostatin receptor imaging scan for the detection of occult carcinoid and metastatic sites of tumor spread. (a) An apparently normal magnetic resonance examination of a 64-year-old man with a several-year history of symptoms suggestive of a carcinoid tumor, although no tumor could be detected by conventional imaging techniques. (b) A somatostatin-receptor scan in which Indium-111–labeled octreilide, an analogue of somatostatin, has been imaged. This scan shows the normal outline of the liver in yellow and blue, although two red spots indicate the site of somatostatin localization; this finding is indicative of hepatic carcinoid metastases. In addition, a yellow region exists beneath the liver, indicating the actual primary gut site of the carcinoid tumor. (c) The somatostatin receptor imaging scan is superimposed on the magnetic resonance image.*

percent of all identifiable abdominal sites of colon cancer as well as additional sites that had not been detected by other technologies.

Therapeutics

This book presents an integrated model of cancer as a somatic genetic disorder of growth and differentiation that arises in association with the diminished genetic stability of the tumor cell. Identification of the specific genes involved in tumorigenesis and knowledge of their physiologic activity have opened totally new avenues of translational research. The most prominent areas of research in cancer therapy include the development of novel agents for the treatment of cancer patients; more efficacious immunotherapies; and new, unanticipated treatment strategies. An appealing aspect of these particular initiatives is that many of them target disseminated cancers, against which currently available therapies frequently lack activity.

The search for cytotoxic drugs and other agents for the treatment of cancer, as well as attempts to develop immunotherapeutic approaches against tumors, have well-known limitations. In both cases, however, the new opportunities afforded by molecular oncology have resulted in an optimistic assessment that more efficacious, less toxic therapies than those currently available can be developed. The basis for this optimism rests in the confidence that new treatment strategies can be developed that address more precise therapeutic goals or target tumor-specific genetic or biochemical alterations. Although major breakthroughs that dramatically affect the survival of cancer patients have not yet been achieved, progress has been made on many different fronts.

NOVEL AGENTS

Cytokines and Mediators of Differentiation   Cytokines are molecules that act physiologically to coordinate and regulate such cellular activities as proliferation, differentiation, and cell death. They are also important mediators of the body's natural defense mechanisms. Few therapeutic studies have evaluated the direct effects of cytokines on tumor cells, although the antitumor activities of some interferons probably include direct effects, such as growth inhibition of tumor cells, in addition to their stimulation of the host immune system. In contrast to many conventional antineoplastic agents, interferons are cytostatic rather than cytotoxic. Although quite toxic at therapeutically active doses, interferon alfa is currently among the most active agents against hairy-cell leukemia, some chronic leukemias, and Kaposi's sarcoma.[26] Tumor necrosis factor is another cytokine whose antineoplastic activity is currently being explored. Although too toxic for systemic administration, the regional administration of tumor necrosis factor for the management of such tumors as melanoma and sarcoma occurring in accessible locations, such as an extremity or the liver, has been explored with some initial success.[27]

The use of cytokines to enhance the natural host immune response against cancer is an active area of clinical investigation. The cytokine that has been most extensively evaluated clinically is interleukin-2 (IL-2).[28] IL-2 administration stimulates the production of numerous other cytokines in T cells, including interleukin-1 (IL-1) and interferon gamma, which themselves alter immune system function. Also, IL-2 can stimulate the proliferation of circulating natural killer cells, which have a direct antitumor effect. IL-2 has proved to be toxic and is an inefficient anticancer agent when it is administered intravenously to cancer patients. IL-2 has, however, been used both in vitro, to expand various autologous immune system effector cell types, which are harvested from individual patients and then reinfused, and in vivo, to augment the activity of these cells after reinfusion. Such therapy has activity against a limited spectrum of tumors but has resulted in prolonged remissions of both melanoma and renal cell tumors. In many cases, it has been possible to show that the biologic activities of different cytokines can be synergistic,[29] and clinical trials are underway to determine whether cytokines can be combined in a manner that will both enhance their activity and diminish their toxicity. Cytokines other than IL-2 that modulate the immune response and are currently being evaluated for antitumor activity in clinical trials include IL-2, interleukin-6, interleukin-7, interleukin-10, interleukin-11, and interleukin-12.

Hematopoietic cytokines that enhance the proliferation of normal blood precursor cells when a patient's bone marrow is compromised by tumor infiltration or toxic chemotherapy have an established role in cancer therapy.[30] Granulocyte colony-stimulating factor, granulocyte-macrophage colony-stimulating factor, and erythropoietin are already in wide clinical use as adjuvants to intensive, high-dose, chemotherapeutic strategies. The recent discovery of thrombopoietin, which is a potent stimulator of megakaryocytic proliferation, will undoubtedly provide the basis for the development of products to alleviate the thrombocytopenia and associated bleeding problems that are significant impediments to the intensive use of cytotoxic antineoplastic agents.[31]

In addition to cytokines, other biologicals are being evaluated as cancer treatments. One of the most interesting lines of investigation involves the use of retinoic acid for the treatment of acute promyelocytic leukemia. Acute promyelocytic leukemia is characterized by a reciprocal chromosomal translocation, t(15;17), that fuses an interrupted retinoic acid receptor-α (RAR-α) with a transcription factor, PML. This rearrangement leads to a functionally altered RAR-α.[32] Introduction of a functional RAR-α into the myeloid leukemia cell line HL-60, in which the endogenous RAR-α gene bears a mutation causing the synthesis of a nonfunctional, truncated RAR-α, renders these cells sensitive to the differentiating effects of all-*trans*-retinoic acid treatment. Patients with acute promyelocytic leukemia whose tumors make an RAR-α–PML fusion mRNA respond to treatment with pharmacological doses of retinoic acid and typically enter a complete, although brief, clinical remission.[33] Retinoic acid is a physiologic mediator of gene expression in many tissues, and the remission observed after the treatment of patients with acute promyelocytic leukemia is associated with cytogenetic and molecular evidence indicating that the leukemic clone of cells undergoes differentiation during therapy.[34] Thus, during remission, mature granulocytes do not exhibit the tumor-specific marker chromosome, a finding suggesting that the malignant clone is suppressed by the retinoic acid–induced differentiation and that a normal program of myeloid differentiation is restored after retinoic acid therapy. Although the precise mechanism of retinoic acid's therapeutic effect remains to be elucidated, these observations provide a strong rationale for evaluating the therapeutic potential of known mediators of differentiation. As additional information emerges regarding the signal transduction pathways over which cellular maturation signals are mediated, additional opportunities to modulate tumor cell differentiation will undoubtedly also emerge.

Monoclonal Antibodies   Monoclonal antibodies that localize to tumor tissue and therefore have diagnostic potential are also being developed as an additional treatment modality for cancer.[35] Antibodies alone can be cytotoxic, killing tumor cells either by a complement-dependent mechanism or by an antibody-dependent cellular toxicity. The antigens against which such antibodies are directed have typically been oncofetal antigens, although in some cases, antibodies that recognize unique cell surface antigens encoded by specific oncogenetic changes have been developed. When such strategies have been undertaken for the treatment of tumors arising in the B cell lineage, it has been possible to develop antibodies against the tumor-specific idiotype of the immunoglobulin expressed on the surface of the tumor cells.[36] The strategy of exploiting the cytotoxic effect of antibodies for cancer therapy has been used with some success in the treatment of patients with hematopoietic tumors, although similar approaches to the treatment of patients with solid tumors have resulted in fewer clinical responses. These studies have, however, formed the basis of ongoing work evaluating the effectiveness of monoclonal antibodies combined with various cytokines. A goal of these studies is to enhance infiltration at the tumor site by mononuclear cells that mediate antibody-dependent cellular toxicity.

Monoclonal antibodies conjugated to radioisotopes, immunotoxins, pro-drug-activating enzymes, and chemotherapeutic agents are likely to be more effective cytotoxic agents than antibodies alone. Radiolabeled antibodies have been developed that recognize oncofetal antigens and proto-oncogenes that are highly expressed on the tumor cell surface. Clinical trials of the latter type have been conducted using radiolabeled antibodies that recognize the highly expressed epidermal growth factor receptor in lung tumors and brain tumors. These antibodies may be useful for other tumors in which this receptor is also highly expressed, such as breast cancer. Other targets for radiolabeled antibodies that are currently being evaluated in clinical trials include the HER-2/*neu* cell surface receptor, which is highly expressed in some breast and ovarian cancers, and the IL-2 receptor, which is highly expressed in several types of lymphoma (unpublished data). Each of these targets has been previously examined in animal models and has been found to be promising. An important conclusion drawn from the current body of human and animal studies has been the recognition that antibody-directed therapy is most likely to play a role in the treatment of minimal residual disease that persists after conventional treatments. For this reason, additional antibodies and closely related therapeutic molecules consisting of radioisotopes and toxins chemically linked to growth factors (or ligands that mimic growth factors by binding to their cognate receptors) that promote tumor growth are being actively explored in animal models.[37]

The propensity of patients who receive murine monoclonal antibodies to develop antibodies against these monoclonals has been a major impediment to the administration of repeated, sequential doses of such antibodies. Patients can only rarely receive even a second course of treatment with murine monoclonal antibodies. Several different strategies for the development of less immunogenic antibodies are being pursued. Most of these involve the use of recombinant DNA technologies to replace nonessential regions of the murine immunoglobulin molecule with the corresponding region of human immunoglobulin. Also, technologies to further facilitate the isolation of human monoclonal antibodies that would not be recognized as foreign are being pursued.[38] An additional approach to the identification of better antibody reagents is based on the screening of immunoglobulin gene libraries constructed in recombinant phage vectors[39] engineered to express and secrete cloned immunoglobulin fragments. Interestingly, these technologies have the capacity to yield exceedingly complex libraries of high-specificity antibodies, including antibodies with structures that may not be present in vivo.

New Drugs Cytotoxic and antiproliferative drugs that affect DNA synthesis, transcription, or mitotic spindle function have been a mainstay of the oncologist's pharmacopeia for disseminated tumors and primary cancers that cannot be surgically removed. Molecular oncology has identified specific biochemical pathways that are essential for the expression of a tumor cell's malignant properties, and the molecules that mediate these pathways are important targets for new antineoplastic drugs. The more closely linked the therapeutic target is to the underlying pathological alteration, the more likely it is that the expected therapeutic action of the agent will be tumor specific and perhaps more effective and less toxic than currently available agents. Ongoing research to identify new therapeutics reflects a variety of ideas regarding how the altered function of tumor cells might best be modulated. These ideas include the interruption of aberrant cellular activities, the identification of molecules to stimulate opposing cellular activities that might balance pathological alterations, and the development of adjuvants for existing nonspecific cytotoxic agents. Some such therapeutic interventions seem likely to induce an apoptotic tumor cell death. Others, in contrast to current cytotoxic treatments, are likely to be cytostatic and require continuous treatment over a prolonged period of time. Such therapies will pose significant pharmacological problems. At the present time, no such initiatives have reached fruition, but some important new drugs are being evaluated in clinical studies.

The search for novel antineoplastic agents is being pursued through two sharply contrasting strategies. Screening programs use high-throughput assays to assess specific biologic activities of many chemicals to find candidate molecules whose structure can be used for the formulation of a series of molecules whose therapeutic activity might be evaluated. Past screening programs sought molecules with antiproliferative activities among compounds that were typically fractionated from natural products, such as plant extracts. More recently developed screening strategies are being used to identify new compounds that have a specific biologic or biochemical activity, which antagonizes the oncogenetic changes promoting tumor cell proliferation. Furthermore, such screening frequently involves the evaluation of very large, in vitro synthesized libraries of molecules. Molecules identified by such screening efforts are in the early stages of preclinical drug development. Other drug discovery programs use biochemical strategies, including so-called rational drug design, to construct molecules that might have a desired therapeutic activity.

The identification of drugs with a specific biochemical activity has resulted in the movement of several new classes of drugs toward clinical evaluation. The most widely heralded targets currently being pursued in drug development are molecules involved in the transduction of growth regulatory signals from the tumor cell membrane to the nucleus. One molecular target is the Ras oncoprotein. Mutations in a *ras* gene are thought to contribute to the pathogenesis of many tumors and occur in greater than 50 percent of tumors arising in some organs of the digestive system.[40] Ras is an important molecule for the transmission of extracellular signals, and its proper functioning depends on its anchorage to the cytoplasmic side of the plasma membrane. This anchorage is mediated by the posttranslational farnesylation of a cysteine residue located near the C-terminal end of the molecule. Farnesylation of Ras is essential for its transforming activity,[41] and farnesyltransferase inhibitors have been shown to block the growth of Ras-transformed cells and Ras-dependent tumors in animal models.[42] Little systemic toxicity was identifiable in these animal studies, and several drugs with this activity are anticipated to reach clinical evaluation soon. Such in vivo studies are of particular importance because proteins other than Ras require farnesylation for biologic activity, raising the possibility that intolerable toxicities would impede the development of these agents as drugs and would require additional strategies to achieve a greater specificity of action.

In addition to drugs such as limonene, which specifically inhibit farnesyltransferase, several other classes of molecules have been identified that inhibit different steps in the metabolic pathway leading to the modification of Ras. Drugs such as lovastatin and phenyl acetate, which inhibit sterol synthesis and the modification of many different cellular proteins, including Ras, are cytotoxic for many different tumor types. The antineoplastic activities of these drugs are currently the subject of a number of ongoing clinical investigations.[43]

Another area of cancer drug development that has emerged as a direct result of our understanding of signal transduction pathways in tumors is tyrosine kinase inhibitors. Tyrosine kinases play a prominent role in tumorigenesis [*see Chapter 7*]. Initially, nonspecific compounds that were reactive against many different protein kinases were identified and evaluated. Genistein and other naturally occurring compounds were among the first such molecules to be examined. Although such molecules can inhibit the proliferation of human tumor cells, they are very toxic to normal cells, presumably because of their lack of specificity. Subsequently, inhibitors of specific tyrosine kinases were identified. The naturally occurring compound erbstatin was among the earliest of such molecules to be examined and found to inhibit the growth of human tumor cells in culture. Erbstatin is a competitive inhibitor of the epidermal growth receptor tyrosine kinase and can retard tumor growth in vivo.

Structurally related inhibitors, tyrphostins, whose activity is similar to that of erbstatin, have been organically synthesized. Tyrphostins are important lead compounds because they have unique structural features that may be manipulated to achieve increased specificity and decreased toxicity. In this regard, the identification of inhibitors that appear to be highly specific for the epidermal growth factor receptor tyrosine kinase has suggested that sufficient structural diversity exists between the different tyrosine kinases to allow the identification of receptor specific inhibitors. To date, herbimycin A, a compound that is structurally related to erbstatin, has been among the most extensively characterized of these agents. It is able to retard the growth of experimental animal tumors in vivo, but its evaluation has not yet reached clinical trials.[44]

Protein serine-threonine kinases also play central roles in the cellular response to many growth regulators [*see Chapter 5*]. In some cells, the predominant activity of these kinases is to mediate proliferation, whereas in others, the kinases are activated during differentiation and in association with growth arrest. One such kinase that is likely to be of particular importance for growth is protein kinase C.[45] Numerous inhibitors of protein kinase C are known, and these can have antineoplastic activities when examined in vivo. One such compound, bryostatin 1, has entered clinical evaluation.[46] A less well-recognized inhibitor of protein kinase C that is already used clinically is tamoxifen. Tamoxifen is an antiestrogen with several different biologic activities, but its inhibition of protein kinase C may well be an important mechanism of its antineoplastic activity.[47]

Antisense Oligonucleotides as Drugs Consistent with the emerging recognition of the key role played by mutated oncogenes and tumor suppressor genes in the development of cancer has been an interest in therapeutic strategies by which these genetic alterations might be "repaired." Systemically administered molecules that specifically target mutated nucleic acids that cause malignant tumor growth have been sought for nearly a decade. Molecules such as highly specific nucleases and proteases may someday become drugs that carry in their primary structure the basis for targeted therapeutic activities. In addition, ribozymes, which can degrade specific RNA molecules and might thereby suppress oncogene expression, may eventually have a role in cancer therapy.[48] At the present time, however, the best known and most extensively characterized agents belonging to this group of "smart" drugs are antisense oligonucleotides.[49]

Antisense oligonucleotides are nucleic acids whose nucleotide sequence is complementary to a known DNA or RNA sequence. The use of antisense oligonucleotides that correspond to genes whose expression is thought to be deleterious to the cell is being pursued as an antineoplastic therapy. The goal of such therapy is to diminish the effective expression of the targeted gene. Although in many cases, the precise mechanism by which such inhibition occurs is unknown, hybridization arrest of translation, inhibition of the splicing of nuclear RNA species into mature mRNA molecules, and ribonuclease (RNase) H enzyme–mediated intracellular RNA degradation have all been demonstrated to be potential contributors to the decreased gene expression caused by antisense oligonucleotides. For such a therapeutic strategy to be effective, the antisense oligodeoxynucleotides must hybridize efficiently to target sequences under conditions that would be encountered in vivo; that is, the association constant of the nucleic acid heteroduplex at body temperature should be favorable, and the complexes should be stable. The antisense nucleotides must also be chemically resistant to nucleases they would encounter after they are administered to a patient. To minimize such degradation, various modifications of oligodeoxynucleotide structure have been examined; these analysis revealed that phosphorothioate oligonucleotide analogues have an increased resistance to nuclease degradation and hybridize to target sequences with only a slightly reduced affinity compared with that of prototypic phosphodiester oligodeoxynucleotides. Other enhancements to this gene-targeting strategy have included efforts to design oligonucleotides that form triple helices with genomic DNA and to conjugate antisense oligonucleotides to antineoplastic agents in order to target them to DNA.

The enthusiasm for this approach to cancer treatment arises both from its potential for specificity and from the results of laboratory studies suggesting that antisense oligodeoxynucleotides added exogenously to cultures can alter gene expression.[49] In such experiments, it was possible to diminish the malignant properties of tumor cells as well as inhibit their tumorigenicity when they were reinoculated back into appropriate animal hosts.[50] It was also possible to inhibit the in vivo expression of a recombinant *myc* gene in B cells of mice treated with antisense oligonucleotides directed against C-*myc*.[51] In addition, infusion of phosphorothioate-modified antisense oligonucleotides that target C-*myb* suppresses the growth of human melanoma and human leukemia xenografts in mice. Interestingly, these antisense molecules seem to have a differential effect on normal versus leukemic hematopoietic cells, although the physiologic mechanisms underlying these differences are not understood.[52] On the basis of these studies, comparable C-*myb* antisense oligonucleotides are being used in clinical trials as infusions for treating patients with chronic myelogenous leukemia in blast crisis. To inhibit the pathogenic effects of mutated *p53*, phosphorothioate oligonucleotides complementary to *p53* mRNA are also being evaluated in clinical trials for the treatment of leukemia.[53] The critical evaluation of antisense strategies for cancer treatment, however, will require additional information regarding the molecular requirements for the successful targeting of oligonucleotides. Furthermore, it will be necessary to develop the means to more easily synthesize large quantities of antisense molecules that are sufficiently stable in vivo so that they can be tested as therapeutic agents both in additional animal models and in humans.

NOVEL TREATMENT STRATEGIES

Antiangiogenesis   Once tumor cell growth can no longer be supported by the diffusion of nutriments, neoangiogenesis is required.[54] Angiogenesis is also a particularly critical step in the establishment of metastases because the development of a vasculature is required for the growth of metastatic tumor foci. The induction and support of blood vessel growth is a complex process that involves molecules produced in normal and neoplastic tissue, both host and tumor-derived molecules, including soluble, angiogenic mitogens and extracellular matrix proteins that must be present in the microenvironment of the tumor [*see Chapter 2*]. Basic fibroblast growth factor, vascular endothelial growth factor, platelet-derived endothelial growth factor, angiogenin, and several of their cognate receptors have been implicated in the regulation of tumor vessel induction, as has the integrin v3, a receptor for vitronectin, fibronectin, and other components of the extracellular matrix found in many tumor types. Antiangiogenic treatment strategies can be expected to result in the suppression of metastases and the prolongation of disease-free remissions induced by other modalities of therapy. Recent evidence indicating that tumor vasculature may "turn over" suggests that antiangiogenic treatment strategies may also be useful in the management of established tumor masses. Although such goals would require long-term treatment, the accessibility of endothelial cell targets via the circulation and the normal genetic characteristics of endothelial cells that make the development of resistance unlikely enhance the appeal of these strategies.

Antiangiogenic agents that have been proposed for the prevention of tumor growth may also inhibit the formation of metastases. Some such agents are physiologic inhibitors of angiogenesis, such as interferon alfa, platelet factor 4, and angiostatin. Angiostatin is a plasminogen fragment that is present in the circulation of tumor-bearing mice and can be isolated from their urine. Angiostatin inhibits endothelial cell proliferation in numerous models and inhibits metastatic growth in mouse models. Other antiangiogenic strategies are targeted to interrupt the activity of known mediators of tumor neoangiogenesis. For example, it may be possible to use soluble receptors for specific endothelial growth factors to bind the ligand and inhibit its mitogenic activity.[55] In another antiangiogenic strategy, gene transfer has been used to inhibit tumor growth in an animal model. In these experiments, retroviruses encoding an inhibiting (dominant-negative) mutant of the vascular endothelial growth factor receptor Flk-1, which is widely expressed in many tumor types, prevented tumor growth in a mouse brain tumor model by inhibiting angiogenesis.[56] Many drugs with known antiangiogenic activities are currently being examined in early clinical trials, and additional, rationally designed interventions will soon follow.

Inhibition of Tumor Cell Invasion   A key pathological characteristic of malignancy is the movement of tumor cells across physiologic boundaries that compartmentalize different tissue components [*see Chapter 8*]. Tumor invasion of normal tissue enhances tumor growth, disrupts normal tissue function, and most importantly is a necessary prelude to metastatic tumor spread. Cells acquire invasive characteristics during the course of their progression to malignancy [*see Chapter 8*]. Invasion is an active, complex process that requires not only tumor cell mobility but also the production of proteases that can digest the extracellular components of the particular tissue type in which a tumor arises. Presumably, the acquisition of these malignant characteristics is the result of tumor cells' expressing a novel "genetic program," rather than the result of specific structural genetic changes in the genes that encode the molecules critical for these processes. Nonetheless, proteases produced by tumor cells, extracellular matrix molecules, and receptors that mediate cell migration provide important targets for the development of novel therapeutics for the inhibition of invasion.

The invasive characteristics of tumor cells are closely correlated with their production of proteases, which may belong to any of the known protease families. Tumor cell production of serine, aspartate, cysteine, and metalloproteinases has been widely documented in many of the common human tumors, but the most extensively studied proteases are the matrix metalloproteinases. Although several different classes of metalloproteinases have been described in tumor cells, they are all inhibited by a family of endogenously occurring inhibitors, tissue inhibitors of metalloproteinase (TIMPs). TIMPs are prototypes for drugs that inhibit metalloproteinases because these enzymes can mediate invasion in many experimental models. Small peptides that mimic the action of TIMPs can also inhibit invasion of tumor cells in an in vitro invasion model,[57] and synthetic compounds that compete for the active site of various metalloproteinases have been examined in animals and found to inhibit tissue invasion by various tumor cell lines.

Another strategy for inhibiting the invasion of normal tissues by tumor cells is the development of synthetic collagen substrate analogues, which presumably bind to the active site of various metalloproteinases. A prototype drug, BB94, has been found to reduce the incidence of metastases in ovarian[58] and colon[59] cancer xenograft models; this difference was associated with prolonged survival of the animals in the treatment group. Although such agents are not yet in clinical trials, these studies provide evidence for the potential importance of anti-invasive therapeutic strategies in the treatment of cancer.

Gene Therapy Strategies   Gene therapy distinguishes itself as a novel modality of cancer therapy in that it involves the therapeutic transfer of new genetic material.[60] The focus of such efforts in cancer medicine has been on somatic cells, both normal cells (e.g., hematopoietic stem cells) and tumor cells, which, even when genetically modified, are not passed on to the patient's offspring. Numerous technologies are currently available for gene transfer, but gene therapy for cancer typically requires efficient transfer strategies.[61] For this reason, most attention has been placed on the use of viral vectors, especially retroviral vectors. Recombinant viral genomes can now be routinely engineered to contain foreign genes that are stably integrated into the host cell genome after infection.[62] Such recombinant viral genomes can be incorporated into retroviral virions after they pass through "packaging cell lines," which produce infectious but replication-defective recombinant viruses that are incapable of further viral propagation beyond the cells they infect. Comparable strategies have been used for the preparation of recombinant adenoviruses.

Recombinant retroviruses result in typical infection efficiencies of approximately 50 percent in tissue culture and less than 10 percent in vivo. Adenoviral vectors have higher transfer efficiencies, but even these are unlikely to be sufficient for cancer gene therapy if the infection of every individual tumor cell is required. Other delivery strategies involving the administration of foreign genes encapsulated in liposomes or some other vehicle that facilitates uptake into the cell (while protecting the administered DNA from nucleases) are similarly inefficient in vivo. These difficulties associated with gene transfer have led to a focus on gene therapy strategies that do not require uniquely efficient in situ transfer of genes to the cells of a tumor. Current strategies typically involve the in vitro transfer of genes to autologous cells from cancer patients, which are then transferred back to the patient.

Several gene therapy strategies currently being pursued reflect our improved understanding of tumor biology. Among these strategies are attempts to enhance the immunogenicity of tumor cells by transferring to them genes that encode cytokines that might be expected to enhance tumor cell antigenicity, enhance the efficacy of host killing by cytotoxic lymphocytes and antibodies, and even alter the malignant behavior of the tumor cells themselves.[63,64] Most commonly, tumor tissue is surgically removed, a cytokine gene is transferred to tumor cells, and these cells are reinjected into the patient, usually after being sufficiently irradiated to block further tumor cell replication. The use of such vaccination strategies in animal models has led to the immune-mediated destruction of tumor cells,[65,66] and several gene therapy trials are currently underway in which tumor cells transfected with one of several different cytokine genes are being used to vaccinate patients with many different tumor types. Recent data have suggested that granulocyte-macrophage colony-stimulating factor will be a cytokine of particular efficacy for such trials because it may be particularly active in enhancing the immunogenicity of tumor cell vaccines.[66] Related strategies involve attempts to enhance tumor immunogenicity by transferring into tumor cells genes that encode major histocompatibility antigens, the B7 accessory antigen, or β_2-microglobulin.

Gene therapy offers other novel possibilities for the development of tumor vaccines. Virus infections are associated with several different human tumors. Viral genes are retained by tumor cells because they are critical for maintenance of malignant cell characteristics and therefore have important potential as tumor-specific antigens. In the case of HPV, which is associated with human genital tract cancer, laboratory experiments have indicated that the transforming potential rests within the viral genes known as *E6* and *E7*. Mouse fibroblasts transfected with a recombinant gene expressing the *E7* encoded protein can immunize mice against the development of tumors after their inoculation with *E7* transformed syngeneic cells.

These findings suggest that tumor-associated viral antigens expressed by such common human tumors as cervical carcinoma (HPV antigens) and hepatoma (hepatitis B virus antigens) might be used as tumor vaccines for protection against the development of certain tumors and perhaps even as an adjuvant to other therapies. Although it is unclear whether the use of oncofetal and other so-called tumor-associated antigens as immunogens will be compromised by unexpected toxicities or diminished antigenicity, viral proteins and gene products encoded uniquely by tumor cells as a result of the genetic rearrangements offer realistic options for vaccine development.

It may also be possible to modify the host immune response to tumors by modifying ex vivo the genome of harvested immune cells that mediate tumor cell killing and then returning these cells to the patient. Because of their tumor-homing potential, TILs (tumor-infiltrating lymphocytes) and NK cells offer a unique vehicle for the mediation of such therapy. Stably modifying the genome of TILs to express exogenously introduced genes may enhance their antitumor activity. TILs modified to carry the *TNF* gene secrete this cytotoxic cytokine at higher levels than can be otherwise achieved. Autologous TILs modified to express *TNF* are being used in an ongoing gene therapy clinical trial attempting to increase the local tumor concentration of this antitumor agent.[67] Such an experiment heralds future approaches in which TILs may be further modified both to enhance their antitumor activities and to facilitate their maintenance and expansion after reinfusion.

Several other distinctive therapeutic approaches using gene therapy for cancer treatment are also being explored. One such strategy is directed at modifying host tolerance for therapy.[68] Considerable evidence suggests that dose intensification of conventional cytotoxic agents may improve the outcome of selected patients with either hematopoietic or solid tissue tumors. Gene therapy may provide an important new opportunity for the administration of doses of conventional antineoplastic agents that are currently too toxic for normal tissues, especially bone marrow. The most straightforward of these approaches involves the transfer of drug-resistance genes to tissues in which the dose-limiting toxicity to commonly used chemotherapeutic agents is first seen [*see Figure 4*]. For example, transfer of the gene that encodes resistance to numerous antineoplastic drugs, the *mdr* gene, to bone marrow hematopoietic precursor cells may make it feasible to administer higher doses of therapy than are currently possible,[69] and this strategy is now being explored in clinical trials. Additionally, several other antineoplastic agents exist for which resistance can be conferred by the activation of even a single gene. For example, dihydrofolate reductase should enhance cellular resistance to methotrexate, topoisomerase mutants may increase resistance to etoposide, and aldehyde dehydrogenase can protect cells from cyclophosphamide. Such genes are candidates for providing normal tissue protection from the toxicities of these agents.

Another novel strategy that uses gene transfer for the treatment of tumors is known as viral-directed enzyme prodrug therapy.[70] This strategy effectively eliminates several different types of experimental tumors,[71] including

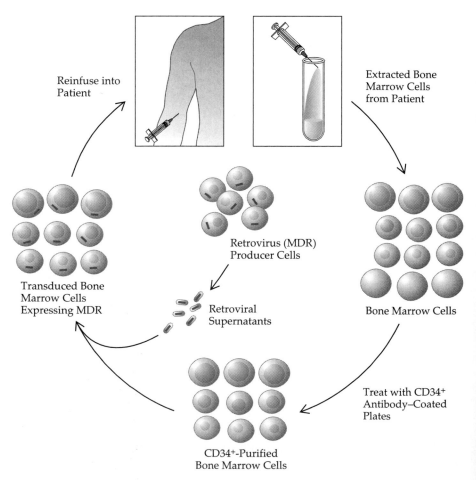

Figure 4 *A gene therapy protocol in which the* mdr *gene that encodes a protein conferring resistance to many chemotherapeutic agents is transferred in vitro into cytokine-treated CD34+ bone marrow precursors. Cells from this patient were infected with a recombinant retrovirus carrying the* mdr *gene (mdr sup) and reinfused into the patient before high-dose antineoplastic therapy was administered. Bone marrow anaplasia is an important side effect that limits the dose of chemotherapy that patients can receive. Enhancing the resistance of bone marrow stem cells to chemotherapy is one method of increasing the amount of chemotherapy that can be administered.*

Reinfuse into Patient

Extracted Bone Marrow Cells from Patient

Retrovirus (MDR) Producer Cells

Transduced Bone Marrow Cells Expressing MDR

Retroviral Supernatants

Bone Marrow Cells

CD34+-Purified Bone Marrow Cells

Treat with CD34+ Antibody–Coated Plates

brain tumors in rodent models.[72] The basis of this approach is straightforward: a viral gene encoding an enzyme that converts an inactive prodrug into a therapeutically active metabolite is transferred selectively into tumor cells, and the prodrug is systemically administered to the patient. This enzyme then mediates a cytotoxic effect in the infected cell. To date, retroviruses have been the vector of choice for such gene therapy. A key feature of this therapy is that the integration of retroviral vector–mediated gene transfers requires dividing cells,[73] and tumor cells tend to be the most actively dividing cells in the area to which such therapies (either retroviruses or retrovirus-producing mouse cells) are locally applied. The most extensively studied viral-directed enzyme prodrug therapy has used a recombinant retrovirus vector into which the gene encoding the enzyme thymidine kinase from the herpes simplex virus (*HSV-tk*) has been inserted. After retroviral vector infection of a tumor cell, the *HSV-tk* gene is incorporated into the host cell genome. The thymidine kinase of mammalian cells does not have a high affinity for certain nucleoside analogues, such as the antiviral drug ganciclovir, that the *HSV-tk* gene avidly phosphorylates. These phosphorylated analogues are then incorporated into the cellular genome during DNA replication, leading to tumor cell death. Because ganciclovir is not a substrate for the mammalian thymidine kinase, this drug does not harm normal cells when it is given in therapeutic doses.

Although it is rarely possible to transfer such genes to even 10 percent of tumor cells, in some tumor models, cell death after infection with the *HSV-tk*–containing retrovirus and treatment with ganciclovir far exceeds the number of cells that express the *HSV-tk* gene. This phenomenon is referred to as the "bystander effect," which is likely to be mediated largely by the intercellular transfer of phosphorylated ganciclovir metabolites through gap junctions formed between cells that express *HSV-tk* and uninfected tumor cells.[74] No evidence of toxicity to the normal brain in animals treated for brain tumors with this gene therapy has been reported, suggesting that the bystander effect, like the gene transfer, is tumor specific. At the present time, such a treatment approach is being evaluated in several clinical trials for the treatment of brain tumors, and a second such prodrug approach, in which the cytosine deaminase gene is used to convert 5-fluorocytosine to 5-fluorouracil, is being examined in preclinical models.

Lastly, attempts are underway to use gene therapy as a strategy to replace tumor suppressor genes that have been inactivated during the formation of a specific tumor type. The major impediment to transduce gene therapies is the inability of current gene transfer strategies to transduce a high percentage of tumor cells in vivo, although vectors derived from adenovirus and liposome-mediated gene transfer may eliminate this problem in the future.

Conclusion

Our emerging knowledge of the pathogenesis of human cancer has provided unique opportunities for the prevention and improved treatment of cancer. In both of these important areas of intervention, the first opportunity for improvement lies in earlier and more accurate diagnosis. When factors contributing to the development of specific tumors are clearly definable, such as papillomaviruses in reproductive tract cancers, a conceptual framework exists in which prevention strategies that are more effective than avoidance can be organized. In other tumors, genetic alterations of etiologic significance can be the targets of prevention efforts.

Enthusiasm for the possibility of devising better cancer therapies rests largely in the belief that such therapies will be directed at tumor-specific alterations and, therefore, be both more effective and less toxic than currently available therapeutic agents. At the present time, the most likely targets for such therapy include activated proto-oncogenes and inactivated tumor suppressor genes. In some cases, it may be possible to target the altered genes themselves. Progress in this area is being made but is stymied by our inability to recognize homogeneous disorders among human tumors. The most common finding in the evaluation of many different specimens from most tumor types is that only a fraction of individual tumor specimens have evidence of any particular genetic alteration that we consider to be of likely etiologic significance. This observation is true among virtually all tumors of any solid tissue, even when such tumors are grouped by important pathological characteristics, such as grade or cell type of origin. Genetic instability and continuous genetic evolution of a tumor may be an inherent aspect of its pathology. Despite this complexity, efforts to build on our understanding of tumor pathogenesis have led to novel undertakings that have resulted in the emergence of important new diagnostic opportunities. More recently, novel therapeutic strategies have emerged that reflect our improved understanding of pathogenesis, and these promise to add significantly to the current clinical armamentarium. Continued therapeutic improvement will require a clearer understanding of the targets of therapy, and defining those targets for specific tumors is an important goal for cancer research.

References

1. Tobi M, Luo FC, Ronai Z: Detection of K-ras mutation in colonic effluent samples from patients without evidence of colorectal carcinoma. *J Natl Cancer Inst* 86:1007, 1994
2. Housman D: Molecular medicine, human DNA polymorphism. *N Engl J Med* 332:318, 1995
3. Cavenee WK, Murphree AL, Shull MM, et al: Prediction of familial predisposition to retinoblastoma. *N Engl J Med* 314:1201, 1986
4. Vail-Smith K, White DM: Risk level, knowledge, and preventive behavior for human papillomaviruses among sexually active college women. *J Am Coll Health* 40:227, 1992
5. Kurman RJ, Henson DE, Herbst Al, et al: Interim guidelines for management of abnormal cervical cytology. *JAMA* 271:1866, 1994
6. Chambers MA, Wei Z, Coleman N, et al: "Natural" presentation of human papillomavavirus type-16 E7 protein to immunocompetent mice results in antigen-specific sensitization or sustained unresponsiveness. *Eur J Immunol* 24:738, 1994
7. National Advisory Council for Human Genome Research: Statement on use of DNA testing for presymptomatic identification of cancer risk. *JAMA* 271:785, 1994
8. Harris NL: Pathology of malignant lymphomas. *Curr Opin Oncol* 3:813, 1991
9. Gauwerky CE, Croce CM: Chromosomal translocations in leukaemia. *Semin Cancer Biol* 4:333, 1993
10. Thiele CJ, McKeon C, Triche TJ, et al: Differential proto-oncogene expression characterizes histopathologically indistinguishable tumors of the peripheral nervous system. *J Clin Invest* 80:804, 1987

11. Thirman MJ, Gill HJ, Burnett RC, et al: Rearrangement of the *MLL* gene in acute lymphoblastic and acute myeloid leukemias with 11q23 chromosomal translocations. *N Engl J Med* 329:909, 1993

12. Pui C-H, Crist WM: Cytogenetic abnormalities in childhood acute lymphoblastic leukemia correlates with clinical features and treatment outcome. *Leuk Lymphoma* 7:259, 1992

13. Seeger RC, Brodeur GM, Sather H, et al: Association of multiple copies of the n-myc oncogene with rapid progression of neuroblastomas. *N Engl J Med* 313:1111, 1985

14. Hynes NE: Amplification and overexpression of the erbB-2 gene in human tumors: its involvement in tumor development, significance as a prognostic factor, and potential as a target for cancer therapy. *Semin Cancer Biol* 4:19, 1993

15. Paik S, Hazan R, Fisher E, et al: Pathologic findings from the national surgical adjuvant breast and bowel project: prognostic significance of erbB-2 protein overexpression in primary breast cancer. *J Clin Oncol* 8:103, 1990

16. Kandl H, Seymour L, Bezwoda WR, et al: Soluble c-erbB-2 fragment in serum correlates with disease stage and predicts for shortened survival in patients with early-stage and advanced breast cancer. *Br J Cancer* 70:739, 1994

17. Reist CJ, Archer GE, Kurpad SN, et al: Tumor-specific anti-epidermal growth factor receptor variant III monoclonal antibodies: use of the tyramine-cellobiose radioiodination method enhances cellular retention and uptake in tumor xenografts. *Cancer Res* 55:4375, 1995

18. Hu E, Trela M, Thompson J, et al: Detection of B cell lymphoma in peripheral blood by DNA hybridization. *Lancet* 2:1092, 1985

19. Ngan BY, Nourse J, Cleary ML: Detection of chromosomal translocation t(14;18) within the minor cluster region of bcl-2 by polymerase chain reaction and direct genomic sequencing of the enzymatically amplified DNA in follicular lymphomas. *Blood* 73:1759, 1989

20. Sidransky D, Boyle J, Koch W: Molecular screening: prospects for a new approach. *Arch Otolaryngol Head Neck Surg* 119:1187, 1993

21. Gribben JG, Neuberg D, Freedman AS, et al: Detection by polymerase chain reaction of residual cells with the bcl-2 translocation is associated with increased risk of relapse after autologous bone marrow transplantation for B-cell lymphoma. *Blood* 81:3449, 1993

22. Larson SM, Schwartz LH: Advances in imaging. *Semin Oncol* 21:598, 1994

23. Allan SM, Dean C, Fernando I, et al: Radioimmunolocalisation in breast cancer using the gene product of c-erbB2. *Br J Cancer* 67:706, 1993

24. Katoh Y, Nakata K, Kohno K, et al: Immunoscintigraphy of human tumors transplanted in nude mice with radiolabeled anti-ras p21 monoclonal antibodies. *J Nucl Med* 31:1520, 1990

25. Martin EW, Mojzisik CM, Hinkle GH, et al: Radioimmunoguided surgery: a new approach to the intraoperative detection of tumor using monoclonal antibody B72.3. *Am J Surg* 156:386, 1988

26. Itri LM: The interferons. *Cancer* 70:940, 1992

27. Fraker DL, Alexander HR: Isolated limb perfusion with high-dose tumor necrosis factor for extremity melanoma and sarcoma. *Important Adv Oncol* 1994:179

28. Rosenburg SA: Karnofsky Memorial Lecture: the immunotherapy and gene therapy of cancer. *J Clin Oncol* 10:180, 1992

29. Leary AG, Ikebuchi K, Hirai Y, et al: Synergism between interleukin-6 and interleukin-3 in supporting proliferation of human hematopoietic stem cells. *Blood* 71:1759, 1988

30. Reed E: The use of colony-stimulating factors as bone marrow support for systemic anti-cancer chemotherapy. *J Natl Med Assoc* 86:459, 1994

31. Schick BP: Hope for treatment of thrombocytopenia. *N Engl J Med* 331:875, 1994

32. de The H, Lavau C, Marchio A, et al: The PML-RAR-alpha fusion mRNA generated by the 5(15;17) translocation in acute promyelocytic leukemia encodes a functionally altered RAR. *Cell* 66:675, 1991

33. Sun GL, Ouyang RR, Chen SJ, et al: Treatment of acute promyelocytic leukemia with all-trans retinoic acid: a five-year experience. *Chin Med J* 106:743, 1993

34. Warrell RP Jr, Frankel SR, Miller WH Jr: Differentiation therapy of acute promyelocytic leukemia with tretinoin (all-trans-retinoic acid). *N Engl J Med* 324:1385, 1991

35. Larson SM, Macapinlac HA, Scott AM, et al: Recent achievements in the development of radiolabeled monoclonal antibodies for diagnosis, therapy and biologic characterization of human tumors. *Acta Oncol* 32:709, 1993

36. Miller RA, Maloney DG, Warnke R: Treatment of B cell lymphoma with monoclonal

anti-idiotype antibody. *N Engl J Med* 306:517, 1982

37. Theuer CP, Pastan I: Immunotoxins and recombinant toxins in the treatment of solid carcinomas. *Am J Surg* 166:284, 1993

38. Winter G, Milstein C: Man-made antibodies. *Nature* 349:293, 1991

39. Marks JD, Hoogenboon HR, Bonnert TP, et al: By-passing immunization: human antibodies from V-gene libraries displayed on phage. *J Mol Biol* 222:581, 1991

40. Barbacid M: Ras genes. *Annu Rev Biochem* 56:779, 1987

41. Willumsen BM, Norris L, Papageorge AG, et al: Harvey murine sarcoma virus p21 ras protein: biological and biochemical significance of the cysteine nearest the carboxy terminus. *EMBO J* 3:2581, 1984

42. Kohl NE, Wilson FR, Mosser SD, et al: A. Protein farnesyltransferase inhibitors block the growth of ras-dependent tumors in nude mice. *Proc Natl Acad Sci USA* 91:9141, 1994

43. Gibbs JB, Oliff A, Kohl NE: Farnesyltransferase inhibitors: ras research yields a potential cancer therapeutic. *Cell* 77:175, 1994

44. Okabe M, Uehara Y, Noshima T, et al: In vivo antitumor activity of herbimycin A, a tyrosine kinase inhibitor, targeted against BCR/ABL oncoprotein in mice bearing BCR/ABL-transfected cells. *Leuk Res* 18:867, 1994

45. Basu A: The potential of protein kinase C as a target for anticancer treatment. *Pharmacol Ther* 59:257, 1993

46. Prendiville J, Crowther D, Thatcher N, et al: A phase I study of intravenous bryostatin 1 in patients with advanced cancer. *Br J Cancer* 68:418, 1993

47. Colletta AA, Benson JR, Baum M: Alternative mechanisms of action of anti-estrogens. *Breast Cancer Res Treat* 31:5, 1994

48. Kashani-Sabet M, Funato T, Florenes VA, et al: Suppression of the neoplastic phenotype in vivo by an anti-ras ribozyme. *Cancer Res* 54:900, 1994

49. Wagner RF: Gene inhibition using antisense oligodeoxynucleotides. *Nature* 372:333, 1994

50. Cotter FE, Johnson P, Hall P, et al: Antisense oligonucleotides suppress B-cell lymphoma growth in a SCID-hu mouse model. *Oncogene* 9:3049, 1994

51. Wickstrom E, Bacon TA, Wickstrom EL: Down-regulation of c-MYC antigen expression in lymphocytes of Emu-c-myc transgenic mice treated with anti-c-myc DNA methylphosphonates. *Cancer Res* 52:6741, 1992

52. Calabretta B, Sims RB, Valtieri M, et al: Normal and leukemic hematopoietic cells manifest differential sensitivity to inhibitory effects of c-myb antisense oligodeoxynucleotides: an in vitro study relevant to bone marrow purging. *Proc Natl Acad Sci USA* 88:2351, 1991

53. Bayever E, Iversen PL, Bishop MR, et al: Systemic administration of a phosphorothioate oligonucleotide with a sequence complementary to p53 for acute myelogenous leukemia and myelodysplastic syndrome: initial results of a phase I trial. *Antisense Res Dev* 3:383, 1993

54. Folkman J: The role of angiogenesis in tumor growth. *Semin Cancer Biol* 3:65, 1992

55. Kendall RL, Thomas KA: Inhibition of vascular endothelial cell growth factor activity by an endogenously encoded soluble receptor. *Proc Natl Acad Sci USA* 90:10705, 1993

56. Millauer B, Shawver LK, Plate KH, et al: Glioblastoma growth inhibited in vivo by a dominant-negative Flk-1 mutant. *Nature* 367:576, 1994

57. Melchiori A, Albini A, Ray JM, et al: Inhibition of tumor cell invasion by a highly conserved peptide sequence form the matrix metalloproteinase enzyme prosegment. *Cancer Res* 52:2353, 1992

58. Davies KB, Brown PD, East N, et al: A synthetic matrix metalloproteinase inhibitor decreases tumor burden and prolongs survival of mice bearing human ovarian carcinoma xenografts. *Cancer Res* 53:2087, 1993

59. Wang X, Fu X, Brown PD, et al: Matrix metalloproteinase inhibitor BB-94 (Batismastat) inhibits human colon tumor growth and spread in a patient-like orthotopic model in nude mice. *Cancer Res* 54:4726, 1994

60. Mulligan RC: The basic science of gene therapy. *Science* 260:926, 1993

61. Vile R, Russell SJ: Gene transfer technologies for the gene therapy of cancer. *Gene Therapy* 1:88, 1994

62. Miller AD, Rosman GJ: Improved retroviral vectors for gene transfer and expression. *Biotechniques* 7: 980, 1989

63. Tepper RI, Pattengal PK, Leder P, et al: Murine interleukin-4 displays potent anti-tumor activity in vivo. *Cell* 57:503, 1989

64. Watanabe Y, Kuribayashi K, Miyatake S, et al: Exogenous expression of mouse interferon gamma cDNA in mouse neuroblastoma C1300 cells: results in reduced tumorigenicity by augmented anti-tumor immunity. *Proc Natl Acad Sci USA* 86:9456, 1989

65. Sanda MG, Ayyagari SR, Jaffee EM, et al: Demonstration of a rational strategy for human prostate cancer gene therapy. *J Urol* 151:622, 1994

66. Dranoff G, Jaffee E, Lazenby A, et al: Vaccination with irradiated tumor cells engineered to secret murine granulocyte-macrophage colony-stimulating factor stimulates potent, specific, and long-lasting anti-tumor immunity. *Proc Natl Acad Sci USA* 90:3539, 1993

67. Rosenberg SA, Anderson WF, Blaese RM: The development of gene therapy for the treatment of cancer. *Ann Surg* 218:455, 1993

68. Gottesman MM, Germann UA, Akskentijevich I, et al: Gene transfer of drug resistance genes: implications for cancer therapy. *Ann NY Acad Sci* 716:126, 1994

69. Mickisch GH, Aksentijevich I, Schoenlein PV, et al: Transplantation of bone marrow cells from transgenic mice expressing the human MDR1 gene results in long-term protection against the myelosuppressive effect of chemotherapy in mice. *Blood* 79:1087, 1992

70. Moolten FL: Tumor chemosensitivity conferred by inserted herpes thymidine kinase genes: paradigm for a prospective cancer control strategy. *Cancer Res* 46:5276, 1986

71. Moolten FL, Wells JM: Curability of tumors bearing herpes thymidine kinase genes transferred by retroviral vectors. *J Natl Cancer Inst* 82:297:1990

72. Culver KW, Ram Z, Walbridge S, et al: In vivo gene transfer with retroviral vector-producer cells for treatment of experimental brain tumors. *Science* 256:1550, 1992

73. Miller DG, Adam MA, Miller AD: Gene transfer by retrovirus vectors occurs only in cells that are actively replicating at the time of infection. *Mol Cell Biol* 10:4239, 1990

74. Fick J, Barker FG II, Daxin P, et al: The extent of heterocellular communication mediated by gap junctions is predictive of bystander tumor cytotoxicity in vitro. *Proc Natl Acad Sci USA* 92:11071, 1995

Acknowledgments

Figures 1 and 2   Seward Hung.

Figure 3   Courtesy of Dr. S. M. Larson, Memorial Sloan-Kettering Cancer Center, New York, New York.

Figure 4   Seward Hung. Adapted from the protocol of Dr. A. Banks, Columbia University, New York, New York.

Index

A

Abelson murine leukemia virus
  abl gene, 64*t*
  transformation by
    of lymphoid cells, 22
    of rat embryo fibroblasts, 19*f*
Abortive transformation, 22
Adenomatous polyposis coli
  APC gene in, 130–131, 135*t*, 157, 161–163, 187, 189, 208*t*
  biomarkers for, 206–207
  clinical features of, 130
  epidemiology of, 130
  genetics of, 130
  molecular pathogenesis of, 188–189
  neoplastic pathology of, 208*t*
  prevention, early intervention in, 212
Adenovirus vector, for gene transfer in gene therapy, 230
Adenylate cyclase, 100, 101*f*
Aflatoxin and cancer, 45, 48, 48*t*
Agammaglobulinemia, 210*t*
AKT8 virus, *akt* gene, 64*t*
Alcohol and cancer, 48, 48*t*
Ames, Bruce, 6, 46, 48
Ames mutation test, 46–47, 47*f*
Amplicon, 145
Anaplasia, 33
Aneuploidy
  definition of, 24
  of tumor cells, 24
Angiogenesis
  cancer treatment directed against, 228–229
  definition of, 27
  tumor, 28, 29*f*, 37, 93–94, 196–201
Angiogenic factor(s)
  activity, 197, 197*f*
  secretion by tumor cells, 28, 29*f*, 37, 94, 197, 201
Angiogenic index, 198
Angiostatin, antitumor activity of, 229
Anogenital tumors, human papillomavirus

and, 210–211
Antiapoptosis protein, 148*t*, 193
Antigen(s)
  cell surface, monoclonal antibodies directed against, 223–224
Antigen receptors, 87*f*
Antineoplastic agents. *See* Drug(s)
Antioxidants, 48
Antisense oligonucleotides, in antineoplastic therapy, 227–228
Apoptosis, 31–32
  escape from, in carcinogenesis, 32, 191–194
  evolutionary conservation of, 32
  p53 gene product and, 125–126
  in tissue homeostasis, 32, 185–186
Arylhydrocarbon hydroxylase, 46
AS42 avian sarcoma virus, *maf* gene, 64*t*
Asbestos and cancer, 48*t*, 181
Astrocytomas
  mutant EGF receptors in, 95
  PDGF dimer and receptor expression in, 93–95
  VEGF-mediated neovascularization of, 94–95
Ataxia-telangiectasia, 210*t*
Autocrine signaling (stimulation), 26, 92
  and aberrant cell proliferation, 92, 191, 192*f*
  in tumorigenesis, 93–95, 191, 192*f*
Avian erythroblastosis virus
  erb-A gene, 64*t*
  erb-B gene, 64*t*
  erythroid cell transformation by, 22
Avian myeloblastosis virus
  erythroid cell transformation by, 22
  myb gene, 64*t*
Avian myelocytomatosis virus, erythroid cell transformation by, 22
Avian reticuloendotheliosis virus, *rel* gene, 64*t*
Avian sarcoma 17 virus, *jun* gene, 64*t*
Avian sarcoma 31 virus, *qin* gene, 64*t*
Avian SK77 virus, *ski* gene, 64*t*

D

Denys-Drash syndrome, 127–128
DHAP-1. *See* 4,5-Dianilinophthalimide
Diagnostic imaging, molecular genetics in, 219–221, 221*f*
4,5-Dianilinophthalimide, 104
Diet
  and cancer, 48
  in cancer prevention, 212
7,12-Dimethylbenz*[a]*anthracene, 43
DNA. *See also* Gene(s); Microsatellites; Molecular cloning
  alterations in cell proliferation, and cellular life span, 16
  amplification, in cancer cells, 25, 25*f*, 26, 69–70, 74–75
  damage
    versus biomarkers of cancer risk, 206
    and cell cycle arrest, 30*f*, 31
  repair
    defects, and carcinogenesis, 10, 25–26
    p53 gene protein product and, 125–126, 133
    tumor suppressor proteins and, 133–134
  replication
    checkpoint controls and, 30*f*, 31
    definition, 28
  as target for carcinogens, 5–7
DNA mismatch repair gene(s)
  *hMLH*1, 135*t*, 173, 189–190, 208*t*
  *hMSH*2, 133–134, 135*t*, 172–173, 189–190, 208*t*
  *hPMS*1, 135*t*, 173, 189–190
  *hPMS*2, 135*t*, 173, 189–190
  and human cancer, 143–144, 170–173
  inactivation, and tumor progression, 143–144
  mutations, and hereditary nonpolyposis colorectal cancer, 133–134, 171–173, 189–190
Dominant inheritance
  definition of, 54–55
  of familial cancer, 54–56
    genes affected in, 56–57
Double minute chromosome(s), 25, 25*f*, 69–70, 145
Down's syndrome, 209
Drug(s)
  antisense oligonucleotides as, 227–228
  development, strategies for, 225
  gene-targeted, 227–228
  host tolerance for, modification of, gene therapy for, 231–232
  novel, 225–228
    screening programs for, 225
  Ras inhibitors, 105
  toxicity to host, reduction of, gene therapy for, 231–232
  tyrosine kinase inhibitors, 104–105
Drug resistance. *See also* Multidrug resistance gene *mdr*
  in cancer cells, genetic basis for, 26, 37–38
Dysplasia
  cervical, human papillomavirus and, 210–212
  as precursor of neoplasia, 186–188, 187*f*, 188–189, 210–21

E

E26 avian erythroblastosis virus, *ets* gene, 64*t*
E-cadherin gene, 170
Elongin complex, 132–133
Endocrine signaling, 86, 94*f*
Endothelial cell growth, regulation by growth factor, 27
Epidemiology
  definition of, 206
  molecular, 206
  and multistep cancer pathogenesis, 180–181, 181*f*
Epidermal growth factor
  activity, 85
    interruption of, as antiangiogenic treatment strategy, 229
  in cell culture, and normal cell growth vs. transformed cell growth, 18*f*
  discovery of, 26
  functions of, 26
  receptors, 87*f*
    activation, 87–89, 88*f*
    oncogenic mutations in, 95
    overexpression, in human cancer, 96
    radiolabeled antibodies directed against, 224
Epithelial cell(s)
  adhesion-dependent growth, 15–16
  culture of, 15
  growth regulation by growth factor, 27
  transformation of, 15
Epstein-Barr virus, 4
  and human cancer, 49*t*, 50, 53, 211*t*
Erbstatin, 226
Erythroleukemia, retroviral oncogenes causing, 64*t*
Erythropoietin, 27
  in cancer treatment, 223
Estrogen and cancer, 45, 48, 48*t*
Ewing's sarcoma
  genetic alterations in, 154*t*, 216*t*
  and retinoblastoma, 119
Experimental oncology
  cell culture in, 13–16
  malignant transformation in, 16–20
Experimental tumor virology, 20–23
Extracellular matrix, in cell culture, 15–16

F

Familial adenomatous polyposis. *See* Adenomatous polyposis coli
Familial cancer, 9, 54–57. *See also* Retinoblastoma; Xeroderma pigmentosum
  cytogenetic studies of, 114, 119–120
  dominantly inherited, 54–56
    genes affected in, 56–57
  evidence for tumor suppressor genes in, 113–114
  genetic counseling in, 212–213
  genetics of, 54*f*, 54–55
  leukocyte karyotype analysis in, 114
  molecular pathogenesis of, 188–189
  recessively inherited, 54, 56
    genes affected in, 56–57
  susceptibility to cancer in, mode of inheritance, 54
Familial syndromes in which malignancy

Kirsten murine sarcoma virus, K-*ras* gene, 64*t*
Klinefelter's syndrome, 209
Knudson, Alfred, 55
Knudson hypothesis, 55–56, 119–121, 135.
See also Two-hit hypothesis
Koch, Robert, 3

L

Laminin binding, in tumor cell invasion, 199*f*
Leucine zipper, dimerization mediated by, 102
and oncogenic activation of *met* receptor tyrosine kinase, 96
Leukemia
acute lymphocytic
B cell, genetic alterations in, 151*t*, 215*t*
genetic alterations in, 151*t*–153*t*, 215*t*
molecular pathology of, 214*f*, 214–215, 215*t*
oncogenic alleles in, 148*t*
Philadelphia chromosome in, 97
pre-B cell, genetic alterations in, 148*t*, 151*t*–152*t*, 215*t*
T cell, genetic alterations in, 148*t*, 151*t*–152*t*, 215*t*
acute myelogenous, genetic alterations in, 153*t*
acute nonlymphocytic, genetic alterations in, 152*t*
acute promyelocytic, 87
genetic alterations in, 152*t*, 223
oncogenic alleles in, 148*t*
treatment, retinoic acid in, 223
acute undifferentiated, genetic alterations in, 153*t*
chromosomal translocations in, 74, 76, 150–155
chronic lymphocytic
B cell, genetic alterations in, 151*t*
molecular pathology of, 214*f*
T cell, genetic alterations in, 151*t*
chronic myelocytic, 6
chronic myelogenous
genetic alterations in, 152*t*–153*t*
oncogenic alleles in, 148*t*
Philadelphia chromosome in, 69, 97
treatment, C-*myb* antisense oligonucleotides in, 228
chronic myelomonocytic, genetic alterations in, 153*t*
deranged differentiation in, 34
juvenile myeloid, 99
molecular pathology of, 214*f*
myeloid
oncogenic alleles in, 148*t*
retroviral oncogenes causing, 64*t*
oncogenic alleles in, 148*t*
prolymphocytic, T cell, genetic alterations in, 151*t*
treatment, antisense oligonucleotides in, 228
Leukemia virus(es), 4
Leukocyte karyotype analysis, in familial cancer, 114
Levi-Montacini, Rita, 26
Life span, cellular, 16
established (immortalized) cell lines and, 16
Li-Fraumeni syndrome
neoplastic pathology of, 208*t*, 209

p53 gene and, 124–125, 135*t*, 159, 189, 208*t*, 209
Ligand(s), 27
radiolabeled, diagnostic imaging and, 220, 221*f*
Limonene, 226
Linkage analysis
in identification of tumor suppressor genes, 146
microsatellites in, 116
Liposarcoma, genetic alterations in, 154*t*
Liver cancer
hepatitis B virus and, 53
hepatitis C virus and, 53
LOH (loss of heterozygosity). *See* Heterozygosity, loss of
Lovastatin, mechanism of action, 226
Lung cancer
biomarkers for, 207
causes of, 3
epidemiology of, 42, 42*f*, 181
genetic alterations in, 216*t*
genetic susceptibility to, 46
loss of heterozygosity in, 118*t*
non–small cell, tumor suppressor gene alterations in, 169*t*
oncogene expression in, prognostic significance of, 217
oncogenic alleles in, 148*t*
small-cell
oncogenic alleles in, 148*t*
proto-oncogene in, 70
tumor suppressor gene alterations in, 168*t*
smoking and, 42, 42*f*, 181
Lymphoid tumor(s). *See also* Leukemia; Lymphoma(s)
B cell, treatment, monoclonal antibodies in, 224
corresponding to recognizable cell types during B cell ontogeny, 214*f*
genetic alterations in, 215*t*
molecular pathology of, 213–215, 214*f*, 215*t*
oncogene lesions in, 150, 151*t*
Lymphokines, functions of, 27
Lymphoma(s). *See also* Non-Hodgkin's lymphoma
B cell
genetic alterations in, 76, 151*t*–152*t*
oncogenic alleles in, 148*t*
chromosomal translocations in, 76, 150–155
cutaneous T cell, genetic alterations in, 215*t*
diffuse large-cell
genetic alterations in, 151*t*
molecular pathology of, 214*f*
diffuse small-cell, molecular pathology of, 214*f*
diffuse small cleaved cell, molecular pathology of, 214*f*
follicular
B cell, oncogenic alleles in, 148*t*
genetic alterations in, 148*t*, 151*t*, 214*f*
small cleaved cell, molecular pathology of, 214*f*
molecular pathology of, 214*f*
pre-B cell, retroviral oncogenes causing, 64*t*
T cell
genetic alterations in, 76, 153*t*
HTLV and, 54
retroviral oncogenes causing, 64*t*
Lynch syndrome II, 133–134

M

Macrophage colony-stimulating factor
 actions, 85
 receptors, 87f
  activation, 87–89, 88f
  oncogenic mutations in, 95
Malignant transformation. *See also*
Fibroblast(s), transformed
 applications to tumor biology, 16–20
 definition, 14, 16–17
 process leading to, 18–19
 by tumor viruses, 5
  viral DNA integration into cellular DNA in,
20–21
Mammary carcinoma virus, 4
Map protein kinase
 activation, 90f, 90–91
 activities, 90f, 90–91
 substrates, 90f, 90–91
Mast cell growth factor, 86
Mastectomy, prophylactic, 212–213
Max nuclear factor
 association with Mad, 102, 103f
 dimerization with Myc protein, 102, 103f
 homodimers, 102, 103f
 as transcriptional repressor, 102, 103f
MC29 avian myelocytomatosis virus, *myc*
gene, 64t
mdr gene. *See* Multidrug resistance gene(s),
mdr
Megacolon, congenital, 157
Mek protein kinase
 activation, 90–91
 as oncogene, 90–91
 Raf protein interaction with, 90, 90f
Melanoma
 genetic alterations in, 154t
 loss of heterozygosity in, 118t
 metastasis, molecular mechanisms of, 201
 tumor suppressor gene alterations in, 169t
MEN. *See* Multiple endocrine neoplasia
Meningioma
 loss of heterozygosity in, 118t
 tumor suppressor gene alterations in, 169t
Merlin, 132
Mesothelioma, epidemiology of, 181
Messenger RNA, 34
Metalloproteinase(s)
 inhibition of, as cancer treatment strategy,
229–230
 production by tumor cells, 229
 tissue inhibitors of, 229
Metastasis, 38, 199f, 200–201
 neuroblastoma, molecular pathology of,
215–216
 process of, 201
 and vascularization, 198, 198f
3-Methylcholanthrene, 43
 as carcinogen, 5
Microcell fusion, 113
Microsatellites
 in linkage analysis, 116
 replication errors in, and human cancer,
133–134, 171–172
Mill Hill-2 virus, *mil* gene, 64t
Mitosis. *See also* Cell cycle
 checkpoint controls and, 30f, 31–32
 definition, 28
Mitotic recombination, and mutational

inactivation of tumor suppressor genes, 115,
117f
Molecular biology
 and cancer prevention, 10–11
 and cancer treatment, 10–11
Molecular cloning, definition, 14
Molecular pathogenesis of cancer, 179–208
Molecular pathology, 213–216
 of hematopoietic tumors, 213–215, 214f,
215t
 prognostic significance of, 216–218
 of tumors arising in solid tissues, 215–216,
216t
Moloney murine sarcoma virus, *mos* gene, 64t
Monoclonal antibodies
 anti–epidermal growth factor receptor,
tumor-specific, in identification of tumor
xenografts, 218
 in cancer treatment, 223–225
 cytotoxic, in cancer treatment, 223–224
 immunogenicity, strategies for reducing, 224
 murine, in cancer treatment, 224
 production, advances in, 224–225
 radioiodinated, in intraoperative tumor
detection, 220–221
 radiolabeled
  in cancer treatment, 224
  diagnostic imaging and, 220, 221f
 tumor-specific, in imaging of tumor cells,
218
Monolayer, cell, definition of, 15
Mouse skin carcinogenesis model, 42–46,
181–182
 tumor induction in
  initiators and promoters in, 43–45, 44f, 57
  as multistep process, 43–45, 49, 181–182
  susceptibility factors, 46
Muller, H. J., 5
Multidrug resistance gene *mdr*
 *mdr*1, 26
 P-glycoprotein product p170, in imaging of
tumor xenografts, 220
 transfer to hematopoietic precursor cells, in
cancer treatment, 232, 232f
Multiple endocrine neoplasia
 gene mutations in, 71, 96–97, 208t
 loss of heterozygosity in, 118t
 ret mutations in, 157
 type I, 208t
 type II, 208t
Multiple mucosal neuroma syndrome, 208t
Multiple myeloma, molecular pathology of,
214f
Multistep model, of carcinogenesis, 43–45, 80,
179–180
 evidence for
  epidemiological, 180–181, 181f
  histopathological, 179–180
  from human tumors, 186–188, 187f
Murine leukemia virus infection, and
tumorigenesis, 184
3611 murine sarcoma virus, *raf* gene, 64t
Mutagen(s)
 Ames test for, 46–47, 47f
 carcinogens as, 5–7, 46–49, 57
  target genes for, 49
 initiators as, 43–45
 oxidants as, 48
Mutagenesis
 assays, 46–47, 47f, 48

transfection into rat embryo fibroblasts, 182, 182*f*

N-*myc*
  amplification of, 102, 155–156
  authentication of, 72
  in human cancer, 148*t*, 155–156
  identification of, 70
N-*ras*
  chromosomal location of, 147
  discovery of, 71
  mutations of, 147–148, 148*t*
  number of, 72
  pathophysiology of, 77–80
  as precursors of cancer genes, 65, 65*f*
  properties of, 111, 112*t*
  protein products, 111
  abnormalities, due to insertion of retroviral DNA, 67–68, 68*f*, 73
    functions of, 121
    serum and urine assays for, 207
  qin, 64*t*
  raf, 64*t*
    structural alterations, 79
  ras family of, 8
    collaboration with other genes, in tumorigenesis, 182, 182*f*, 183–185
    in human cancer, 71, 75, 129, 147–149, 187, 187*f*
    point mutations, 75, 76*f*, 76–77, 79, 99–100, 147–149, 148*t*, 149*f*
    transfection assays for, 71
    transfection into rat embryo fibroblasts, 182, 182*f*
    transformation of NIH3T3 cells, 182
  rel, 64*t*
  ret
    activation by point mutations, 75–76, 79
    discovery of, 75
    in heritable endocrine cancer, 71, 76, 96, 111, 147, 156–157, 208*t*
    in human cancer, 75, 147, 156–157
    retroviral, 7, 61
  RNA production by, increase in, by insertion of retroviral DNA, 67–68, 68*f*
  ros, 64*t*
  sea, 64*t*
  sis, 64*t*
  ski, 64*t*
  structural alterations, 78–79
  tissue specificity of, 72
  transduction of, 7
    retroviral, 61, 73*f*, 73–74
    into retroviruses, 65*f*, 65–66
  transforming activity, transfection assay for, 70*f*, 70–71
  trk, in human cancer, 148*t*
  ttg, in human cancer, 148*t*
  in tumor virology, 20
  Wnt-1, in chromosomal translocation studies, 68*f*
  yes, 64*t*
Provirus
  definition, 21
  integration into cellular DNA, 20–21, 66
PTK receptors. *See* Receptor protein-tyrosine kinase

Q

Quiescent cells, 17, 103

R

Radiation
  ionizing, as carcinogen, 3, 23
  ultraviolet, as carcinogen, 3, 23, 45, 48
Radiolabeling
  diagnostic imaging and, 220, 221*f*
  of monoclonal antibodies, 224
Raf protein
  interaction with Mek protein kinase, 90, 90*f*
  interaction with Ras, 89
  as oncogene, 90–91
Ramón y Cajal, Santiago, 14
rasGAP. *See* GTPase-activating proteins (GAPs)
Ras inhibitors, and cancer treatment, 105
Ras protein(s)
  activation of, 89–90, 90*f*
  in cell signaling, 98–100, 129
  farnesyltransferase, inhibitors, 106, 226
  GTPase activity, 98–99, 129
  GTP-bound, 89–90, 90*f*
    constitutive activation, 98–99
    inactivation, 98–100, 129
    oncogenic variants, 99–100
  PTK receptor coupling to, 89–90, 90*f*
  Raf protein interaction with, 89, 98
    inhibition of, therapeutic implications, 105
  site-directed mutagenesis in vitro, 100
  structure of, 89, 91*f*
  as target for drug development, 225–226
Receptor protein-tyrosine kinase
  Abl, genetics of, 97
  activation, 87–89, 88*f*
  autophosphorylation, 88*f*, 89
  chimeric, 148*t*
  constitutive activation, 97–98
  coupling to Ras proteins, 89–90, 90*f*
  cytoplasmic, 97–98
  genes
    amplification, 88*f*
    oncogenic mutations in, 88*f*, 95–96, 148*t*
    rearrangements in human cancer, 96
  growth factors and, 86
  intracellular, 97
  mitogenic signaling pathway activated by, 89–90, 90*f*
    and nuclear events, 90*f*, 90–91
    oncogenic mutations and, 92
  oncogene, inherited, 96–97
  overexpression, 88*f*
  and proto-oncogene mutation, 78–79
  signal transduction pathways, 86–87, 87*f*
  Src, genetics of, 97
  transmembrane, 97
Recessive inheritance
  definition of, 54
  of familial cancer, 54, 56
    genes affected in, 56–57
  of susceptibility to familial cancer, 54*f*, 54–56
Recombinant DNA technology. *See* Molecular cloning
Renal cell carcinoma
  loss of heterozygosity in, 118*t*
  tumor suppressor gene alterations in, 169*t*
  in von Hippel-Lindau disease, 132, 166
Restriction fragment length polymorphism analysis
  of loss of heterozygosity, 115, 117*f*
  in retinoblastoma, 120

87–89, 88*f*
  intracellular, 98–101
Simian sarcoma virus
  sis gene, 64*t*
  in tumorigenesis, 93
Sipple's syndrome. *See* Multiple endocrine
neoplasia, type II
SM feline sarcoma virus, *fms* gene, 64*t*
Smoking
  and cancer, 48, 48*t*
  and lung cancer, 42, 42*f*, 181
Smooth muscle cells, growth regulation by
growth factor, 27
Somatic cell hybrid experiments, 112–113
Somatic cells
  life span, in culture, 16
  senescence, 16, 194–195, 195*f*
Somatostatin receptor imaging scan, 221*f*
Sos protein, 89, 98–99
Src homology 2 domain. *See* SH2 domains
Staging. *See* Cancer, staging
ST and GA feline sarcoma virus, *fes* gene, 64*t*
Steel factor, 86
  receptors, oncogenic mutations in, 95
Stem cell(s)
  cell production from
    deranged, 32–34, 33*f*
    normal, 33*f*
  pluripotential, differentiation, 15
Stem cell factor, 86
Stomach cancer. *See* Gastric cancer
Sunlight and cancer, 48*t*. *See also* Radiation,
ultraviolet
  in xeroderma pigmentosum, 56
SV40 virus, 4
  cytopathic effects, 22
  large T antigen
    and apoptosis, 193–194
    binding to retinoblastoma protein,
122–123

T

Tamoxifen, 227
T antigen activities
  in nonpermissive cells, 23
  in normal cells, 23
Target genes, in carcinogenesis, 49
T cells
  antigen receptor genes, in identification of
proto-oncogenes, 69
  tumors. *See* Leukemia; Lymphoid tumor(s);
Lymphoma(s)
Telomerase
  in established (immortalized) cell lines, 16,
195*f*, 195–196
  regulation of, 196
Telomere shortening, and cellular senescence,
195*f*, 195–196
12-*O*-Tetradecanoylphorpbol-13-acetate, 43
Therapeutics. *See* Cancer, treatment
Thrombopoietin, 223
Thrombospondin, 201
Thyroid cancer
  papillary
    gene rearrangements in, 96
    oncogenic alleles in, 148*t*
    ret mutations in, 154*t*, 157
Thyroid hormone receptor, 86–87

TIMPs. *See* Metalloproteinase(s), tissue
inhibitors of
Tobacco and cancer, 3, 45, 48*t*, 181
Transcription factors, 34, 86–87
  AP-1, 102
  chimeric, in cancer, 148*t*, 154–155
  E2A-Pbx1, 154–155
  E2F, interaction with retinoblastoma
protein, 124
  fos, 102
  functions of, 101
  jun, 102
  Myc, 102–103, 103*f*
  oncogenic, 101–103, 148*t*, 154–155
  in PTK/Ras/Map signaling pathway, 90*f*,
90–91
  regulation of, 101–102
Transduction
  definition of, 7, 61
  of proto-oncogenes, by retroviruses, 7, 61
    activation by, 73*f*, 73–74
  of *src* gene, 7
Transfection, gene transfer by, 179–180
  in assay for cancer genes, 70–71
  process of, 70, 70*f*
Transformation. *See* Malignant
transformation
Transforming growth factor-β, cell cycle
arrest induction by, 123–124
Transgenic mice, tumorigenesis in
  angiogenesis in, 198–199
  oncogene collaboration in, 183–184, 185*f*
Treatment. *See* Cancer, treatment; Patient
management
Trisomy 21. *See* Down's syndrome
trk gene, rearrangements, 96
Tuberous sclerosis, 210*t*
Tumor(s)
  capillary density in, visualization of, 198,
198*f*
  classification of, 213
  clonal analysis of, 35
  hematopoietic
    molecular pathology of, 213–215, 214*f*,
215*t*
    oncogene lesions in, 150, 151*t*
    prognostic markers in, 216–217
  lymphoid
    genetic alterations in, 215*t*
    molecular pathology of, 213–215, 214*f*,
215*t*
    oncogene lesions in, 150, 151*t*
  metastases. *See* Metastasis
  monoclonal, 35
  polyclonal, 35
  solid
    chromosomal translocations in, 150–155
    molecular pathology of, 215–216, 216*t*
    prognostic markers in, 217
    proto-oncogene expression in, therapeutic
implications of, 215–216
Tumor cell(s)
  acquisition of malignancy, 35–38
  anchorage-independent growth, 21, 22*f*
  aneuploidy of, 24
  chromosomal instability of, 24–26
    and cancer treatment, 26
  clonal evolution of, 36*f*, 37–38
  clonality, 2, 9
  deranged differentiation in, 32–35